Textbook of Community Health for Health Inspectors

Textbook of Community Health for Health Inspectors

GN Prabhakara MD
Principal and Professor of Community Medicine
SDM College of Medical Sciences and Hospital
Manjushree Nagar, Sattur
Dharwad, Karnataka, India

JAYPEE BROTHERS MEDICAL PUBLISHERS (P) LTD

New Delhi • Ahmedabad • Bengaluru • Chennai • Hyderabad
Kochi • Kolkata • Lucknow • Mumbai • Nagpur • St Louis (USA)

Published by

Jitendar P Vij
Jaypee Brothers Medical Publishers (P) Ltd

Corporate Office
4838/24 Ansari Road, Daryaganj, **New Delhi** - 110002, India, +91-11-43574357

Registered Office
B-3 EMCA House, 23/23B Ansari Road, Daryaganj, **New Delhi** 110 002, India
Phones: +91-11-23272143, +91-11-23272703, +91-11-23282021
+91-11-23245672, Rel: +91-11-32558559, Fax: +91-11-23276490, +91-11-23245683
e-mail: jaypee@jaypeebrothers.com, Website: www.jaypeebrothers.com

Branches

- 2/B, Akruti Society, Jodhpur Gam Road Satellite
  Ahmedabad 380 015, Phones: +91-79-26926233, Rel: +91-79-32988717
  Fax: +91-79-26927094, e-mail: ahmedabad@jaypeebrothers.com
- 202 Batavia Chambers, 8 Kumara Krupa Road, Kumara Park East
  Bengaluru 560 001, Phones: +91-80-22285971, +91-80-22382956, +91-80-22372664
  Rel: +91-80-32714073, Fax: +91-80-22281761, e-mail: bangalore@jaypeebrothers.com
- 282 IIIrd Floor, Khaleel Shirazi Estate, Fountain Plaza, Pantheon Road
  Chennai 600 008, Phones: +91-44-28193265, +91-44-28194897
  Rel: +91-44-32972089, Fax: +91-44-28193231, e-mail: chennai@jaypeebrothers.com
- 4-2-1067/1-3, 1st Floor, Balaji Building, Ramkote Cross Road
  Hyderabad 500 095, Phones: +91-40-66610020, +91-40-24758498, Rel:+91-40-32940929
  Fax:+91-40-24758499, e-mail: hyderabad@jaypeebrothers.com
- No. 41/3098, B & B1, Kuruvi Building, St. Vincent Road
  Kochi 682 018, Kerala, Phones: +91-484-4036109, +91-484-2395739, +91-484-2395740
  e-mail: kochi@jaypeebrothers.com
- 1-A Indian Mirror Street, Wellington Square
  Kolkata 700 013, Phones: +91-33-22651926, +91-33-22276404, +91-33-22276415
  Rel: +91-33-32901926, Fax: +91-33-22656075, e-mail: kolkata@jaypeebrothers.com
- Lekhraj Market III, B-2, Sector-4, Faizabad Road, Indira Nagar
  Lucknow 226 016, Phones: +91-522-3040553, +91-522-3040554
  e-mail: lucknow@jaypeebrothers.com
- 106 Amit Industrial Estate, 61 Dr SS Rao Road, Near MGM Hospital, Parel
  Mumbai 400012, Phones: +91-22-24124863, +91-22-24104532, Rel: +91-22-32926896
  Fax: +91-22-24160828, e-mail: mumbai@jaypeebrothers.com
- "KAMALPUSHPA" 38, Reshimbag, Opp. Mohota Science College, Umred Road
  Nagpur 440 009 (MS), Phone: Rel: +91-712-3245220
  Fax: +91-712-2704275, e-mail: nagpur@jaypeebrothers.com

USA Office
1745, Pheasant Run Drive, Maryland Heights (Missouri), MO 63043, USA, Ph: 001-636-6279734
e-mail: jaypee@jaypeebrothers.com, anjulav@jaypeebrothers.com

Textbook of Community Health for Health Inspectors

First Edition: 2009

ISBN 978-81-8448-644-5

Typeset at JPBMP typesetting unit
Printed at

To

My Parents

Late Smt Sharadamma Narayana Sastry

and

Late Shri GR Narayana Sastry

Who brought me to this world

PREFACE

Paramedical staff particularly Health Inspectors are indispensable entity in the care of the sick and injured people as well as in giving preventive care for a healthy community in the society. Because of remarkable changes in Health Sciences and Social Sciences, their role has attained high level duties and responsibilities in the following areas:

- City corporation limits
- Primary health centres
- Subcentres
- Railway hospitals
- District health activities
- Epidemic control
- International travel
- Seaport, airport and land areas
- CGHS and ESIC activities
- Public health engineering
- Public health laboratory services

An effort is made to incorporate information on all theoretical, practical and field aspect of Health Inspector Training (HIT) course as per Paramedical Board; which was wanted in the field both by trainers and trainees; all based on three decades of teaching and training to HITs.

The book covers in-depth information about the present areas of interest like malaria smear staining, first aid, essential drugs, treatment of minor ailments, basic legal medicine, Paramedical Board (PMB) syllabus, inspection of factory, management of fair and festival, Orientation Training Centre (OTC) camps, sanitary survey, drugs of other systems of medicine, scientific procedure of killing of stray dogs, hospital waste management and emergency public health measures.

The text covers Section I for first year course, Section II for second year course as per the syllabus and an outline of Municipality Act.

I hope that this book will definitely serve the present requirement of Health Inspector Training course.

GN Prabhakara

ACKNOWLEDGEMENTS

I thankfully acknowledge the blessings from Rajarushi Padmabhushana, Dr D Veerendra Heggade, Dharmadhikari of Dharmasthala.

I acknowledge the guidance and encouragement by Dr Niranjan Kumar, Medical Director and Dr YS Rai, Dean of SDM College of Medical Sciences and Hospital, Manjushree Nagar, Sattur, Dharwad, Karnataka.

I acknowledge the opportunity given for Health Inspector Training and Teaching by all Directors of Medical Education and all District Health and Family Welfare Officers from Karnataka State during the period 1974 to 2004.

I acknowledge the help received from Director Professor, PSM, JIPMER, Puducherry; Professor and HOD, PSM at Government Medical Colleges, Mysore, Bengaluru, Hubli and Bellary in Karnataka State.

I appreciate the guidance, correction, encouragement and thorough help of my life partner Mrs Malathi Prabhakara, Scientist (Retired), Technology Transfer, Industrial Development and Consultancy Services, CFTRI (CSIR), Mysore.

I remember the source of inspiration of my son Dr Bharat M Prabhakara, Junior Faculty, Department of Radio Diagnosis and Imaging at SDM College of Medical Sciences and Hospital, Manjushree Nagar, Sattur, Dharwad, Karnataka.

I cannot forget to mention and appreciate the efforts of Shri Jitendar P Vij (Chairman and Managing Director), who is always there with authors through Author's Meet with all his encouragement words and Mr Tarun Duneja (Director-Publishing) of M/s Jaypee Brothers Medical Publishers (P) Ltd, New Delhi in giving a good shape to my modest work as *Textbook of Community Health for Health Inspectors,* which is a unique textbook solely written for Health Inspector Training course.

CONTENTS

Section 1: Basics of Public Health

Section 2: Application of Public Health

Plate 1

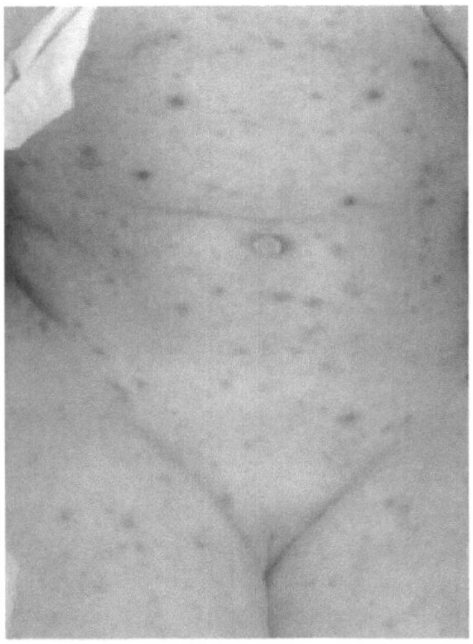

Fig. 15.2: Chickenpox rash in a child

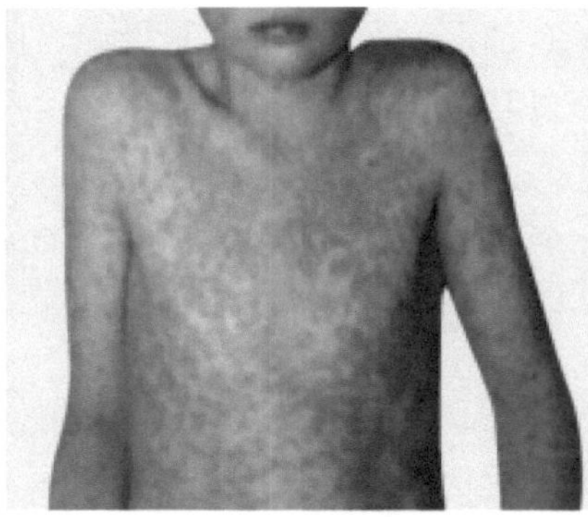

Fig. 15.3: Measles rashes on the chest

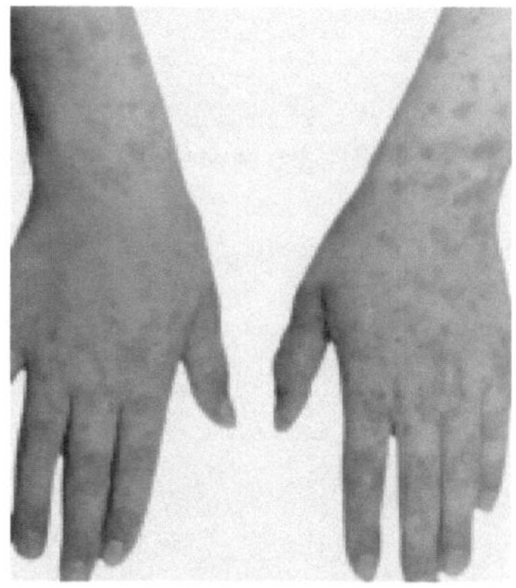

Fig. 15.4: Measles rashes on the hand

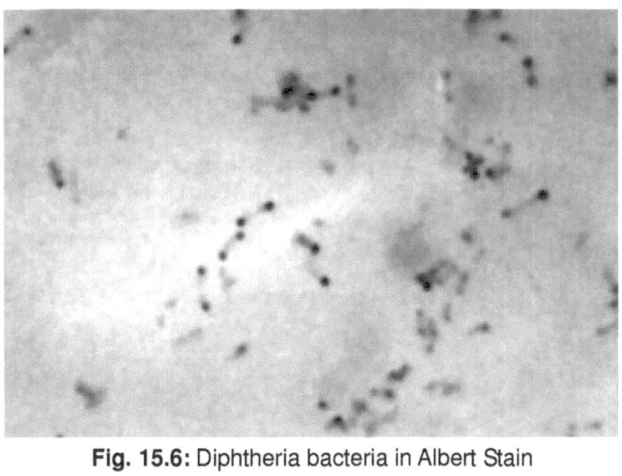

Fig. 15.6: Diphtheria bacteria in Albert Stain

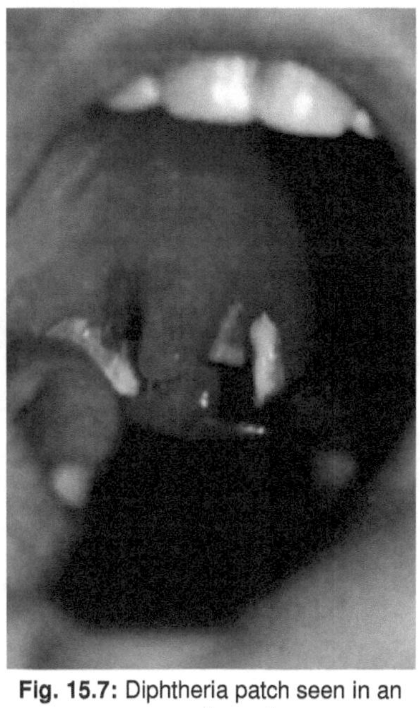

Fig. 15.7: Diphtheria patch seen in an opened mouth

Plate 2

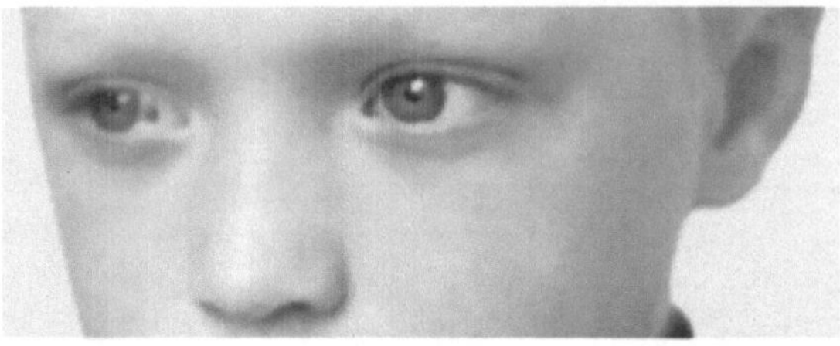

Fig. 15.8: Case of whooping cough showing bleeding in eye

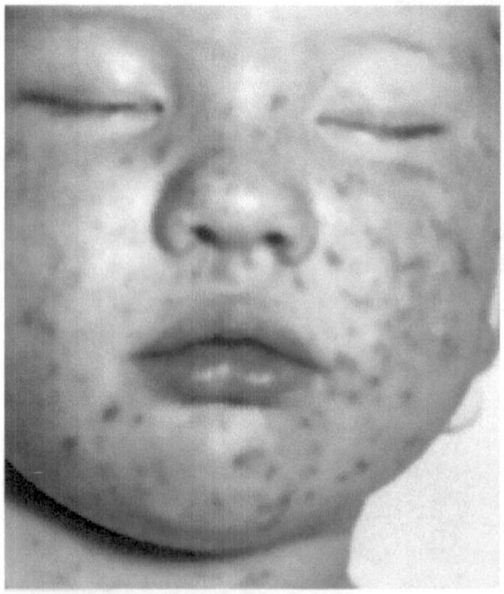

Fig. 15.11: Face of a child in meningitis showing skin bleeding

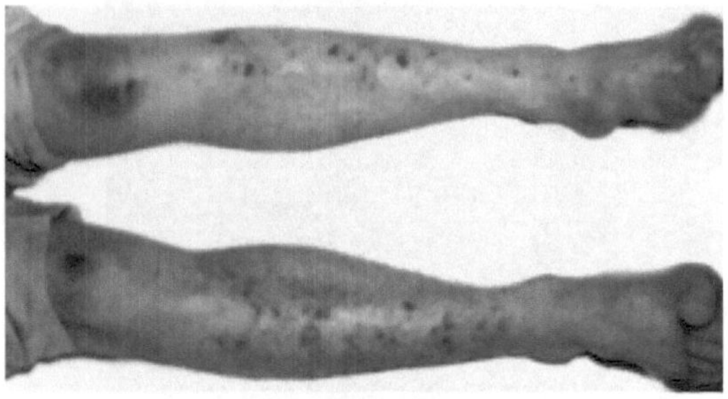

Fig. 15.12: Legs of meningitis case showing bleeding rash

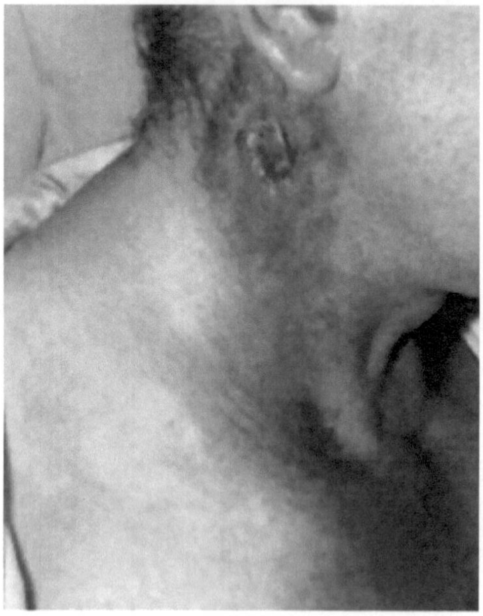

Fig. 15.21: Anthrax ulcer below the ear

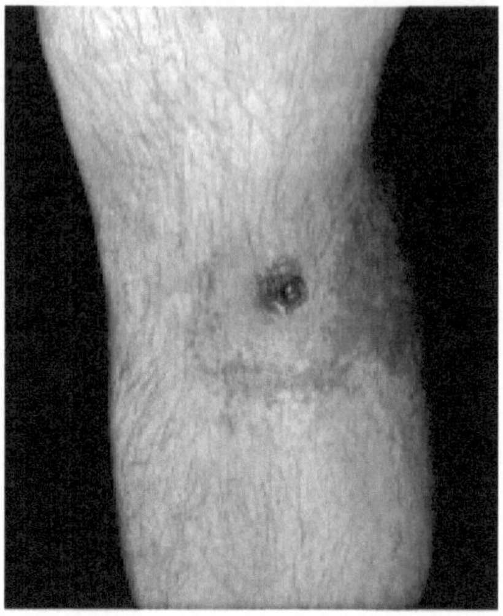

Fig. 15.22: Anthrax ulcer on leg

SECTION

1

Basics of Public Health

1. Elementary Concept of Applied Anatomy and Physiology
2. Sociological Concept of Health and Disease
3. Behavioural Science and its Importance
4. Concept of Community Health
5. Elementary and Vital Statistics
6. Elements of Medical Microbiology and Parasitology
7. Nutrition
8. Environmental Health
9. Personal Hygiene
10. Basic Epidemiology
11. Dynamics of Disease Transmission
12. Concept of Disease Prevention and Control
13. Medical Entomology
14. Concept of Primary Health Care

1 Elementary Concept of Applied Anatomy and Physiology

ANATOMY AND PHYSIOLOGY

Man is different from animals, which is observed by his ability to talk, to think and to make judgement. This is made possible by working together of cells, organs or body fluids.

Anatomy is concerned with structure of human body (Fig. 1.1).

Physiology is concerned with functions of human body.

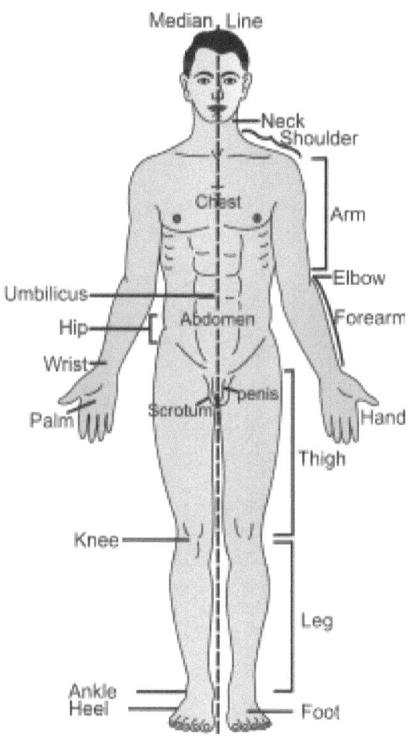

Fig. 1.1: Parts of human body

Systems

Human body is made up of many systems. A system is an arrangement of organs closely related to one another.

These are:

- Skeletal system
- Muscular system
- Nervous system
- Circulatory system
- Endocrine system
- Respiratory system
- Digestive system
- Excretory system
- Reproductive system

Organs

An organ is a member of a system, which is made up of tissues, which perform some specific function.

Digestive system: It is made up of the following organs:

- Tongue
- Salivary glands } Oral cavity
- Teeth
- Pharynx
- Oesophagus
- Stomach
- Duodenum
- Jejunum } Small intestine
- Ileum
- Caecum
- Colon } Large intestine
- Rectum
- Anal canal

Tissues

Many cells together go to form tissue. There are different types of tissues depending upon their functions. They are:

- Skin tissue
- Connective tissue
- Muscle tissue
- Nervous tissue, etc.

Cells

They are structural and physiological units of human body (Fig. 1.2). Human body is multicellular consisting of enormous cells. In human body, cells are not directly in contact with air or food. They excrete waste material. The cells depend on circulating body fluids to carry oxygen, food and waste material.

A cell is made up of cytoplasm, nucleus with a covering cell wall. Cytoplasm contains mitochondria and Golgi apparatus. Mitochondria exist near nucleus.

The portion of the protoplasm composing the nucleus is called *karyoplasms.* Nucleus consists of granules of a material called *chromatin*. At cell division, these chromatins get aggregated into chromosomes. Human cell is specific and contains 46 chromosomes of which 22 pairs of ordinary chromosomes and a pair of sex chromosomes.

Ribonucleic acid (RNA) is found in the cytoplasm, the nucleus and chromosomes. Deoxyribo-nucleic acid (DNA) is present only in chromo-somes.

Building up of living materials within the cell is called *anabolism.* Breaking down of such material is called *catabolism.* The above processes (anabo-lism and catabolism) are called *metabolism.*

Functions of a Living Cell

They are:

- Support by cohesiveness
- Cell respiration
- Food is oxidised for energy
- Motion is exhibited
- Distribution of oxygen and nutrition
- Excretes waste products
- Responds to external stimuli
- Cell division

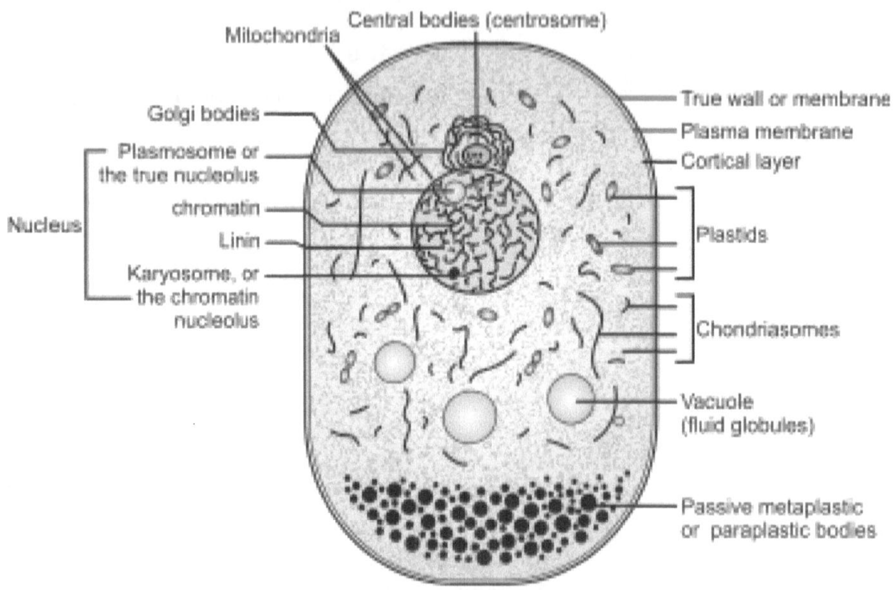

Fig. 1.2: Structure of a cell

BODY CAVITIES

Main body cavities are (Fig. 1.3):

- Thoracic cavity (chest)
- Abdominal cavity
- Pelvic cavity
- Open cavities like orbital, nasal and buccal cavities

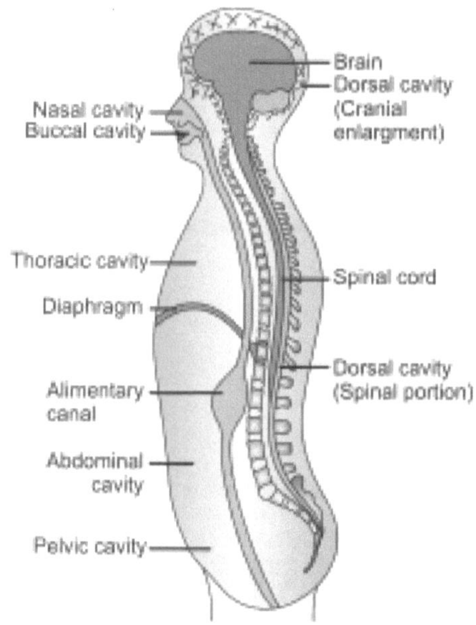

Fig. 1.3: Body cavities

SKELETAL SYSTEM

The skeletal system consists of a large number of bones held together by the ligaments and muscles to form a supporting framework for the body (Figs 1.4 and 1.5).

The skeletal system helps to protect more delicate organs of human body. By its joints, it permits one bone to move on the other.

Other functions are passive instruments of locomotion. Blood cells are formed in bone marrow.

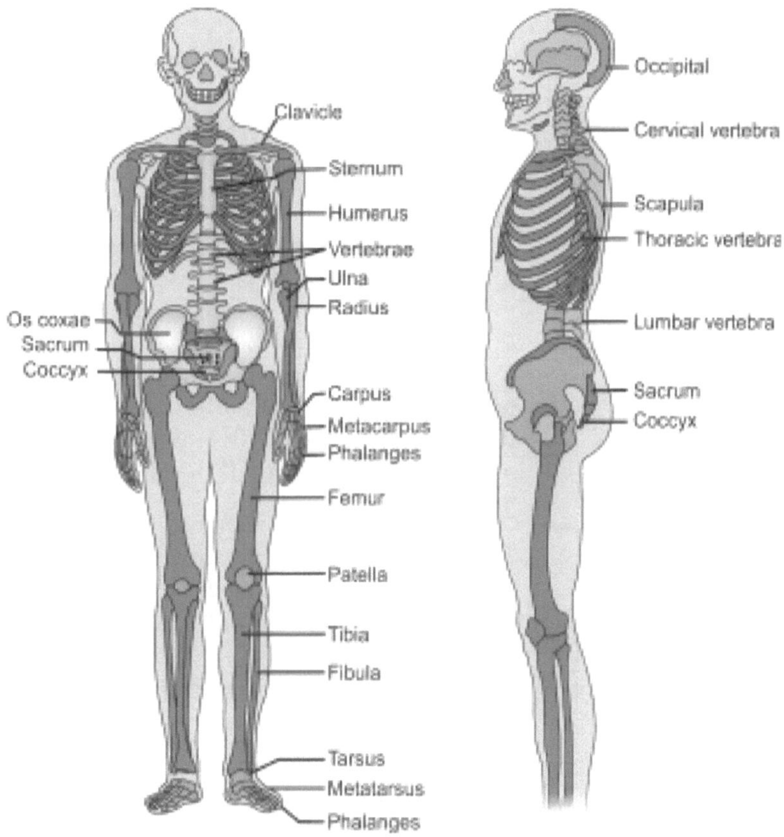

Fig. 1.4: Skeletal system

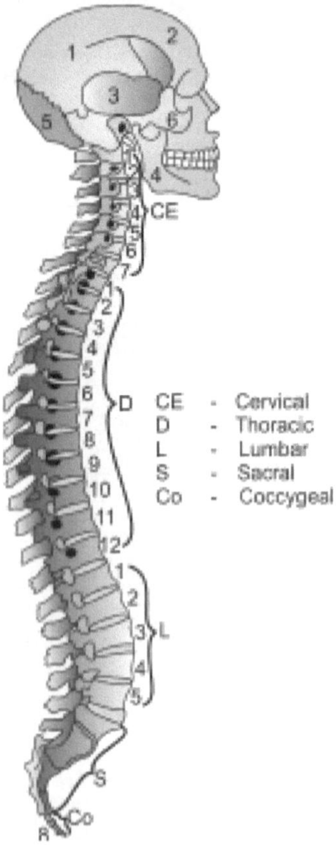

Fig. 1.5: Vertebrae

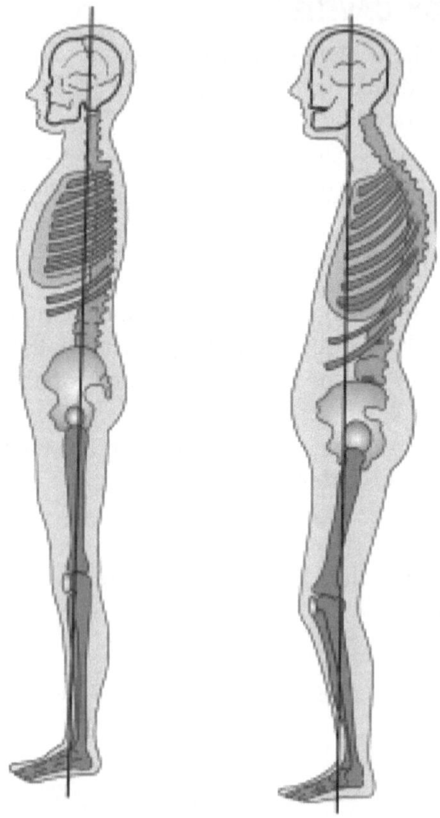

Fig. 1.6: Good and bad body posture by individual skeletal system

The adult skeleton consists of total 206 named bones. They are:

• Upper limbs	—	64
• Lower limbs	—	62
• Chest bone and ribs	—	25
• Vertebral column	—	26
• Hyoid bone	—	1
• Ear bones	—	6
• Face bones	—	14
• Skull bones	—	8

Stature and movement is determined by bones of our body (Fig. 1.6)

Common conditions that are to be noted by Paramedical are:

- Fractures of bone (accidents)
- Bone cancers
- Skeletal fluorosis (bone softening by fluorosis)
- Osteoarthritis (bone softening)

MUSCULAR SYSTEM

By muscle contraction human has good motion of the body. Muscles also help in breathing, heartbeat, bowel movement, etc.

The chemical changes take place in muscle contraction are shown in Flow chart 1.1.

Human body has innumerable number of muscles (Figs 1.7 and 1.8).

Muscular system consists of muscles which are attached to the bones by strong fibrous cords called *tendons*.

Flow chart 1.1: Chemical changes in muscle contraction

1. Adenosine triphosphate (ATP) – Actomyosin ⟶ Adenosine diphosphate (ADP)–Actomyosin + Phosphate ion + Energy

2. Phosphocreatine + ADP ⟶ Creatine + ATP

3. Glycogen ⟶ Pyruvic acid + CO_2 + Water + energy

   Glycogen ⟶ Lactic acid + energy ⟵ Pyruvic acid + CO_2 + Water + energy

   Lactic acid + energy ⟶ Reformed to glycogen in liver

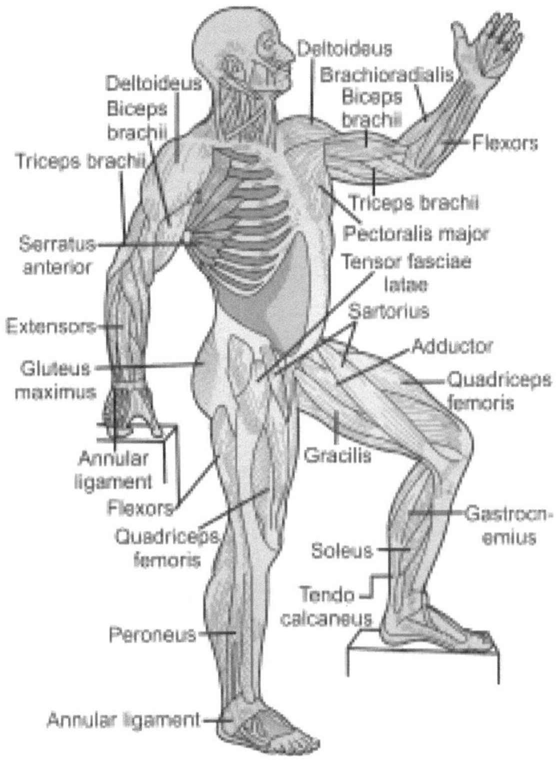

Fig. 1.7: Muscles of our body

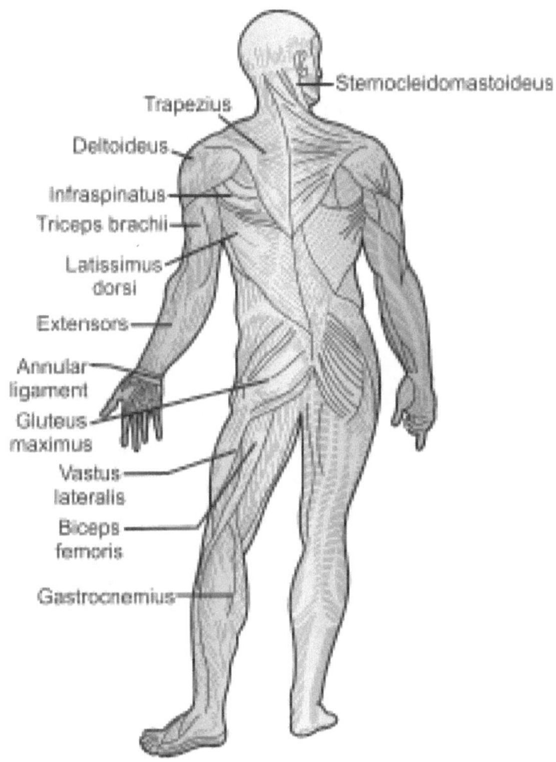

Fig. 1.8: Back muscles of our body

During immunisation, Deltoid muscle in upper limb and Gluteus maximus muscle in lower limb (loin) are commonly selected for injections. Hence, identification of these two muscles is to be done properly by Health Inspectors in:

- Anatomical models
- Living models

Common conditions that a paramedical person should note in this system are:

i. Muscle sprains
ii. Muscle tears
iii. Muscle spasm due to infection (tetanus)
iv. Muscle paralysis due to infection (polio)

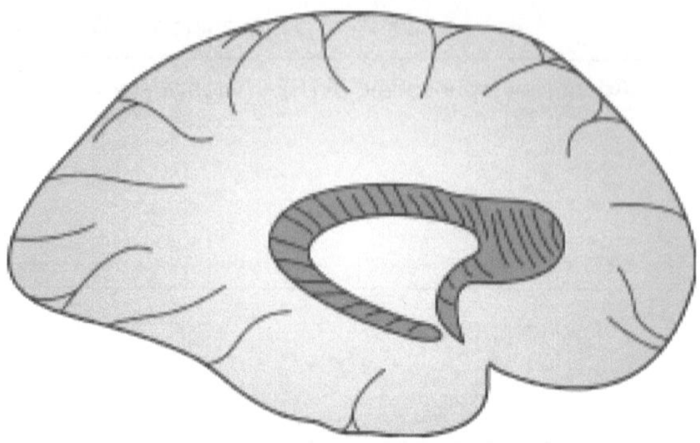

Fig. 1.10: Inner white matter (contains fibres for transmission)

NERVOUS SYSTEM

This system is the main controlling system of our body. The centre of nervous system is the brain (Figs 1.9 and 1.10). The brain can be compared to a telephone exchange containing billions of telephone connections.

The brain is connected to the spinal cord and further with spinal nerves (Fig. 1.11).

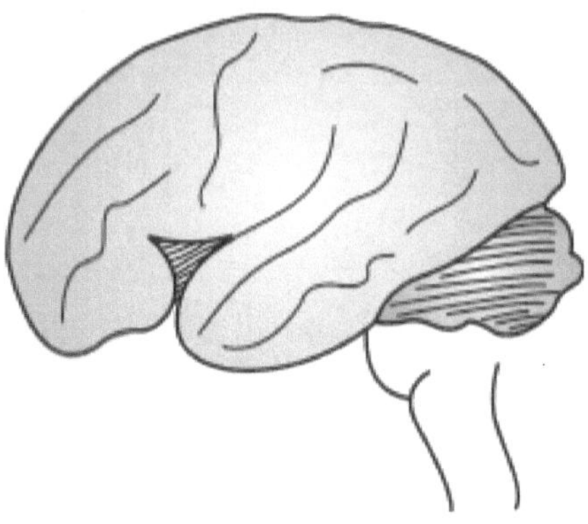

Fig. 1.9: Outer grey matter (contains special cells)

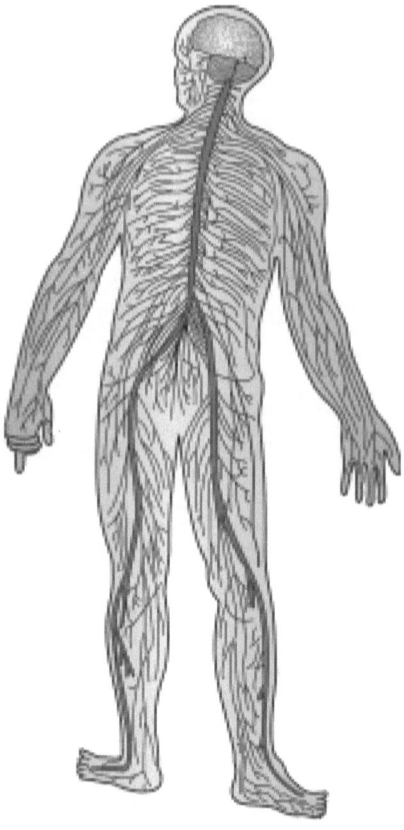

Fig. 1.11: Nervous system containing brain, spinal cord and spinal nerves

Spinal Nerves

There are 31 pairs of spinal nerves, which can be grouped under each region of the vertebral column. They are:

- Cervical nerves — 8 pairs
- Thoracic nerves — 12 pairs
- Lumbar nerves — 5 pairs
- Sacral nerves — 5 pairs
- Coccygeal nerves — 1 pair

Brain

It is a complex mass of nervous system, which has the distinctly connected parts. (Figs 1.12 A and B).

Cranial Nerves

There are 12 pairs of cranial nerves. They emerge from the under surface of the brain. They are **sensory**, **motor** and **mixed** nerves (Table 1.1).

Clinical conditions that are to be noted by a paramedical person:

- Speech loss in a stroke patient
- Loss of consciousness after major epilepsy (fits)

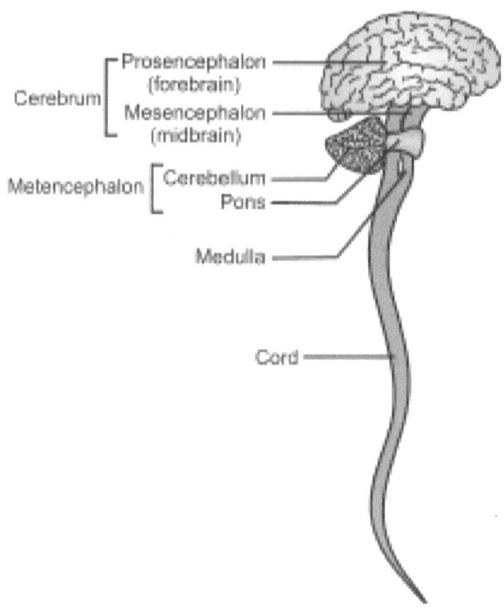

Fig. 1.12A: Divisions of brain

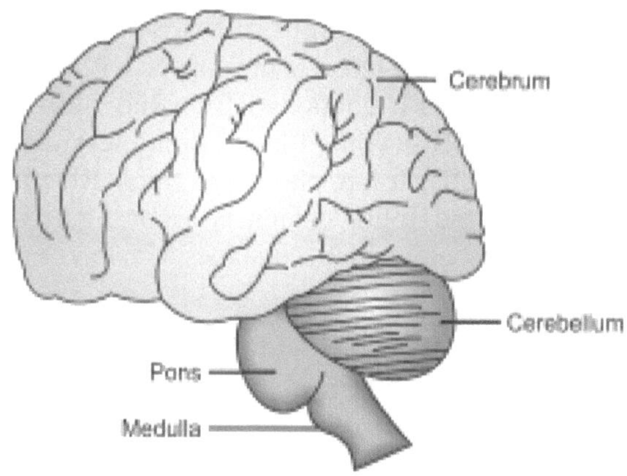

Fig. 1.12B: Parts of brain

Table 1.1: Twelve cranial nerves

Sensory	*Motor*	*Mixed*
1. Olfactory nerve (smell)	3. Oculomotor nerve (eye movement)	5. Trigeminal nerve (face, teeth)
2. Optic nerve (vision)	4. Trochlear nerve (eye movement)	7. Facial nerve (facial muscles)
8. Acoustic nerve (hearing)	6. Abducens nerve (eye movement)	9. Glassopharyngeal nerve (tongue, pharynx)
	11. Accessory nerve (neck muscles)	10. Vagus nerve (viscera, heart, lung)
	12. Hypoglossal nerve (tongue)	

- Tubercular meningitis (headache, vomiting, convulsion)
- Brain fever (mosquito-borne viral infection of brain)
- Polio (infantile paralysis by viral infection)
- Paraplegia (by compression of spinal cord)
- Psychosis and neurosis (anxiety, hysteria, etc.)

CIRCULATORY SYSTEM

The organ of circulation is called heart. Heart pumps approximate quantity of 6 litres of blood continuously around human body. Arteries convey pure blood. Veins carry impure blood. Interchange of oxygen takes place at capillaries. A separate circulation occurs in lung where oxygen is taken up by the blood.

Blood

Human body has the blood to the tune of 1/12th of his body weight. It contains RBC (Red Blood Corpuscles), WBC (White Blood Corpuscles) and platelets as cells. It has plasma as fluid. Blood contains haemoglobin, which is a conjugated protein. Haemoglobin (Hb) combines with oxygen and carries it to the tissues.

Normal Blood Values

They are as under:

- RBC count — 5 million per cubic mm
- WBC count — 5 to 9 thousand per cubic mm
- Platelets count — 3 lakh per cubic mm.
- Hb % — 11.5 to 19 g%

The white cells (WBC) are usually:

- 20 to 25 lymphocytes
- 3 to 8 per cent monocytes
- 60 to 70 per cent leukocytes

Blood Group

There are four types of blood groups in man. They are:

1. Blood group O
2. Blood group A
3. Blood group B
4. Blood group AB

The Rhesus (Rh) factor is important in giving blood transfusion and in conditions like pregnancy. The condition *erythroblastosis* is caused by production of anti-Rh in mother's blood. If mother is Rh –ve, father is Rh + ve, the child may be Rh +ve.

Figure 1.13 gives picture of general blood circulation and human vascular system.

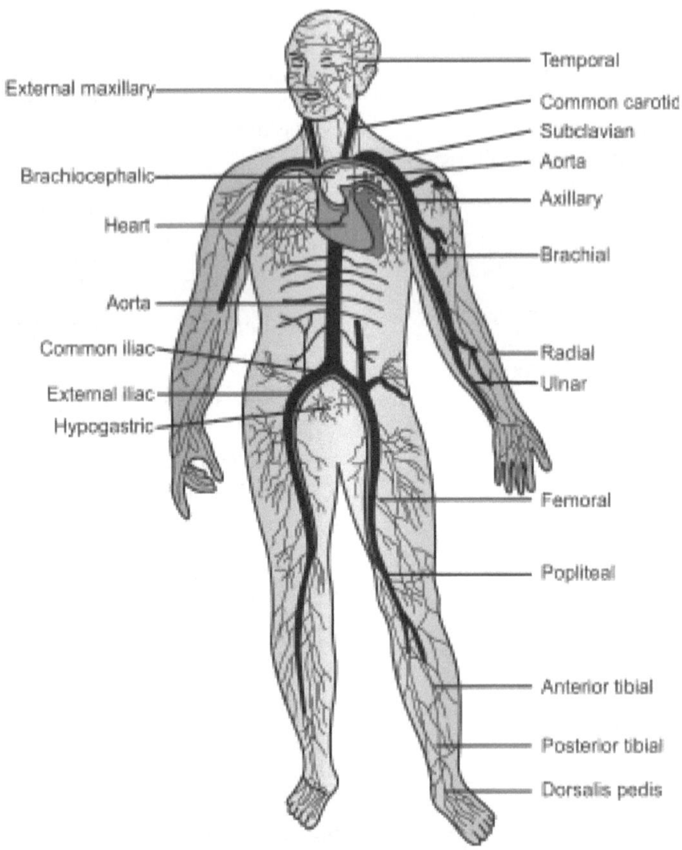

Fig. 1.13: Human circulation and vascular system

Pulse

This denotes heart-rate. Normally, it is about 65 to 70 per minute in men and about 70 to 80 per minute in women. Factors which influence heartbeat can influence the pulse. Hence, recording of pulse is important as a duty of health inspector in the field.

The pulse is best felt with tips of fingers. The patient's forearm is pronated (make forearm to see that palm comes upside at examination). The wrist is slightly flexed (bent) (Fig. 1.14).

The pulse is counted for one minute. If it is more than 80 or less than 60, the person is referred to health centre for further examination.

Blood Pressure

Blood pressure (BP) is defined as pressure the blood exerts against the wall of blood vessels where it is flowing. Systolic BP is pressure exerted when the heart contracts. Diastolic BP is pressure exerted when the heart relaxes. It is normally seen as:

- 120 mm of mercury systolic BP
- 80 mm of mercury diastolic BP

and hence it is written as 120/80 mm Hg.

Method of Recording BP

Support the arm on a table. You can adjust books for height. The arm is to be supported to make the arm muscles relaxed, since relaxed muscle gives correct BP. All tight clothes are removed from the arm (Figs 1.15 to 1.17).

Wrap the cuff firmly around the upper arm (1 inch above the elbow) (Figs 1.18A and B).

Pump up the bulb until radial pulse or brachial pulse is no longer felt (Fig 1.19) and Hun slowly release till pulse is felt. It is systolic BP.

If stethoscope is used, then pump up the bulb till pulse is no longer felt. Keep stethoscope over brachial artery area, slowly release till sound becomes quieter. It is diastolic BP.

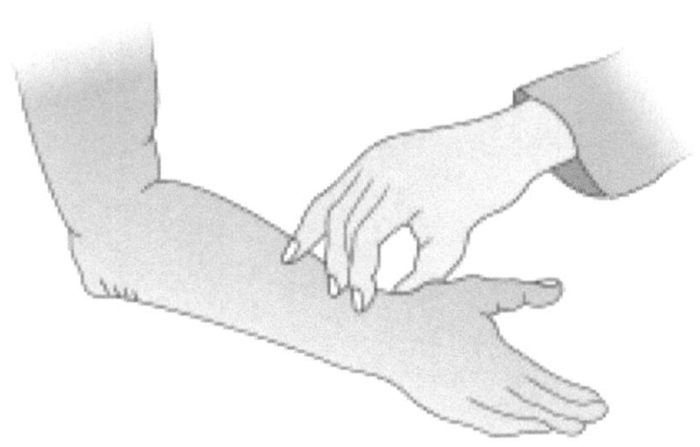

Fig. 1.14: Pulse feeling to record pulse rate

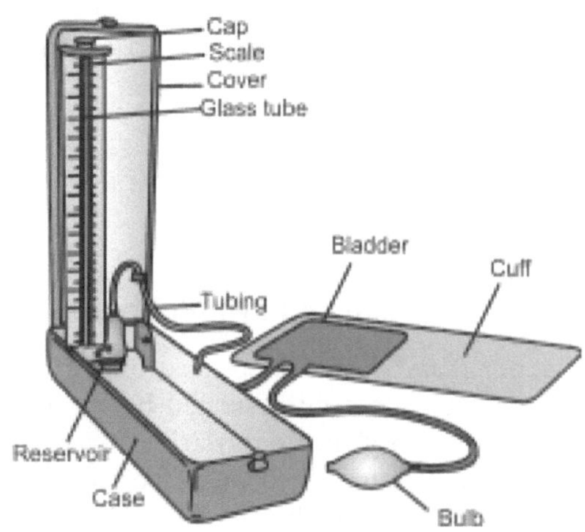

Fig. 1.15: BP apparatus (mercury)

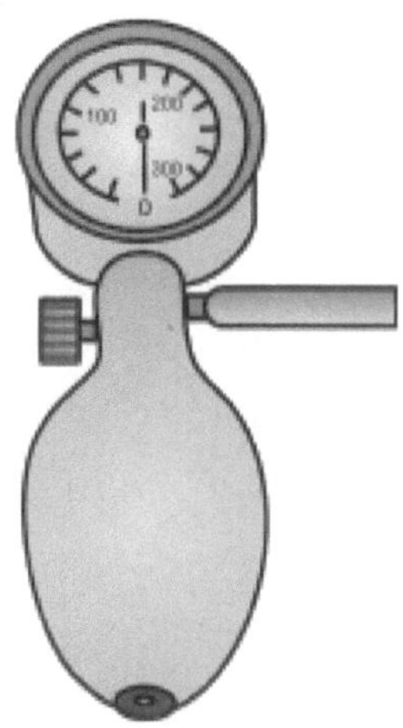

Fig. 1.16: BP apparatus (aneroid)

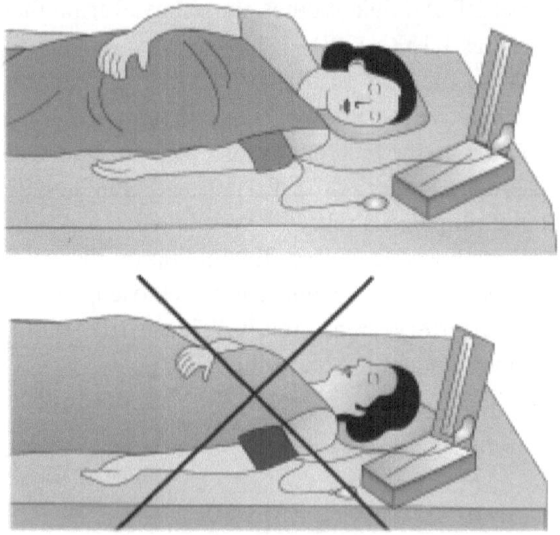

Fig. 1.17: Method of recording BP by mercury sphygmomonometer

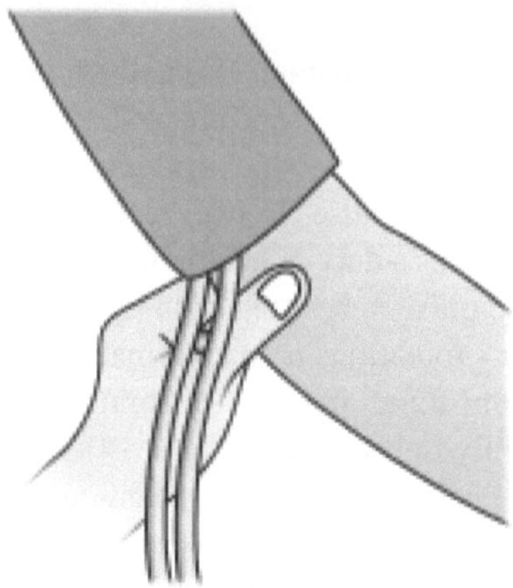

Fig. 1.19: Pulse feeling

Lymphatic System and Lymph Nodes

It is middleman between blood and tissue fluid. Material that cannot be collected by blood is collected by lymphatic capillaries for waste disposal. Lymph nodes function in the protection mechanism of human body.

Conditions to be noted by a Paramedical person:

- Iron deficiency anaemia
- Rh incompatibility
- High BP (Hypertension)
- Heart attack (MI)
- Rheumatic heart disease in children
- Thrombophlebitis (injury of inner wall of vein by inflammation like complication of oral contraception).

ENDOCRINE SYSTEM

There are exocrine glands (glands of external secretions) like pancreas, liver, sweat gland, mammary gland, salivary gland, etc.

There are endocrine glands (glands of internal secretions and which do not have ducts to pour their secretions to tissues) like pituitary gland, thyroid gland, adrenal gland, ovary and testes.

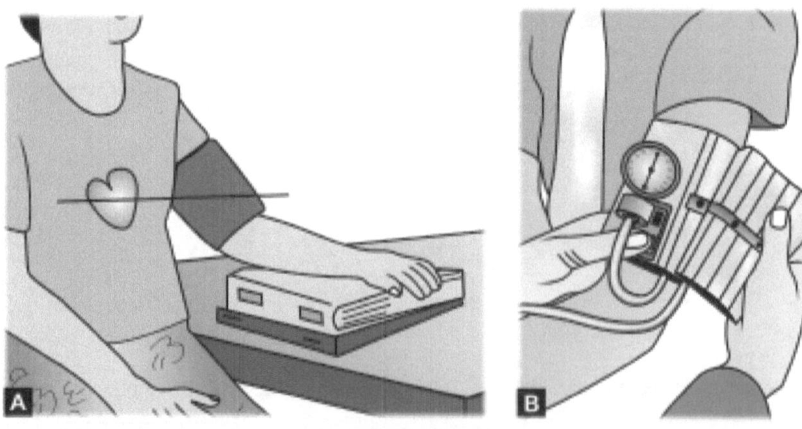

Figs 1.18A and B: Method of recording BP by aneroid monometer

Conditions that are to be noted by the Paramedical worker:

- Dwarfism (lowered function of pituitary and thyroid glands)
- Goitre (lowered function of thyroid gland)
- Tetany (low serum calcium)
- Diabetes (a non-communicable disease).

RESPIRATORY SYSTEM

Respiratory system helps in providing oxygen to tissues and eliminates CO_2 from cells. This is evident by the following observations (Table 1.2).

Table 1.2: Amount of air taken in and breathed out

	Air taken in (Inspiration)	*Air breathed out (Expiration)*
Oxygen	20%	16%
Carbondioxide	zero	4%

Structure of respiratory system is shown in Figure 1.20.

Respiratory illnesses that need to be noted are:

- Common cold (viral infection)
- Influenza (viral infection)
- Chronic bronchitis (infection of bronchi)
- Bronchial asthma (allergy causing difficulty in breathing)
- Acute respiratory infection (ARI)
- Pulmonary tuberculosis
- Pneumoconiosis due to dust inhalation.

Respiratory Rate

It is normally 14 to 18 per minute. Increased respiratory rate is possible in pulmonary diseases

Taking a breath and breathing out the air taken constitute one respiratory rate. It is to be counted for one minute.

DIGESTIVE SYSTEM

This system consists of food canal, which starts from mouth to anus. This leads through whole body. Total length is about 9 metres long, which includes oesophagus, stomach, small intestine and large intestine (Fig. 1.21).

Digestive system disorders that are to be noted by a Paramedical worker are: (Fig. 1.22)

- Peptic ulcer (gastric ulcer, duodenal ulcer)
- Food poisoning
- Gastroenteritis (G and E)

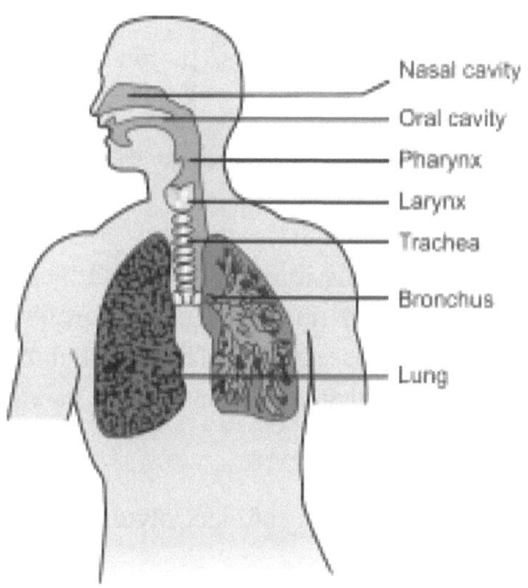

Fig. 1.20: Structure of respiratory system

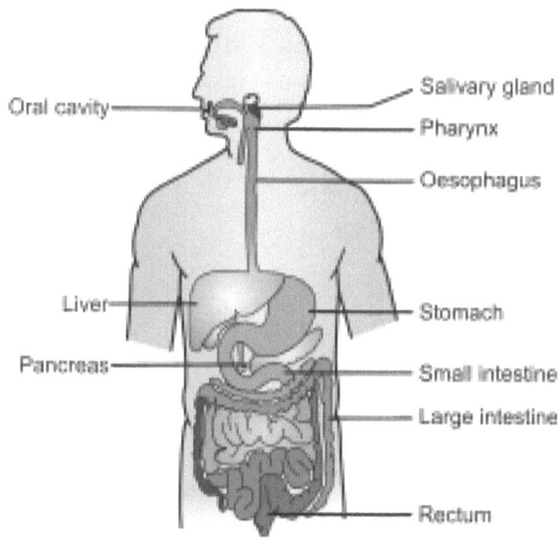

Fig. 1.21: Digestive system

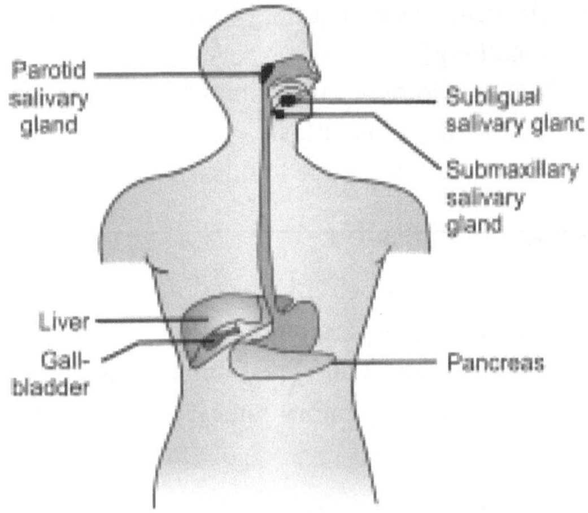

Fig. 1.22: Glands connected with digestive system

- Bacterial infections like cholera, typhoid
- Malabsorption causing malnutrition
- Amoebiasis (protozoal infection)
- Diarrhoea and dysentery
- Jaundice (infective hepatitis)
- Cirrhosis of liver (alcoholic)
- Gallstones
- Diabetes due to lack of insulin by pancreas

EXCRETORY SYSTEM

This system is concerned with the removal of waste products from the blood (Fig. 1.23). Main organs of excretory system are:

- Kidneys
- Connecting ureters
- Urinary bladder
- Urethra.

Electrolytes

Electrolytes are acids, alkalies and salt. Since these items conduct an electric current in water, they are called *electrolytes.*

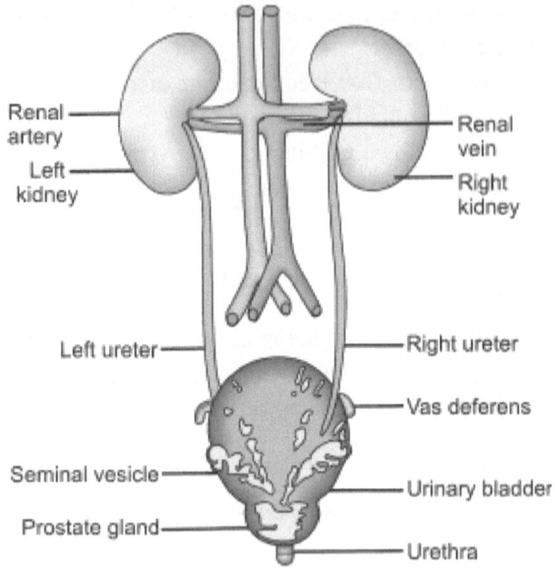

Fig. 1.23: The excretory system

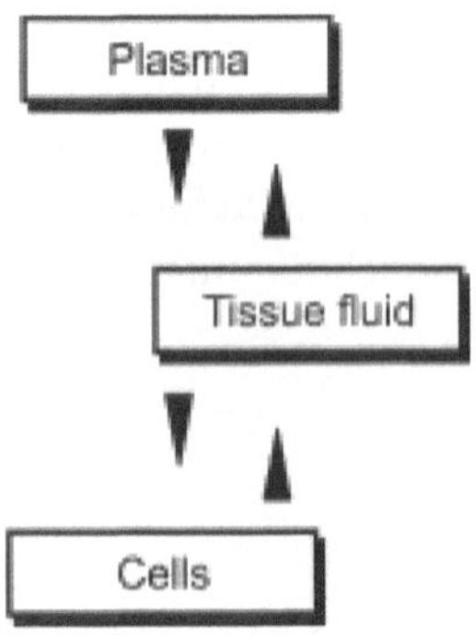

Fig. 1.24: Movement of fluid between compartments

Sodium, potassium, chloride and bicarbonate function to hold fluid within compartments and maintain acid-base balance (Figs 1.24 and 1.25).

Conditions that need attention by a Paramedical worker:

- Renal stones
- Dehydration (loss of electrolytes and water).

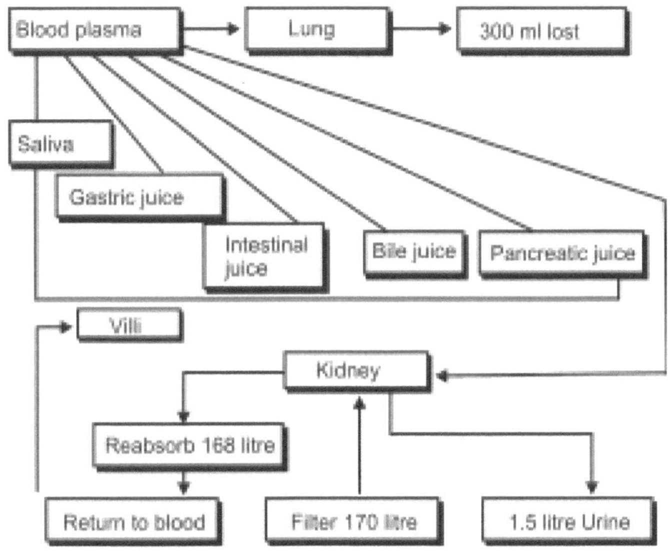

Fig. 1.25: Fluid exchange during 24-hour period in man for acid and base balance

REPRODUCTIVE SYSTEM

Human race is propagated by reproduction, which is carried out by fertilisation of female germ cell with male germ cell (ovum and sperm) (Figs 1.26 and 1.27). The fertilised ovum gets embedded in

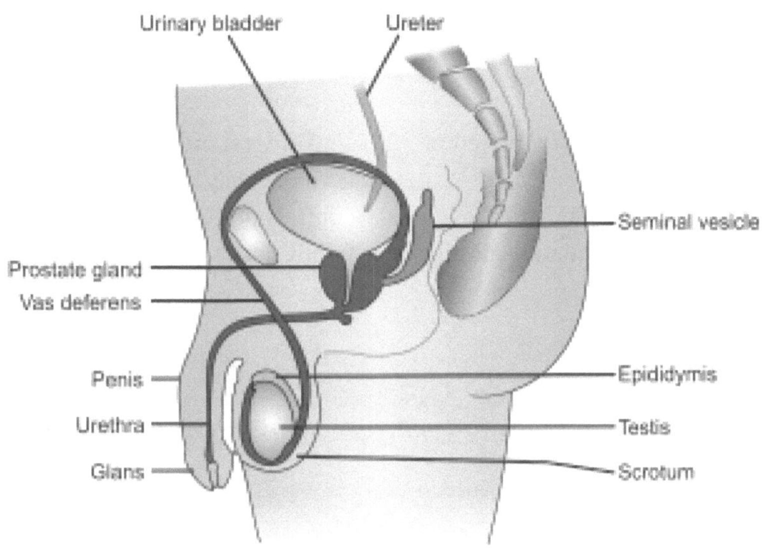

Fig. 1.26: Male sex organs

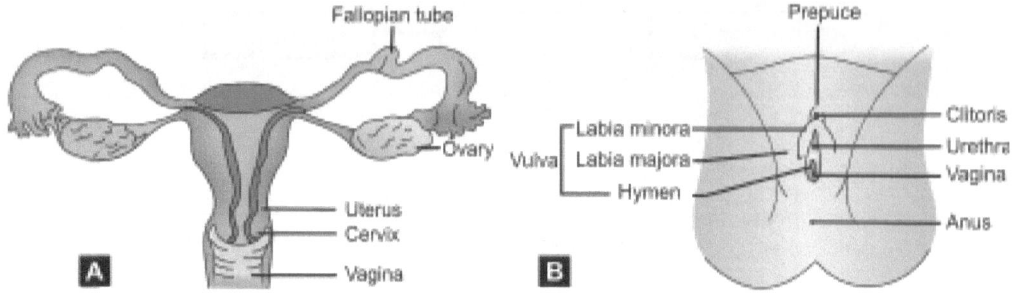

Figs 1.27A and B: Female sex organs

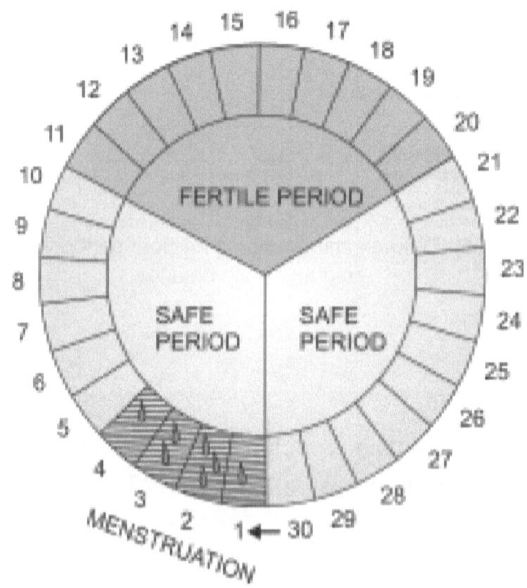

Fig. 1.28: Menstrual cycle

womb, develops into a foetus over a period of 32 weeks as gestational period.

Understanding of female menstrual cycle is necessary for advice on fertility control and also on family planning (Fig. 1.28).

Understanding of menstrual cycle and sex hormones have helped in advice and adoption of oral contraceptives, sterilisation operations for small family norms.

2

Sociological Concept of Health and Disease

Sociology is the study of human beings and their groups like family, society and community. How man behaves as a person and as a member in society is studied. It can be represented as under (Fig. 2.1).

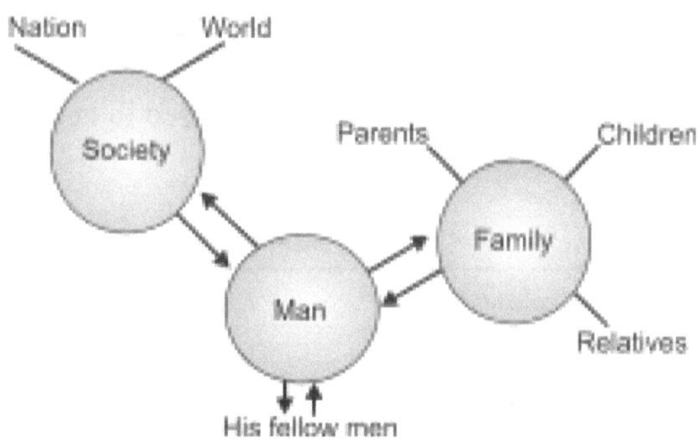

Fig. 2.1: Study of relationship in man

FAMILY

Family Structure

Family is defined as a group of individuals who are biologically related to each other and live together. They eat from a common kitchen.

Family lives in home. Home is a social environment which is shared by all family members. Hence, family is called a *social unit.* Each family has a culture and hence it is also called a *cultural unit.*

When unrelated people live together, it cannot be called a family. It is called a *household.*

Family Types

• Single family	— Married couple and their children
• Joint family	— More than one married couple live together
• Three-generation family	— Married couple, their parents, and their children live together
• Extended family	— When old generation and unmarried children are included

Relationship

Family relationship is important for physical and mental health. Many social and economic problems lead to disturbed relations among members of a family. Common disturbed family relations are seen in the following situations:

- Infertility
- Marital disharmony
- Broken family
- Divorce
- Alcoholism
- Chronic illness in family

Responsibilities of individuals:

- Child rearing
- Socialisation
- Social support
- Economic support
- Role play and job responsibility

COMMUNITY

Community Structure

In a defined place when a group of individuals and families live together, it becomes a community. Common examples are villages, towns and cities.

Functioning of the Community

Community is grouped under different categories based on their occupation. Primary occupations like agriculture, fishing, mining; secondary occupations like fabricating, auto, industry production; tertiary occupations like education and recreation are known in the present society.

Community functioning is determined by:

- Literacy
- Standard of living
- Population movement

In the community, role-play as son, father, uncle, leader, minister, collector, inspector, etc. demarcate our relations within the community. By virtue of our age and sex, we have certain responsi-bilities. By virtue of our education and experience, we have another set of responsibility in the community. For example:

- An elderly person becomes head of a family or leader of a religion.
- By education, a person becomes a doctor or a nurse and serves the community in their illness as well as in health conditions.

Maintenance of Law and Order

In every community, there are a set of rules and regulations for the maintenance of authority or subordination. At home, we have social rules and regulations. Similarly, in the community, we have law as a social control mechanism. They are necessary to maintain health of a community. For example:

- Food adulteration is controlled by PFA Act.
- Prostitution is controlled by Suppression of Immoral Traffic Act.
- Spread of disease (epidemic) is controlled by Municipalities Act.

Community has problems of poverty, crime, disease, alcoholism, STD, drug addiction. They are to be tackled through law and order.

Law and order are required under the following circumstances:

- Civil unrest
- Crime
- Unemployment
- Overgrowth of population

Our house is situated in a community; our children are educated in the community. Human basic needs are thus met in the community.

Collection and Expenditure of Revenues, Services Provided

A community needs different types of services. Let us take the examples of community need in health care services (Table 2.1).

Table 2.1: Community need in health care services

Health care services	*Revenue*
i. Treatment and control of diseases like malaria, tuberculosis, diarrhoea, ARI, leprosy, filaria, AIDS and others	i. Individual tax ii. Group tax iii. Occupation tax iv. Entertainment tax v. Corporation cess
ii. Services to tackle malnutrition, anaemia, LBW, blindness, iodine deficiency and others	vi. Licence fees vii. Collection of public fund viii. International help
iii. Providing protected water supply and environmental sanitation	
iv. Running hospital, health centres, speciality centres	
v. Employment, education and housing	

NATION

Nation has drafted the national health problems. To tackle these problems, national health policies are made. Through various national health programmes, the health care services are taken care of.

The government of India has launched Health Scheme based on the principles of Primary Health Care through community participation.

Collection of revenue is done and expenditure is planned through the Five-Year Plans and Annual Plans. At present, India is spending 3 per cent of gross national product (GNP) on health and family welfare (FW) services for the development of community health.

Religion

India is a democratic country and its community welcomes and respects all religions. Certain rules and sanctions of a religion define influences health of the community.

Social Institutions

Social institutions are:
- Family
- School
- Church
- Temple
- Masjid
- Club
- Hospital
- Political parties
- Indian Medical Association (IMA)
- Gram Panchayat.

They define the rights and duties of each member of the social institution. Social institutions stipulate a set of rules for man in his birthright, social right, marriage and inheritance of property.

In primitive social institutions, stringent regulation was there which lead to revolutions. In advanced social institutions, many changes are brought out for the welfare of man in his family, country and nation. Certain examples of modern social institutions which are the result of social revolution in human welfare activities are:
- Widow marriage
- Abolition of sati system
- Social rehabilitation of tuberculosis and leprosy
- Inter-caste marriage
- Reservations for minorities, SCs, STs in a community
- Compulsory primary education of children.
- Welfare of the girl child.

Responsibilities of a Citizen

A person by birth acquires citizenship of a country. This provides certain birthrights like:
- Becoming a member of a community
- Acquiring property
- Voting and electing a leader
- Helping the nation in its development
- Helping the co-citizens for education, health and living.

Social Attitude, Ideal and Ability

Positive attitude, good ideology and leadership ability are the main requisites of a person in a society. These bring out definite positive changes in economic, political, educational and religious outlook for the betterment of the country.

In the current trend, there is a need for social support, employment opportunity and lowered stress to the community. This is possible by appreciable social attitude, noble ideology and creative ability.

Health outcome is influenced by many factors:

i. Current circumstance (family life, income, etc.)
ii. Individual predispositions (illness, malnutrition, etc.)
iii. Ecological predispositions (community value, lifestyle, etc.)
iv. Opportunities available (education, food, sanitation, etc.)

The desired social attitudes, ideals and abilities help in the development of the community.

Owning and controlling wealth by the government, and democratic by people are two major changes that are seen in modern society.

Self help and cooperative activities are extended in almost all spheres of life. In the field of Health and Family Welfare, it is seen in the following areas:
- Health insurance
- Minimum need programme
- District industry centres (DIC).

Urban Society and Rural Society

In India 78 per cent of population constitute urban society and remaining 22 per cent rural society. Rural society is self-sufficient and mainly agriculture is taken up for livelihood. Urban society is not self-sufficient with business, education and industry as main source of livelihood.

Urban and rural societies differ on the following aspects:
- Socio-economic character
- Demographic character
- Health manpower
- Health status
- Health problems

Table 2.2 gives the difference between urban and rural societies.

Table 2.2: Difference between urban and rural societies

	Rural society	*Urban society*
Doctors Paramedical	Shortage is seen	They are surplus
Common health problems	Diarrhoea, ARI, skin infection, malnutrition, communicable diseases	Obesity, diabetes, heart problems, other NCD
Demographic pattern	Children are more High birth rate High death rate High growth rate High IMR High MMR Low life span	Old people are more Low birth rate Low death rate Low growth rate Low IMR Low MMR High life span
Social pattern	Rural Joint family Mainly agriculture Low literacy	Urban Single family Mainly industry High literacy
Economic pattern	Low standard of living Low access to health care Low income Low per capita income Very poor Less possessions (Cycle, bullock cart, etc.)	High standard of living More access to health care High income High per capita income More wealthy More possessions (Car, house, property, etc.)

Improvement in Life Standards and Life Expectancy

It is possible to raise the health standard and life expectancy through provision of basic needs and primary health care services.

Basic needs are minimum education, housing, protected water, provision of food which can provide required calories and nutrition.

Health care services are:

For individual:
- Treatment of illness
- Rehabilitation

For group:
- RCH
- School health

Social Customs and Norms

Society lays the foundation for the norms and customs from which no person can escape. Many norms are laid down in a society for the purpose of social regulations like:
- Marriage is a norm for procreation
- Man should earn and support all members of the family
- Women holds the key position in the child rearing practices
- Rich man should extend economic support to the poorer sector of the society

Folkways

Similarly, customs are laid down which are described as right way of doing things. Routine customs seen in a family are called *folkways,* which disciplines a person. Examples are:

- Take bath everyday
- Do prayer in the morning
- Distribute small portion of eatables (before eating) to the poor
- Respect elders and help them in need
- Do not trouble the weaker section of the society like women and children
- Do not steal other's property
- Be vegetarian and protect animals.

Folkways normally come through convention. This is followed by the younger generations observing elders who follow certain customs. On the contrary, there are certain customs, which are strictly followed called *mores.* In case of mores, public takes severe action on individuals who do not follow such customs. Common examples are:

- A man and woman living together without marriage is forbidden and penalised.
- A person involved in gambling is punished.
- A person who commits sexual offence is punished.
- Polygamy and polyandry are prohibited and punishable.
- Inter-caste marriage allows the public to boycott and do not allow acquiring property in some communities.

Resistance to adoption of new practices and new ways of life: Science and technology has brought many advantages to keep us healthy and maintain longevity. But traditional communities do not accept easily such new practices and new ways of life which largely depend on:

- Level of their knowledge
- Whether they have positive or negative attitude
- Whether the practice came by convention (passed on from generation-to-generation)

Common causes of resistance to new practices and new ways of life are:

- Illiteracy
- Ignorance
- Poor knowledge
- Negative attitude
- Innate fear of getting into trouble
- No motivation
- Stringent custom in the family

MAJOR AREAS OF NEW HEALTH PRACTICES

Major areas of new health practices that need emphasis in day-to-day practice of health care delivery system are:

i. Practice of exclusive breast-feeding.
ii. Growth monitoring of baby in well-baby clinic.
iii. Feeding colostrums to the new born as first feed.
iv. No cradle near mother for proper rooming in and prevention of hypothermia.
v. Use of women hygiene kit (sanitary napkin) to prevent urinary tract infection and RTI among adolescence girls and reproductive age group.
vi. Weaning and supplementation of child is started after 4 months without waiting for ceremony of *annaprashana.*

Specialities in Sociology

They are:

- Medical sociology
- Rural sociology
- Urban sociology
- Industrial sociology
- Educational sociology
- Hospital sociology

Socialisation

Man learns to acquire custom, belief and tradition by day-to-day interaction. It is called socialisation.

- Primary socialisation — a baby learns from his/her mother
- Secondary socialisation — a child learns at school
- Re-socialisation — a person learns when he visits a foreign country

Culture

Man acquires the knowledge and proper behaviour in a society is called culture. It is always acquired from surroun-dings.

Standard of Living

It is a scale that measures the purchasing power of a person and fulfils the mode of living by getting all requirements like food, cloth, education, entertainment, etc.

Social Problems

- Poverty
- Malnutrition
- Alcoholism
- STD
- Mental illness
- Drug addiction
- Divorce
- Juvenile delinquency.

Field Study

It is observation and data collection on public health aspect by visiting the social unit "family".

This gives total picture and in-depth knowledge on health status, nutrition status, morbidity status and mortality status.

Social Defence

It is a type of social security where the society is protected from antisocial, criminal and mentally deviated elements. Common examples are:

- Control of alcoholism
- Control of prostitution
- Control of beggary

Functions of a Family

1. Provides place to live
2. Provides role to play for each family members
3. Procreation
4. Helps to acquire culture
5. Gives economic support
6. Gives social care
7. Protects the family members.

Problem Family

When backwardness, mental illness, and marital disharmony exist, the family is said to be a problem family. It is common in slums and shantytowns. Such families will be lagging behind others. Rehabi-litation of problem family is to be taken up by the paramedical worker of the area.

Broken Family

When death of either mother or father occurs, when parents are separated by divorce, the family is a broken family. This lowers the mental development of a child in the family. Such children become deviants, e.g., juvenile delinquent.

Cultural Factors

Table 2.3 shows the common cultural factors influencing health of the community.

Table 2.3: Common cultural factors influencing health of the community

Type of culture	*Examples*
Supernatural	Chickenpox is caused by wrath of Goddess Amma
Physical	Sunstroke causes heart attack
Human excreta	Latrine is not constructed at home prefer open field defecation
House waste	Thrown indiscriminately
River water	Commonplace for worship, waste throwing and ablution
Food habit	Jaggery and sugar are hot foods Curd and lemon are cold foods
Child care	Female child is not welcome in the family
Personal hygiene	Reverse smoking is a custom

Social Class

Commonly, income, education and occupation are to group people under a given social class.

Types of Social Classifications

They are:

Occupational grouping:

i. Profession
ii. Intermediate occupation
iii. Non-manual skilled
iv. Manual skilled
v. Partly skilled
vi. Unskilled

Kuppuswamy's grouping: This considers income, occupation and education.

Scale grouping: This considers possession of a person with movable property (car, cycle, TV), immovable property (land, house), family size, etc.

Technique of Interviewing

It is a device to interview people. Interviewing us in research. By personal contact the information is collected, either by proforma, questionnaire or oral interrogation. The technique involves:

- Contact establishment
- Started with general discussion
- Rapport is kept-up
- Should help in their recall
- Continuous encouragement is given
- On-the-spot recording is done
- Should be closed casually.

3

Behavioural Science and Its Importance

BEHAVIOURAL SCIENCE

Behaviour is important in public health because it influences illnesses and also positive health of an individual, family and society. To study behaviour scientifically there are many subjects that are listed by social scientists. But the following subjects are specifically called *behavioural science* because they deal with human behaviour directly.

a. Sociology
b. Psychology
c. Anthropology
d. Psychiatry

Sociology

Sociology deals with human relationships and interaction of a person with other person, with family and with community. This aspect is highlighted in Chapter 2.

Psychology

Psychology is the study of human mind to differentiate normal and abnormal from mental health point of view. Understanding of psychology helps to take measures in community psychiatry.

Psychological Implication

Examples of psychological implication in health and disease are as follows.

Health behaviour: Good health behaviour is that practicing monogamy prevents STD/HIV/AIDS.

Illness behaviour: Bad illness behaviour is that a patient suffering from tuberculosis comes to PHC at a late stage of disease.

Treatment behaviour: Good treatment behaviour is that a leprosy patient takes regular MDT regimen till cure and follows.

The above examples illustrate how human psychology has implication on health and disease. Fear, anger and anxiety are some known specific emotions that deal with abnormal behaviour. Disturbed emotion can lead to certain diseases like asthma, peptic ulcer and hypertension which are called psychosomatic disorders. Man needs motivation (as an inner force) to get positive attitude.

Personality

Adjustment of a person to his surroundings which are characteristic of a given individual is called personality. If a person is dashing in nature and mixes easily, he will be called an extrovert. If a person is reserved and does not mix easily with others, he will be branded as an introvert.

The personality is determined by human development during man's life cycle, main stages of which are depicted as under:

- Infancy and childhood
- School age
- Adolescent period

- Adult age
- Old age.

Intelligence

Intelligence is an ability to see meaningful relationship between things. This also conveys motor ability, adoptive nature and language. This is expressed by IQ (Intelligent Quotient), which is calculated by:

$$IQ = \frac{\text{Mental age}}{\text{Chronological age}} \times 100$$

Table 3.1 shows IQ levels to be learnt for child examination in the field.

Table 3.1: IQ levels

Level	*IQ*
Idiot	0 to 24
Moron	50 to 69
Borderline	70 to 79
Normal	90 to 109

Human Anthropology

This branch of behavioural science deals with physical stature of human beings, types of social life they lead and their thinking capacity. In other words, human anthropology deals with total study of man from different angles.

Table 3.2 shows components of anthropology in the study of human behaviour.

Table 3.2: Components of anthropology in the study of human behaviour

Type	*Example*
Physical anthropology	Erect posture of man is responsible for hernia, piles and varicose veins
Social anthropology	Changes in social life bring illness like diabetes and heart attack
Cultural anthropology	Changes in food culture leading to intestinal disturbances by low fibre diet

Psychiatry

This branch of behavioural science deals with mental illness, diagnosis and treatment. This highlights the following causes of illness called *mental illness:*

- Disturbances in crucial point of life cycle like pregnancy, under five children, etc.
- Family and society interactions leading to psychosis.
- Neurosis and personality disturbances.

Community Psychiatry

With the help of health workers and with minimum essential drugs like chlorpromazine, phenobarbitone and imipramine common clinical conditions like psychosis, depression, epilepsy and mental retar-dation are tackled.

PUBLIC HEALTH AND BEHAVIOURAL SCIENCES

Behavioural scientists help public health professionals in the study of natural history of diseases and risk factors in certain diseases. They are helping medical professionals by giving relevance of social and behavioural system in health, disease and health care delivery. Particularly, attention is given to the interaction of health personnel and community in health management and health care services.

4

Concept of Community Health

COMMUNITY HEALTH

The community health is depending on our understanding of health by community diagnosis. All categories of people like Administrators, Science specialists. Paramedicals and social scientists help in the development of the health of a community.

Community health depends on:

- Germs or pathogens around us
- Man's surrounding, which is called *ecology*.
- Socio-psychological influences.

In other words, many dimensions in life determine the health status of man.

Health

World Health Organisation (WHO) has defined health as:

"Health is a state of complete physical, mental and social well-being and not merely an absence of disease or infirmity."

Physical Quality of Life

If there is no death in early productive age, if a person lives longer say up to 100 years (at least 64 years in developing countries like India) and if a person has attained good education, we say the person has good physical quality of life.

It is measured by a scale and it is called Physical Quality of Life Index (PQLI) (Table 4.1).

Table 4.1: An example of PQLI

Scale	*Inference*
Zero	Worst quality of life
50	Medium quality of life
100	Best quality of life

Health Spectrum

At a given point of time, we come across all categories of people. Majority of them are healthy, but a small proportion are sick who may be mild sick, severe sick, dying or dead. This picture of all categories is called *spectrum of health* (Fig. 4.1).

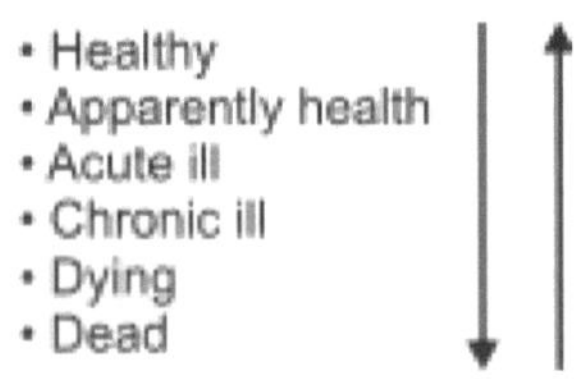

Fig. 4.1: Spectrum of health

Community Responsibilities

For positive health of a community, community is responsible on several occasions. People should understand ill health and should involve in helping the sick and also participate in all health-related activities. Hence, responsibilities of a community in community health care are:

- Pre-planning
- Planning
- Implementation
- Use
- Health care service promotion
- Cross-check the utility of health care service.

Health Indicators

Health is measurable. To measure the health, we have developed some health indicators. They are commonly used in survey, screening, and surveillance and health care services.

The health indicators can be grouped into the following categories:

- Death (mortality)
  - Crude death rate
  - Life expectation
  - IMR
  - MMR
- Sickness (morbidity)
  - Incidence and prevalence
- Handicap (disability)
  - Days admitted in a hospital
  - Work loss by illness
- Nourishment (nutrition)
  - Height
  - Weight
  - Birth weight
- Service givers (health care delivery)
  - Doctor population ratio (Dr : Pop)
  - Doctor nurse ratio (Dr : Nurse)
- Use (Utilisation)
  - Fully immunised
  - Deliveries by TBA

Health System

This contains organisations and management for health care service (Table 4.2).

Table 4.2: Health system—organisation and management

Health system of a big hospital	*Health system of a district health care*	*Health system of a city corporation*
Superintendent	DH & FWO	City Health Officer
RMO	AH & FWO	Regional Health Officer
Doctors	PHC Medical Officer	Asstt. Health Officer
Paramedicals	Staff of PHC	Health Inspectors
Other Class III	Sub-centre staff	Assistants
Class IV staff	Community Health Guide	Sanitary workers

In health system, we have three levels of health care. They are *primary*, *secondary* and *tertiary*. This is depicted in Table 4.3.

Table 4.3: Levels of health care

Primary	*Secondary*	*Tertiary*
Close to people	District hospital	Super specialty hospital
First contact PHC and Sub-centre	Specialist	

Health for All

This is a social goal of all Governments in the world. Opportunity given to all to enjoy good health is called Health For All (HFA).

MULTIFACTORIAL CAUSE OF DISEASES

Instead of one cause like bacteria or virus, the disease is caused by many (multiple) factors. These factors are:

- Social
- Economic
- Cultural
- Genetic
- Psychological

Risk Factors

The cause of a disease is strongly associated with some known influencing factors. They are called *risk factors*. Examples are depicted in Table 4.4.

Table 4.4: Examples of risk factors

Risk factors	*Illness*
High BP Fat body Chronic smoking	Stroke
Alcoholic No seat belt or helmet High speed driving	Accident
Drinking habit	Liver failure
Type A personality Lack of exercise	Heart problem

The Iceberg in Disease

In Figure 4.2, we see a small portion of illness and a major portion of iceberg (disease) is not seen. Here, illness is compared with an ice floating in the water where the tip is seen and the major portion is not seen. This is called *iceberg phenomenon* of disease.

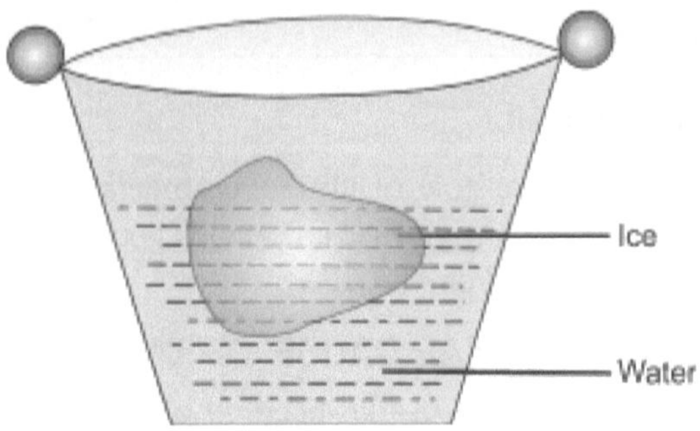

Fig. 4.2: The Iceberg

Table 4.5 shows control, elimination and eradication of disease.

Table 4.5: Control, elimination and eradication of disease

Control	*Elimination*	*Eradication*
Incidence is reduced to make that it is not a public health problem, for example, cholera control	Transmission of disease is interrupted, for example, measles elimination, polio elimination	Removing illness by cutting at the root of illness, for example, polio eradication

Surveillance

Continuous scrutiny and monitoring of illness in a community is called *surveillance.*

For example, STD surveillance and HIV/AIDS sur-veillance.

Prevention

It is a process to see that diseases do not occur in a community. They are done at four levels.

First Level *(Primordial prevention)* : This is possible by preventing harmful lifestyles by the community.

Second Level *(Primary prevention)* : It is an action taken prior to the onset of illness, which removes the possibilities that illness never occur.

Third Level *(Secondary prevention)* : Early diagnosis and prompt treatment constitute secondary prevention

Fourth Level *(Tertiary prevention)* : This involves measures to limit impairment and disabilities of a person.

Health Intervention

When we intervene to halt a disease or to prevent its occurrence, the measure taken is called *inter-vention*. The intervention can be any one of the following:

- Giving health education
- Providing safe water

- Providing sanitary RCA latrines
- Nutrition feeding programmes
- Diagnosis
- Treatment
- Limitation of disabilities
- Rehabilitation

Health interventions can also be grouped under five categories:

1. Health promotion, e.g. good nutrition, change in lifestyle
2. Specific protection, e.g. immunisation, helmet to driver
3. Early diagnosis and prompt treatment, e.g. blood pressure, cancer
4. Disability limitation, e.g. reconstructive surgery in leprosy
5. Rehabilitation, e.g. artificial limb to polio case.

Terminologies in Community Health

Hygiene: It is a science of health.

Public health: It is a science and art of preventing disease, prolonging life and promoting health by organised community effort.

Community diagnosis: Illness detected at community level is called community diagnosis. This requires the collection of health data.

Community treatment: It is the community health action for giving positive health to the community.

5

Elementary and Vital Statistics

STATISTICS

Statistics is science of figures. This is a useful tool to a Health Inspector in his day-to-day activities like:

- Surveys
- Surveillance
- Screening
- Reporting
- Reviewing

When you say that you have examined 100 fever cases, took 100 malaria smears under active malaria surveillance and that 4 were MP positive, you mean that:

- 100 per cent is smear collection.
- 4 per cent is positive rate.

Here, you express in numbers and it is definite that you know what you are speaking. This is the advantage of knowing statistics, speaking statistics and reporting statistics.

All PHC activities are recorded which form data. This is analysed by tabulation. Later, it is presented by picture or graph.

When biological events are collected, tabulated and analysed, it is called *biostatistics*.

When data on health, disease and preventive medicine are collected, tabulated and analysed, it is called *medical statistics*.

When data on the births, deaths and marriages are collected, tabulated and analysed, it is called vital statistics.

There are two types of data in day-to-day public health activities. They are:

I. *Type*: When we cannot count or measure properly, it is called *qualitative data*. For example,

- Sex—male, female
- Result of treatment—died, survived
- Race—Indian, American
- Malaria smear—positive, negative

II. *Type*: When we can count or measure properly, it is called *quantitative data*. For example,

- Body weight — 55 kg, 14 kg,
- Hb% — 14g%, 12 g%
- Pulse — 72, 68, 70

Uses of Statistics

- It is a guide for the Health Inspector's health care services.
- It measures health status of the community.
- It helps to find out health needs of the community.
- It helps to compare:
  - Person to person
  - PHC to PHC
  - District to District
  - Country to Country
- It helps in health planning.
- It helps in good health administration.

Importance

- Helps in decision taking on Public Health Measures.
- It identifies the community as health or sick.
- It is a bases for report preparation.
- It is necessary for health policy making.
- It measures the impact of National Health Programmes.

Parameter

Parameter measures and describes the characteristics of a population.

For example,

Size of family = 5.3
IMR = 71

Data

When you collect information like age, sex, fever, births, operations done, etc., these are data. These do not give any meaning.

To get meaning, the data must be tabulated and presented in the form of a table.

Tabulation

On a particular day, when you visit a village, you come across 16 fever cases. You collect the information and also collect the blood smear. It will be as depicted in Table 5.1.

Table 5.1: Collected information and blood smear of 16 fever cases

Date: __________ Village/Area: __________

Sl. No.	*Name*	*Age*	*Sex*	*MP smears Tallies*	*PT given*
1	Govinda	38 years	M	√	√
2	Singla	41 years	M	√	√
3	Bose	60 years	M	√	√
4	Maria	10 years	M	√	√
5	Janaki	22 years	F	√	√
6	Baby	8 months	F	√	√
7	Ranjit	51 years	M	√	√
8	Punekar	50 years	M	√	√
9	Mahanta	42 years	M	√	√
10	Banu	17 years	F	√	√
11	Chitra	27 years	F	√	√
12	Reshma	30 years	F	√	√
13	Dara	40 years	M	√	√
14	Dakshayani	21 years	F	√	√
15	Ali	18 years	M	√	√
16	Peter	9 years	M	√	√

Let us tabulate above data, to get distribution of cases according to age (Table 5.2).

Table 5.2: Distribution of above discussed cases according to age

Age interval	*Frequency*	*Members*
0 – 1 years	I	1
1 – 5 years	—	—
5 – 14 years	II	2
14 – 45 years	~~IIII~~ ~~IIII~~	10
45 + above	III	3
	Total	16

Data is tabulated for the distribution of sex in Table 5.3.

Table 5.3: Distribution of cases according to sex

Sex	*Frequency*	*Members*
Male	~~IIII~~ ~~IIII~~	10
Female	~~IIII~~ I	6
	Total	16

Presentation of Data

When data tabulated is represented to give a full meaning, we call it as presentation of data. The Health Inspector is expected to know two common types of data presentation.

They are:

i. Bar diagram
ii. Pie diagram

Let us take, the example of fever cases mentioned earlier, where MP smear was taken. The bar diagram is presented as in Figure 5.1.

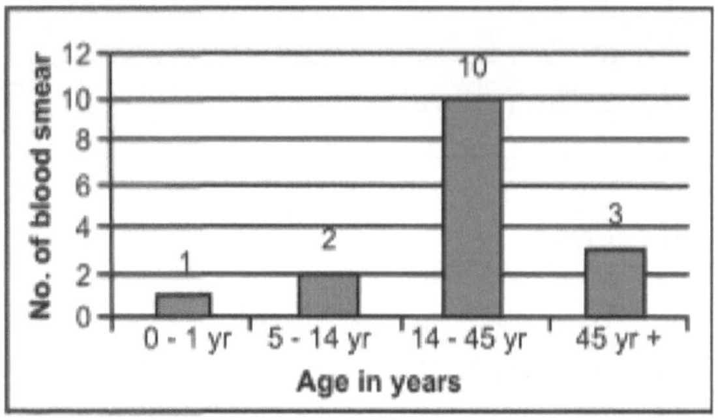

Fig. 5.1: Bar diagram showing age distribution of fever cases in whom MP smear was taken

The same fever cases where MP smear was taken, if the data tabulated for sex distribution is presented as under (Fig. 5.2):

$\frac{10}{16} \times 360 = 225° = 10$ cases

$\frac{6}{16} \times 360 = 135° = 6$ cases

Total = 360°

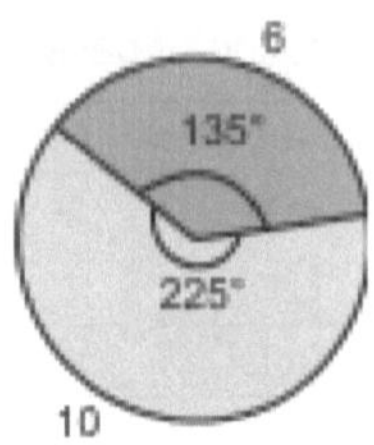

Fig. 5.2: Pie diagram showing the distribution of sex among fever cases on whom MP smear was taken

Finding Average

Average is called *arithmetic mean* in statistics. When you check pulse or body temperature of a group of people, the average helps us to understand that how many are nearer to average.

Let us take pulse and body temperature of 16 fever cases, when a Health Inspector visited the villages and took the MP smear (Table 5.4).

Table 5.4: Pulse rate and body temperature of 16 fever cases

Sl. No.	*Pulse rate*	*Temperature*
1	74	99
2	77	99
3	80	99.5
4	73	100
5	78	100
6	96	99.5
7	82	100.5
8	82	100
9	76	99
10	77	98.5
11	78	99
12	80	99.5
13	82	99
14	87	99
15	88	98.5
16	90	99.5

To find out mean or average, we have to total the value and later should divide the total value by number of cases.

We get the value as under:

$$\text{Mean of pulse rate} = \frac{\text{Total pulse rate}}{16}$$

$$= \frac{1300}{16} = 81.25$$

$$\text{Mean of temperature} = \frac{\text{Total temperature}}{16}$$

$$= \frac{1589.5}{16} = 99.3$$

Their average pulse rate of fever cases is 81 and average body temperature of fever cases is 99.

When we do not have body temperature (i.e., fever) normally average pulse rate is 72 and average body temperature is 98.4°F.

Since all 16 cases have shown above the average of normal person, it is an indication of fever, may be due to malaria. Hence, presumptive treatment (PT) is given to all fever cases.

Spot Map

To show distribution of gastroenteritis (GE) cases or any other diseases, a dot is marked to indicate the cases in a map of the area where it is studied. For example, on a given day 42 cases of GE are identified in Gujarat. When they are spotted on the map of Gujarat, it showed that more cases were seen near Porbandar and Rajkot (Fig. 5.3). This helps us to draft Public Health Measures to be taken.

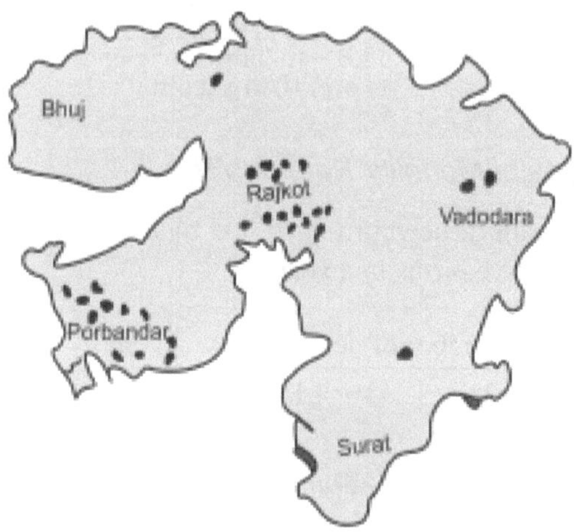

Fig. 5.3: Gujarat map showing thedistribution of GE cases (spot map)

VITAL STATISTICS

This aspect of statistics deals with human life events like, births, deaths, sickness, marriage, divorce and migration, etc., which are called *vital statistics.*

Health Inspectors should know about these vital events, which are to be collected, compiled and reported to higher authorities. They are in simple words events occurring in a community.

Definition: Data collected and analysed on vital events of a community is called *vital statistics.*

Value: The vital statistics gives us leading cause of death, important cause of illness in the community, whether a particular disease is increasing or not, what is the composition of a population and priority for the National Health Programme.

Objectives

To help Health Inspectors to apply vital statistics knowledge in:

- Their job responsibilities
- Proper reporting
- Adjusting workload in supervising activities
- Apply legal measures wherever public health problem arises.

Population Census

The collective study of mankind is called *demography.* The vital statistics are important tool for demography. Population census is not a vital event. But it gives clear picture of vital events of a country.

Census is a big national level process where data collection, data compilation and data publishing are done on social data, economic data, and demographic data once in 10 years (Table 5.5).

In India, the first census was done in 1872 and continued on 1881. From then, it is done once in 10 years. The latest census was done in 2001. It is done at one given time covering all persons in the country. This helps in National Planning and National Programmes on Health.

Table 5.5: Census data

	2001
Population of India	1027 million
Density of population	324 per sq km
Total fertility rate	3 per cent
Literacy rate	65.38 per cent
Life expectation	62.8 for men 63.8 for women
Birth rate	26.1
Death rate	8.7
Growth rate	1.93 per cent
IMR	70
MMR	4

Estimation of Population

Commonly, arithmetic progression method is used to estimate population. Let us take the following example:

Population of a city in 2001 = 4,00,000
Population of a city in 1991 = 3,30,000

Increase in 10 years = 70,000
Increase in 1 year = 5,833

Therefore, population in 2005 of that city could be:

$$4,00,000 + (5833)\frac{1}{3} = 4,23,332$$

(The illustration is a simple method of calculation. But for mid-year population (MYP) estimation, we have to add 4 more months of population because census will be taken on first March of first year of the decade. The mid-year population should be up to first July of 2005. So the period from first March to first July is to be added up).

Rates

Rate, ratio or proportions express magnitude of a disease, of a problem or of an event. They are basic tools in health indicators.

Common Indicators

Birth Rate (BR)

It is the number of live births (LB) during a year per 1000 mid-year population.

$$\text{BR} = \frac{\text{Number of births in 1 year}}{\text{Mid-year population (MYP)}} \times 1000$$

Death Rate (DR)

It is the number of deaths per 1000 mid-year population in 1 year.

$$\text{DR} = \frac{\text{Number of deaths in 1 year}}{\text{Mid-year population (MYP)}} \times 100$$

Infant Mortality Rate (IMR)

It is the ratio of infant deaths registered in 1 year to the live births of the same year.

$$\text{IMR} = \frac{\text{Number of deaths below 1 year or in 1 year}}{\text{Live births (LB)}} \times 1000$$

Stillbirth Rate

It is death of a foetus weighing 1000 g or more occurring during 1 year in every 1000 total births (Total births include live births and stillbirths).

$$\text{Stillbirth rate} = \frac{\text{Foetal death weighing over 1000 g at birth}}{\text{Total LB + stillbirths weighing over 1000 g at birth}} \times 1000$$

Neonatal Mortality Rate (NMR)

It is death of newborn-aged less than 28 days out of total live births in a year.

$$\text{NMR} = \frac{\text{Number of deaths below 28 days}}{\text{LB}} \times 1000$$

Maternal Mortality Rate (MMR)

It is death of women while pregnant or within 42 days of delivery per 1000 live births.

$$\text{MMR} = \frac{\text{Number of mothers dying due to pregnancy, childbirth within 42 days of delivery}}{\text{Number of LB}} \times 1000$$

Morbidity Rates

Incidence

It is the number of new cases occurring in a defined population during 1 year and prevalence is the prevailing status at a given point of time which include old and new cases, are common morbidity rates used in Public Health practice.

$$\text{Incidence} = \frac{\text{Number of new cases in 1 year}}{\text{Population at risk}} \times 1000$$

$$\text{Prevalence} = \frac{\text{Number of old and new cases in 1 year}}{\text{Population at risk}} \times 1000$$

Apart from these, bed occupancy rate and bed turn-over ratio explain the extent of morbidity of a community.

Significance

By above rates, Health Inspectors can assess the impact of health measures adopted by the country. *For example*,

- Typhoid epidemic in a village can be brought down by:
  - Personal hygiene
  - Milk hygiene
- Literacy rate can bring down birth rate
- Protected water supply can reduce gastro-enteritis (GE) in a locality.

IMPORTANCE AND USE OF VITAL STATISTICS

- Helps to know local health problems.
- Identifies cause of death.
- Helps to know whether a disease is coming down or not.
- Identifies as to who are affected most.
- It can project population pattern and family pattern.

Informants, Collection and Compilation

In India, over the many years Revenue Agency, Police Agency, Panchayat Agency and Health Agency are reporting and have been informants. But this showed no uniformity. Since 1970, the central Births and Deaths Registration Act 1969, came to power. This has fixed responsibility for reporting. Parents and relatives are expected to report the events that occurred in their houses. With regard to hospital, health centre, nursing home, hotel, jail, and dharamshalas, the head of the organisation should report the vital event.

Birth must be informed within 14 days and death must be informed within 7 days. A fine of Rs 50.00 attends any default.

Village health guide and local leaders are expected to be lay informants. They are non-professionals.

Survey data and hospital registers also give information on vital events.

Registration—Rural, Urban, Objects, Machinery and Checking (Figs 5.4 and 5.5)

Health workers attached to PHC or City Corporation do cross-check. Weekly report and fortnightly report are submitted to district authorities. Further, monthly and quarterly reports reach the government.

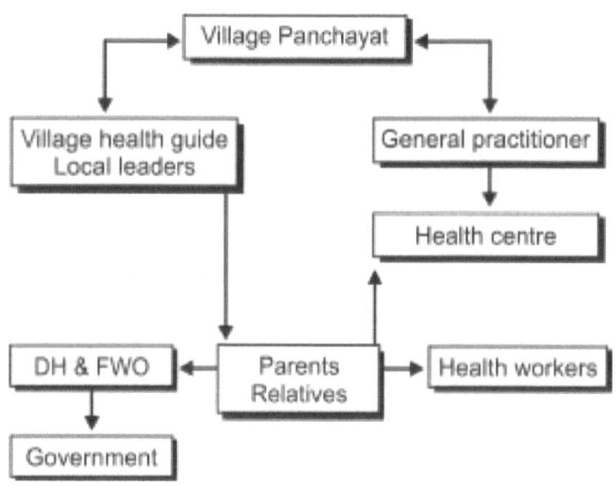

Fig. 5.4: Registration (Rural)

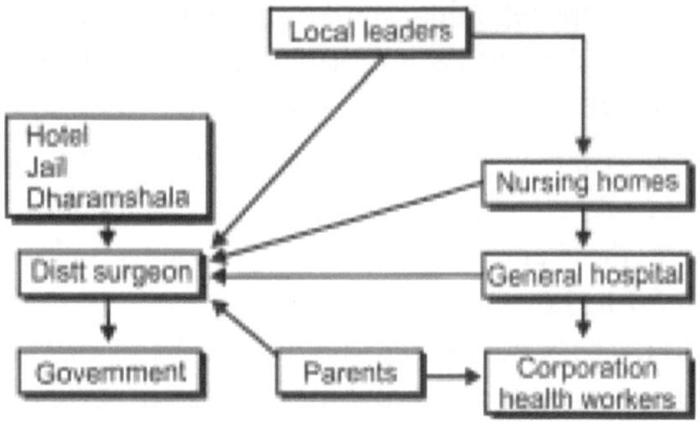

Fig. 5.5: Registration (Urban)

Uses of Notification and Records

Notification is an important source of epidemiological and public health information. It helps in detection of outbreak of diseases.

Notification is done by attending doctors, health workers, public, religious leaders, political leaders and teachers.

According to International Health Regulations, cholera, plague and yellow fever are notifiable diseases. They are major diseases because they are controlled under quarantinable diseases (Quarantine disease is not allowed to spread to other countries).

Notifications under the WHO and Govt. of India Surveillance are existing for polio, malaria, influenza, relapsing fever and typhus.

Main uses of notification are:

- Prevention of diseases
- Control of infections
- Serves as source of data
- Identifies disease fluctuation

At present, the Government of India has made it mandatory to certain conditions and non-communicable diseases like:

- Handicapped persons
- Stroke
- Mental illness
- Birth defects
- Cancer.

Record Keeping

Definition

Hospitals, health centres and all health workers have to maintain specified registers and ledgers for OPD, in-patient, notifiable diseases, ANC registration, PNC follow up, ICDS service, growth monitoring immunisation done, etc., which are sources of data for a check to the ongoing health activities and health programmes.

Reporting

Day-to-day activities mentioned under definition are to be reported at specified period of time to the designated authorities. A Health Inspector for having collected and sent a food sample for test, blood smear collected for MP smear, chlorination of water done in the wells of village, etc., are to be compiled and are to be reported to PHC Medical Officers, who in turn will report to District health authorities.

Purpose and Application

It is a systematic method of entry of health statistics. It helps to compare with past and helps to take measure to check future. Regular administrative machinery and health workers are assigned the responsibility of record keeping.

Record keeping is taken up for review in regular monthly staff meeting at PHC, CHC and District level meetings.

Appreciation of record keeping comes to the picture when it serves as a guideline for action or measures during public health emergencies like epidemics and calamities.

Classification: Depending on the source, we have hospital records, nursing home records, health centre records, supervisory records, survey records, research records and experiment records.

Service

Hospital records and health centre records are mandatory and separate section headed by Medical Record Officer or in–charge officer of records are seen throughout the country.

Methodological approach like ICD (International Classification of Diseases) classification is followed in the established service departments.

Modern methods of computer recording and record keeping have revolutionised the medical record system. This revolution has gone beyond and is called *information system* and *documentation centre*.

Sanitation Data

Recording of availability of water supply, provision for sanitary method of disposal of human excreta, methods available for refuse or garbage have been taken-up under the National Health Programme to prevent water-borne diseases, soil-borne diseases and vector-borne diseases.

Village Health Record

This is a new form, which has replaced earlier form MF-1 in PHC area. Health workers should fill it during baseline survey of villages covered by a subcentre. It is to be updated every three years.

The information gives overall picture of village like:

- Number of households
- Population distribution (age, sex)
- GP available (general practitioners)
- Health guides of the areas
- Depot holders of the areas
- *Dais* of the areas
- Community resource and agencies
- Public facilities of village
- Number of eligible couples
- Water supply
- Sanitation facility
- Present confirmed cases of specified disease.

Sanitation

This is a specific area of a Health Inspector who has to handle recording, reporting and implementing public health measures.

Specified activities under sanitation are:

- Chlorinate public water source at regular intervals.
- Educate community on the method of disposal xof liquid waste.
- Help community to construct soakage pit, kitchen garden.
- Educate community about method of disposal of solid waste.
- Help community to construct compost pit or manure pit.
- Create awareness on sanitary latrine and help to construct a sanitary latrine.
- Health education on home sanitation.
- Educate public on public health hazards and about personal hygiene.

Sanitary Survey Forms

Sanitary survey of an area, a village or extension consists of the following:

- Topography of the area
- Communication facility
- Water facility
- Provision for disposal of
  - Liquid waste
  - Solid waste
  - Human excreta

- Market sanitation
  - Vegetable market
  - Mutton/fish market
- Drainage system
- Special provisions like soakage pit, kitchen garden, manure pit, compost pit and sanitary latrine.

Spot Maps

During an investigation, survey of epidemic, the current status of conditions or cases or events is put down to represent their occurrence according to geographical area.

Their use and illustration are given in earlier unit.

6

Elements of Medical Microbiology and Parasitology

MICROSCOPE

Elementary knowledge of *microscope* is necessary for Health Inspectors in field examination of microbes and parasites. Figure 6.1 illustrates parts of microscope.

The piece through which we look into the microscope is called *eyepiece*. Near the slide, three objectives namely low power, high power and oil immersion are there which magnify the microbes and parasites.

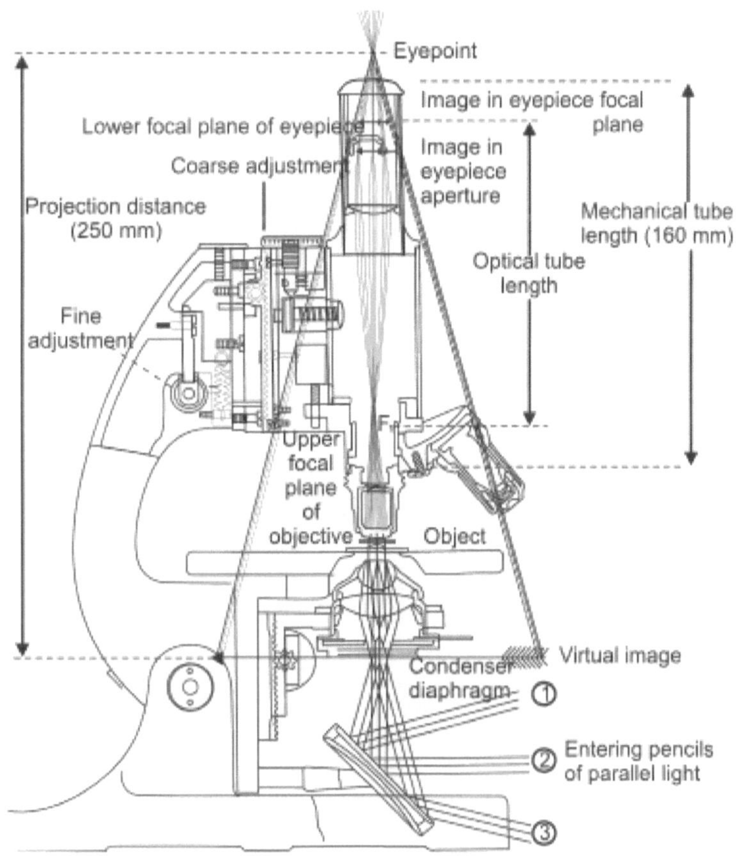

Fig. 6.1: Parts of microscope

Microscope is set up to a convenient position. Slide is put on a platform. Low power is adjusted to observe. Later, high power is turned and specimen is examined. For oil immersion, one-drop cedar wood oil is placed on the slide below the objective.

For oil immersion (e.g. Malaria parasite smear), condenser is raised, diaphragm is opened, mirror is adjusted and focused for examination.

Hanging Drop Preparation

One loopful of material is placed in the centre of cover slip. Another clean depression slide with a Vaseline ring is inverted over it. After turning, direct examination is done. This is useful to demonstrate motility of *Vibrio cholerae.*

Stool Examination

Stool sample diluted with normal saline is taken on a slide. After putting a cover slip, it is examined under microscope. A Health Inspector is expected to identify ova or cyst of the following:

- Amoeba (Amoebiasis) (Fig. 6.2)
- Roundworm (Ascariasis) (Fig. 6.3)
- Hookworm (Ankylsostomiasis) (Fig. 6.4)
- Threadworm (Fig. 6.5).

Gram's Stain

- Thin film of suspension is prepared, dried, and fixed.
- Stained with gentian violet for 3 minutes.
- Washed with gentle stream of water, slide is drained; Gram's iodine is put, allowed for 1 minute.

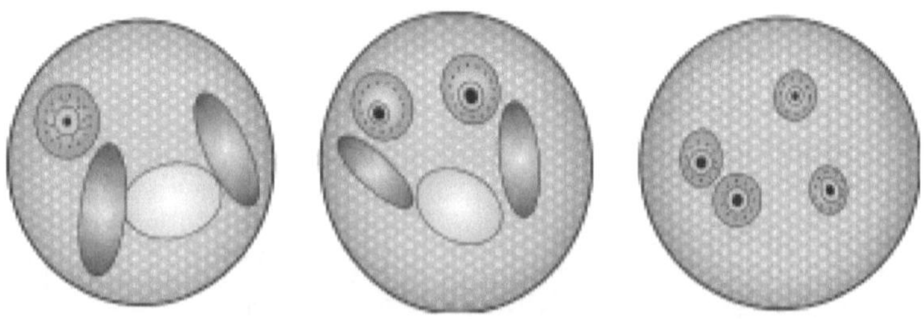

Fig. 6.2: Amoebic cyst under microscope

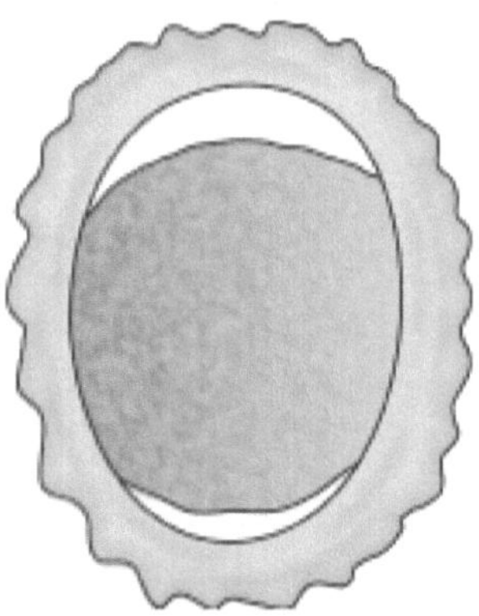

Fig. 6.3: Egg of roundworm under microscope

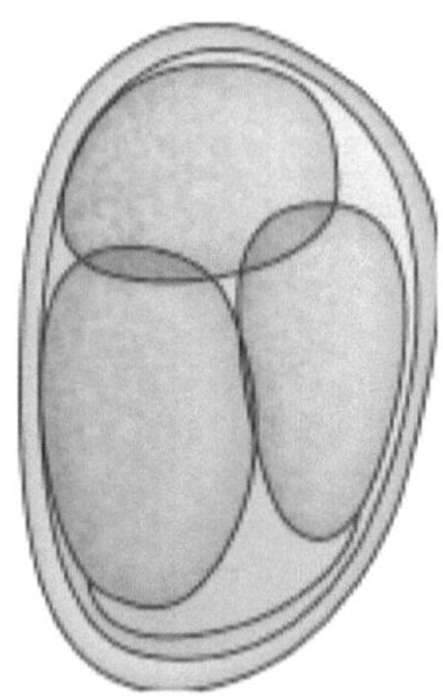

Fig. 6.4: Egg of hookworm under microscope

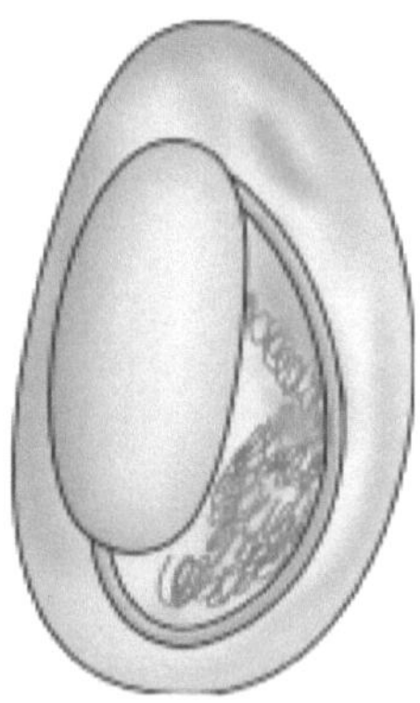

Fig. 6.5: Egg of threadworm under microscope

- Washed and dried.
- Slide is flood with alcohol with gentle rocking. Repeated till it is no longer coloured by dye. Alcohol is allowed for 2 minutes, washed with water.
- Counterstained with dilute carbolfuchsine for 1 minute.
- Washed, blotted and allowed to dry.

Inference

- If violet, it is gram-positive.
- If red, it is gram-negative.
  For example,
- Gram-positive *cocci*:
  - *Streptococci*
  - *Staphylococci*
  - *Pneumococci*
- Gram-negative cocci:
  - *Gonococci*
- Gram-positive bacilli:
  - Diphtheria
  - Tuberculosis
- Gram-negative bacilli:
  - Salmonella (typhoid)
  - Pasturella (plague)
  - Cholera

Albert's Stain

For Diphtheria

- Throat smear is prepared, dried and fixed.
- Stain with Albert A for 5 minutes
- Wash in water
- Blot
- Stain with Albert B for 1 minute
- Blot

Inference

Light green dumb-bell shape bacteria.

Ziehl-Neelsen (ZN) Stain

For Acid-fast Bacillus

- Sputum material is taken, dried and fixed
- Slide is placed on rack
- Carbolfuchsine is poured; heated to steam, allowed 5 minutes, heated at interval
- Wash with water
- Immerse slide in 20 percent sulphuric acid for 1 minutes. Repeat it till decolouration is complete
- Five percent alcohol poured and allowed for 2 minutes
- Wash with water
- Counter stain with Loffler's methylene blue for 1 minute.
- Wash, blot, dry, mount and exam.

Inference

Brighter red AFB seen

Slit and Scrape Method of Skin Smear

Leprosy Case

- Skin is cleaned with soap and detergent
- A slide is taken and marked with name and number of patient
- Three smears are taken from any one of the following sites:
  - Right ear
  - Left ear
  - Forehead
  - Chin
  - Buttock in men
  - Thigh in women
  - Arm
  - Back
  - Front of chest
- Pinch a fold of skin, make a 5 mm. Cut with scalpel
- Scrape a bit of tissue by tip of scalpel blade
- Scrape is taken on to slide
- Cut is dressed.

Skin smear technique and nasal mucosal smear technique are shown in Figures 6.6 and 6.7.

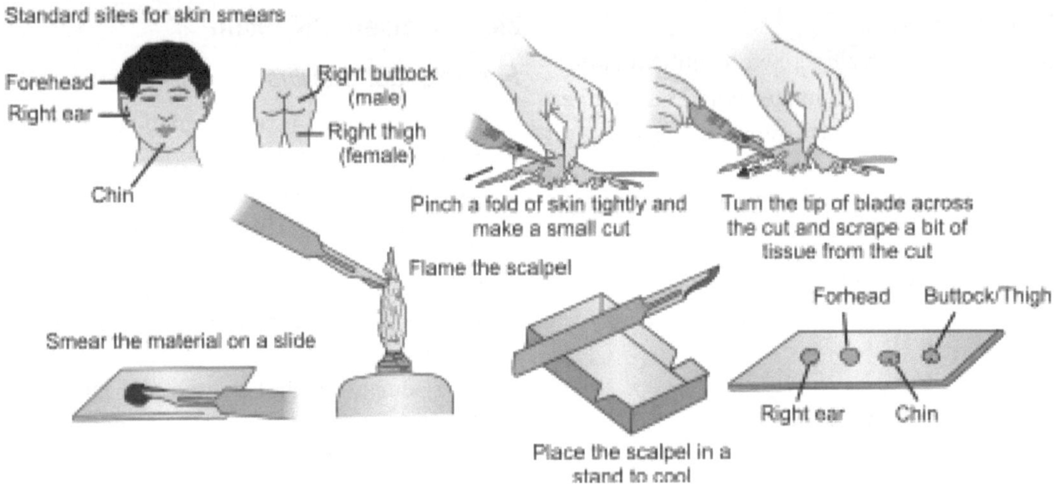

Fig. 6.6: Slit and scrape technique

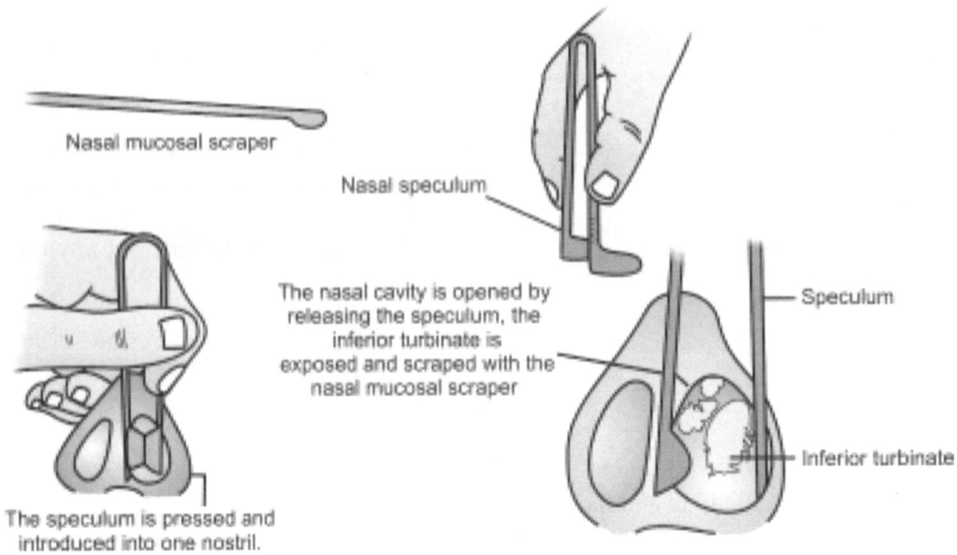

Fig. 6.7: Nasal mucosal smears technique

MICROBES

Aerobes and Anaerobes

Aerobes are bacteria, which require oxygen for their growth.

Anaerobes are bacteria, which do not grow if oxygen is present.

In between aerobe and anaerobe, there is a group called facultative anaerobes, which can grow both in the absence and presence of oxygen.

Methods of Sterilisation

To kill pathogens and to stop the growth of pathogens, there are many methods. They are called *sterilisation methods*. They are:

- Dry heat
- Moist heat
- Chemicals
- Filtration

Common chemicals used to disinfect medical items are:

- Phenol
- Lysol
- Dettol
- Hypochlorite

Bacteriological Analysis of Water

This is done in many tubes and hence it is also called "multiple tube method". By doing this test, most probable number (MPN) of coliform in 100 ml of sample of water is found out (Table 6.1). It is commonly known as presumptive coliform test (PCT).

Table 6.1: Field guideline for bacteriological analysis of water

MPN value	*Result*
Zero / 100 ml	Excellent
1 to 2 / 100 ml	Satisfactory
3 to 10 / 100 ml	Suspicious
10 + / 100 ml	Unfit

Other common tests done under microbiology are:

- VDRL test for syphilis
- Widal test for typhoid
- HIV test for HIV/AIDS
- Pregnancy test for diagnosis of pregnancy
- Coomb's test for Rh incompatibility.

Immunity

When a person is infected with bacteria or virus, his body fights with organisms to destroy or to eliminate them. If the person succeeds in destroying organisms, he is said to have body immunity.

Types of Immunity

They are:

Active immunity: If a person gets immunity by way of infection or by immunisation.

For example,

i. A boy gets chickenpox. After natural cure, he gets immunity.
ii. OPV given to child. It develops active immunity.

Passive immunity: After infection, man and animal develop antibiotics. Such blood is taken and given to other persons who develop immediate protection called passive immunity.

Herd immunity: This is the body protective mechanism shown by a group of people.

Immunisation Agents

They are grouped under three categories (Table 6.2)

- Vaccines
- Immunoglobulins
- Antisera

Table 6.2: Immunisation agents

Vaccines	*Immunoglobulins*	*Antisera*
DPT	Rabies	ADS
DT	Tetanus	ATS
OPV		
BCG		
Measles		

National Immunisation Schedule (Table 6.3)

Table 6.3: National immunisation schedule

		Vaccines
a. For infants		
	At birth	BCG and OPV 0 dose (for institutional deliveries)
	At 6 weeks	BCG (if not given at birth) DPT 1 and OPV 1
	At 10 weeks	DPT 2 and OPV 2
	At 14 weeks	DPT 3 and OPV 3
	At 9 months	Measles
b. At 16 and 24 months		DPT and OPV
c. At 5 to 6 years		DT—the second dose of DT should be given at an interval of one month if there is no clear history or documented evidence of previous immunization with DPT
d. At 10 and at 16 years		TT—the second dose of TT vaccine should be given at an interval of one month if there is no clear history or documented evidence of previous immunisation with DPT, DT or TT vaccines
e. For pregnant women		Early pregnancy—TT 1 or booster One month after —TT 1 or TT 2

Other vaccines given in Public Health Practice:

- Cholera vaccine
- Typhoid vaccine

Vaccines for International travel:

- Cholera
- Meningitis
- Yellow fever

Quarantine

Restriction on suspected healthy contacts to prevent disease entry to another country.

It holds good with cholera and plague to Indian conditions.

Adverse Reaction Following Immunisation

All vaccines are tested for safety of 100 per cent. Reactions are very mild when compared with health benefit of vaccination.

Monitoring of adverse reaction is done for:

- Check at programme error
- To avoid public fear
- To give moral support to health workers

RCH officer investigates all vaccines reactions within 48 hours. Experts from the department of community medicine, microbiology and paediatrics are considered in the investigation.

Types of reactions are:

- By vaccine—only mild reaction, fever, irritability
- By programme error—abscess sepsis, etc.
- Coincidental—aspiration

Disinfection

Killing the germs by germicide is called *disinfection.* A substance which inhibits growth of microbe is called *antiseptic.*

Types of Disinfections (Table 6.4)

Table 6.4: Types of disinfections

Type	*Germicidal method*
Concurrent disinfection	Urine, stool, vomit, cloth etc., of patient is disinfected.
Terminal	When patients are discharged or died after infectious diseases
Prophylactic	Water chlorination Milk pasteurisation Washing the hands

Common disinfections in hospital and PHC use:

- Burning – Incineration
- Boiling – Instruments, rubber glove
- Autoclaving – Dressings, linen, non-sharp instruments
- Chemical – Phenol, cresol, dettol, savlon, bleaching powder, sodium hypochlorite

Recommended disinfection procedures:

- Stool – 10 per cent phenol, 8 per cent bleaching powder
- Urine – 10 per cent phenol, 8 per cent bleaching powder
- Sputum – Burning
- Dead body – Covered with bedsheet soaked in 10 per cent formalin
- Syringe – Boiling
- Urinals – Hypochlorite solution
- Bedpan – Lysol

MICROBES OF PUBLIC HEALTH IMPORTANCE

Infections

Respiratory Infections

- ARI – Bacteria and virus
- Chickenpox – Varicella virus
- Diphtheria – *Corynebacterium diphtheriae*
- Measles – Myxovirus
- Tuberculosis – *Mycobacterium tuberculosis*
- Whooping cough – *Bordetella pertussis*

Intestinal Infections

- Cholera – *Vibrio cholerae*
- Diarrhoea – Virus and bacteria
- Hepatitis – Hepatitis A virus
- Polio – Polio virus
- Typhoid – *Salmonella typhi*

Arthropod-borne Infections

- Dengue – Viral infection
- Filaria – *Wuchereria bancrofti*
- Malaria – Plasmodium parasite

Others

- Plague – Bacteria
- Rabies – Virus
- JE – Virus
- KFD – Virus
- Tetanus – *Clostridium tetani*
- STD – Spirochete, bacteria, virus
- Leprosy – *Mycobacterium leprae*
- AIDS – HIV virus

PARASITOLOGY

It is the study of animal species, which live at the expense of other living organisms.

Parasites

Types of Parasites

Ectoparasite: When they live outside the body of the host.

Endoparasite: When they live inside the body of the host.

Definite host: When adult parasites are seen and where there is sexual reproduction in the host, that host is called definitive host.

Intermediate host: When larval form of parasite is found.

Classification

They are classified as under:

Unicellular

- *E. histolytica* – cause amoebiasis
- *Trypanosoma* – cause sleeping sickness
- *Leishmania* – cause kala azar
- *Plasmodium vivax*, *P. malariae*, *P. ovale* and *P. falciparum* – cause malaria.

Multicellular

- *Taenia solium and taenia saginata* – cause tapeworm infection
- *Fasciolopsis hepatica* – liver fluke
- *Dracunculus medinensis* – guinea worm infection

- *Ascaris lumbricoides* – roundworm
- *Enterobius vermicularis* – threadworm
- *Trichuris trichura* – whipworm
- *Ancylostoma duodenale* – hookworm
- *Wuchereria bancrofti* – filarial worm

Entamoeba Histolytica

Morphology (Table 6.5, Figs 6.8 and 6.9)

Table 6.5: Trophozoites and cysts

Trophozoites	*Cysts*
• Big size, oval	• Small and round
• Show ectoplasm and endoplasm	• No ectoplasm or endoplasm is seen
• Spherical nucleus (single)	• Quadrinucleate nucleus (four)

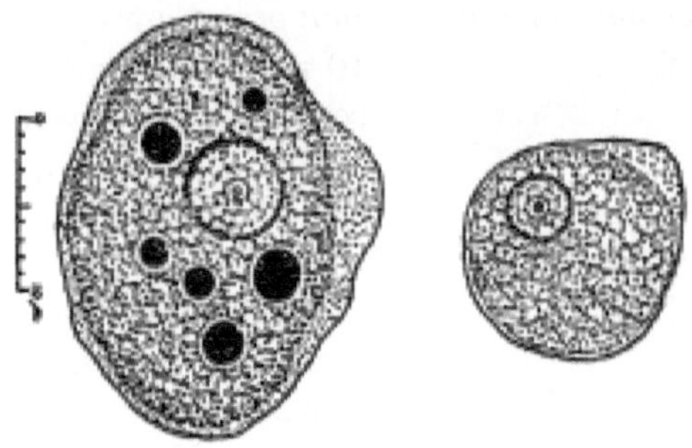

Fig. 6.8: Morphology of *E. histolytica*

Plasmodium Malariae Parasite

Morphology

Schizonts (Fig. 6.10)
- 42 microns in diameter
- Contain many merozoites
- Develop in liver and blood

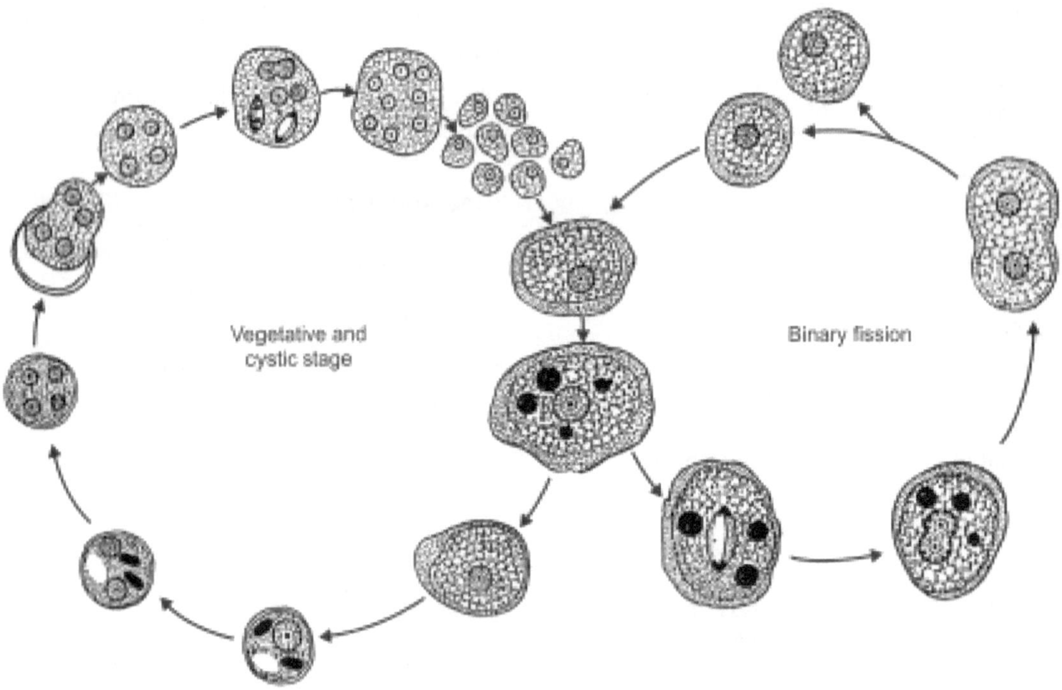

Fig. 6.9: Life cycle of *E. histolytica*

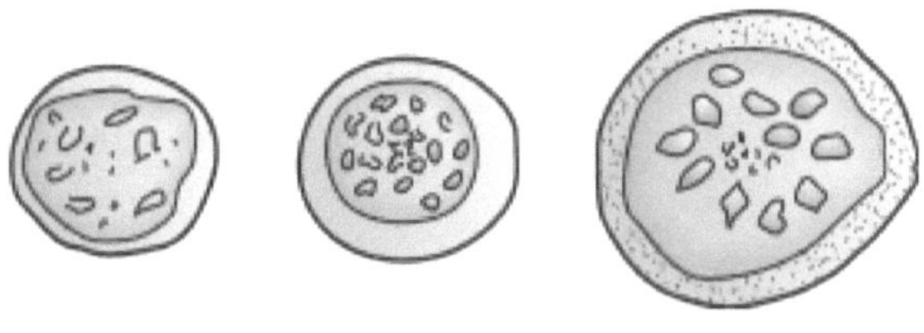

Fig. 6.10: Schizont

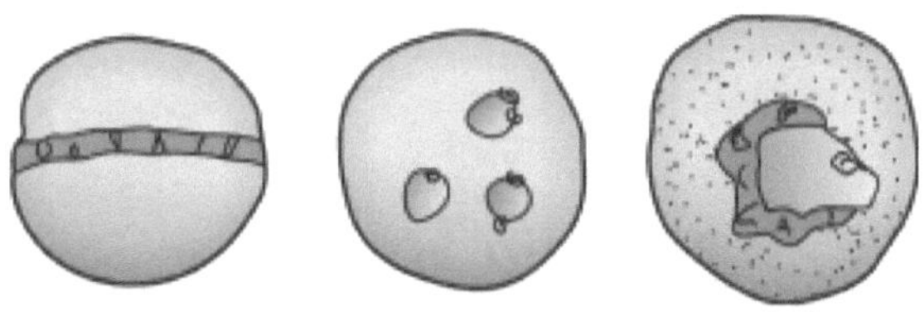

Fig. 6.11: Trophozoite

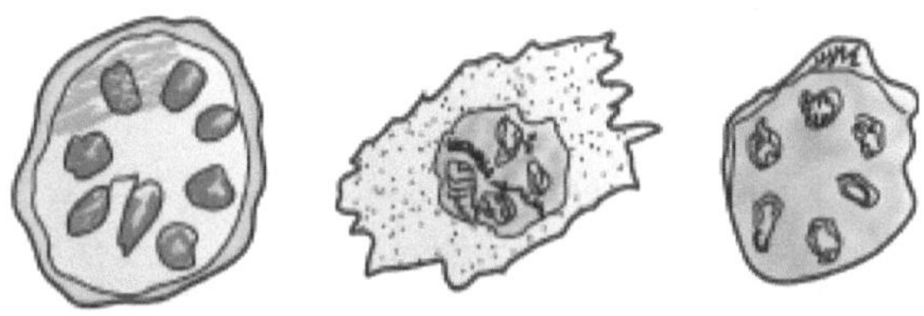

Fig. 6.12: Merozoite

Trophozoites (Fig. 6.11)
- 3 microns in diameter
- Show amoeboid movement
- Show pigments
- Develop in RBC

Merozoites (Fig. 6.12)
- Oval mass
- Central nucleus
- Attack red cells

Gametes

They are sexual forms of malaria parasite (Figs 6.13 and 6.14, Table 6.6).

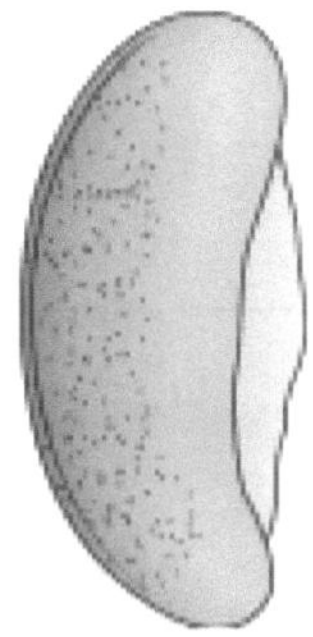

Fig. 6.13: Male gamete

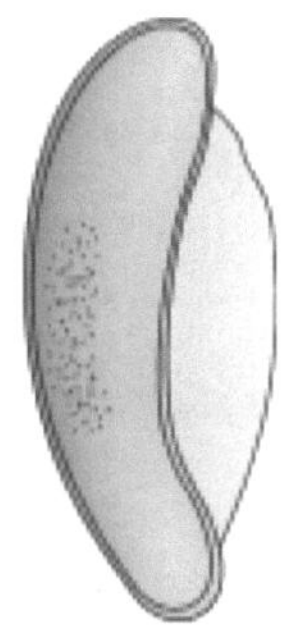

Fig. 6.14: Female gamete

Table 6.6: Male and female gametes

Male gamete	*Female gamete*
• Microgametes	• Macrogametes
• Size 10 microns	• Size 12 microns
• Stain light blue	• Stain deep blue
• Large nucleus, diffuse	• Small nucleus, compact

Pathogenicity

- *P vivax* – vivax or BT (benign tertian) malaria
- *P malariae* – quartan malaria
- *P ovale* – ovale or benign tertian mala-ria
- *P falciparum* – MT (malignant tertian) malaria

In Mosquitoes

When mosquito sucks blood, it also sucks male and female gametocytes. These gametocytes develop further to sporozoites, which are infective to man. This period of development is called *extrinsic incubation period* (Fig. 6.15).

In Man

When it sucks blood, infected mosquito introduces sporozoites to man. They enter liver and blood and develop to schizonts and later to gametocytes.

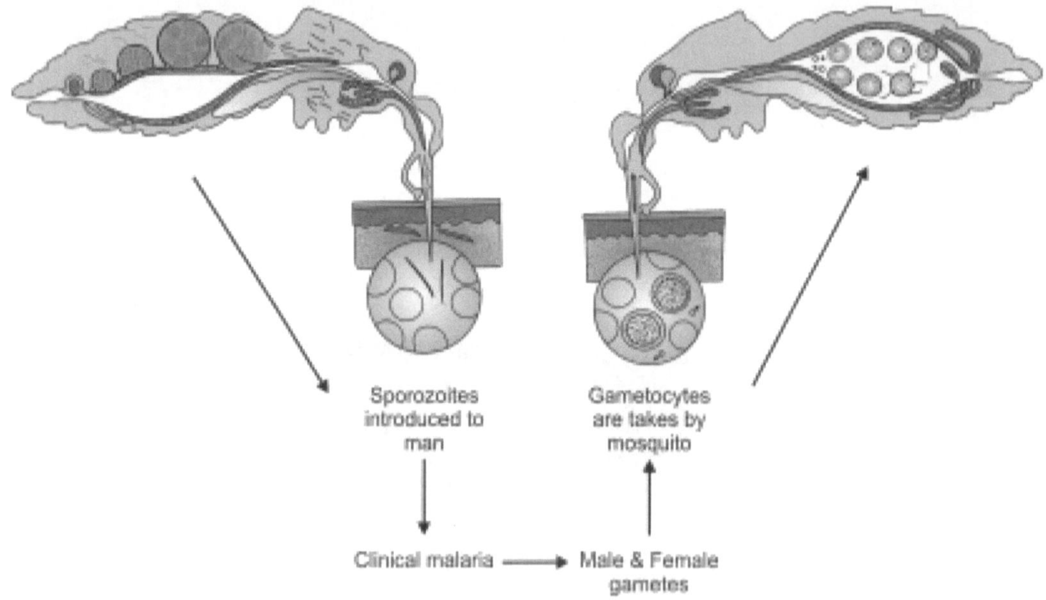

Fig. 6.15: Life cycle of malaria parasite

Roundworm (*Ascaris Lumbricoides*)

Morphology (Fig. 6.16 and Table 6.7)

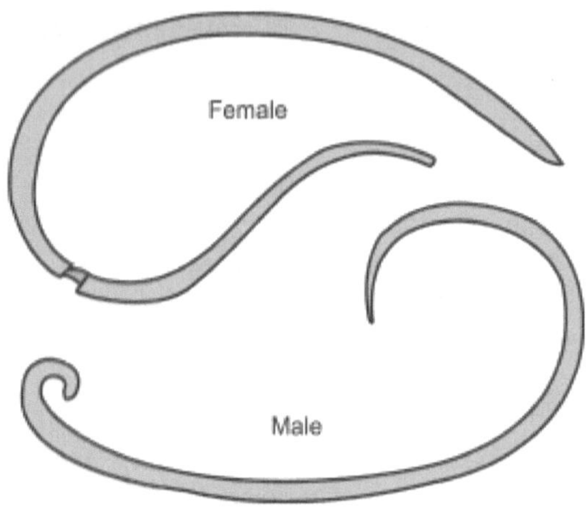

Fig. 6.16: Adult roundworm

Table 6.7: Male and female roundworms

Male roundworm	*Female roundworm*
• 25 cm long	• 40 cm long
• 3 mm diameter	• 5 mm diameter
• Tail end form a hook	• Tail end is conical

Eggs (Fig. 6.17 and Table 6.8)

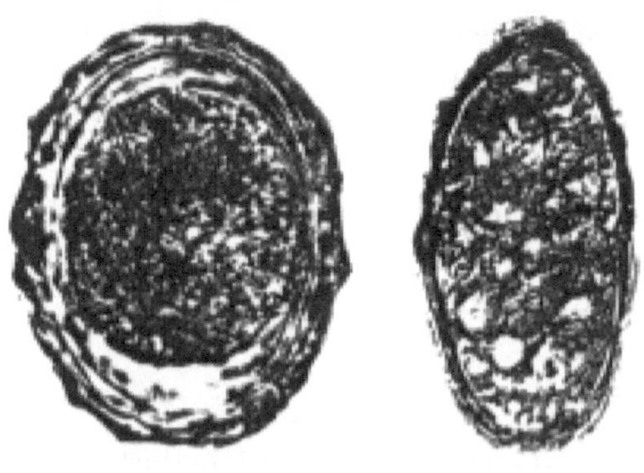

Fig. 6.17: Fertilised and unfertilised eggs of roundworm

Table 6.8: Eggs of roundworm

Fertilised	*Unfertilised egg of roundworm*
1. Round, oval	1. Narrow, long
2. Golden brown colour	2. Brown colour
3. Outer coat shows mamillation	3. No mamillation
4. Contains ovum	4. Only granules, no ovum
5. Floats in salt solution	5. Does not float in salt solution

Life Cycle of Roundworm (Figs 6.18 and 6.19)

Hookworm (*Ancylostoma Duodenale*)

Morphology

Egg is oval, colourless and it is surrounded by shell membrane which contains four blastomeres (segmented ovum). It floats in saturated solution.

Man is the only host. Eggs are passed in stool. When they reach soil, they develop to infective stage of larva called *filariform larva* (Fig. 6.20).

When man walks barefooted—in open field defaecated area, these filariform larvae enter another man through skin.

After entry through skin, they enter circulation, lung, later to duodenum where they stick by teeth of their buccal capsule.

They localise in small intestine, develop to adult, copulate and produce eggs.

Chronic blood loss occurs because:

- Hookworms drink blood as their food
- They cause bleeding at punctured wound.

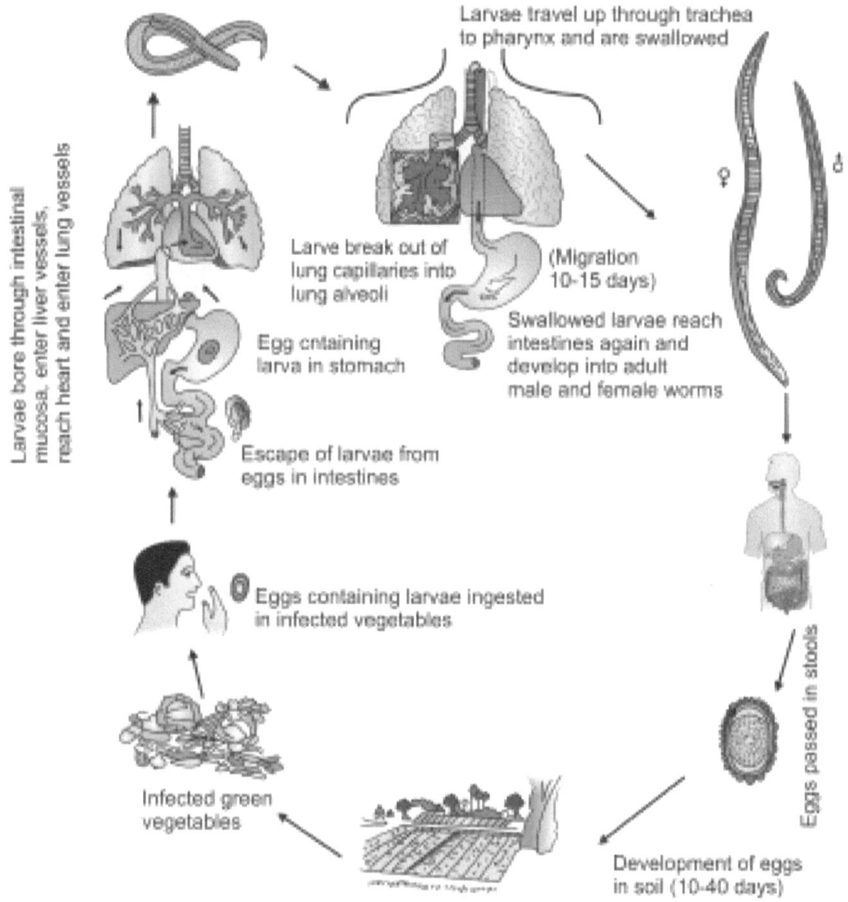

Fig. 6.18: Life cycle of roundworm (pictorial)

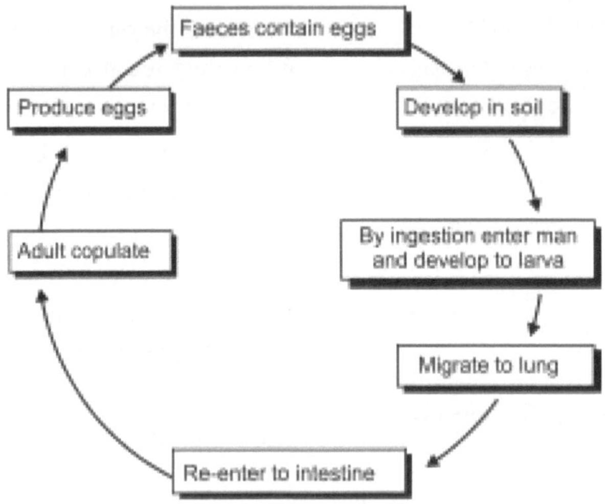

Fig. 6.19: Life cycle of roundworm (diagrammatic)

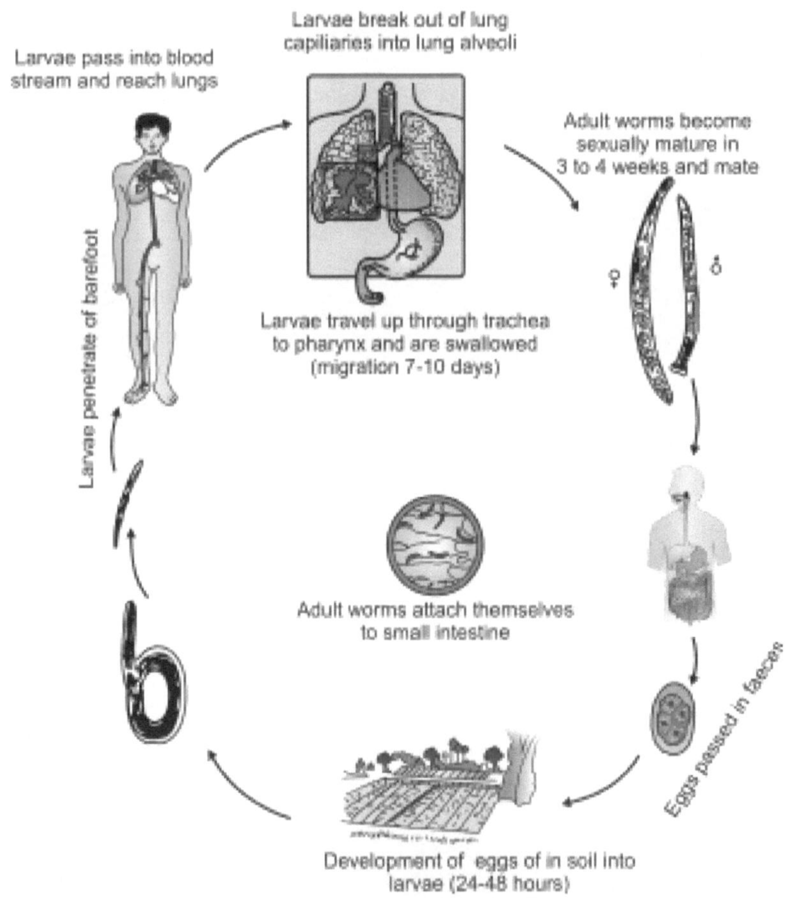

Fig. 6.20: Life cycle of hookworm

Threadworm (*Enterobius Vermicularis*)

Morphology

They are common infection among children. Eggs containing infective larvae carried on fingers and swallowed. When adult worms copulate, female worm liberates eggs in the intestine.

Eggs are discharged on the perianal skin and cause itching. Hence, autoinfection is common (Fig. 6.21).

Perianal itching and child is made devoid of food taken are the health problems by threadworm infection.

Personal hygiene and specific drug are very effective in the control of threadworm.

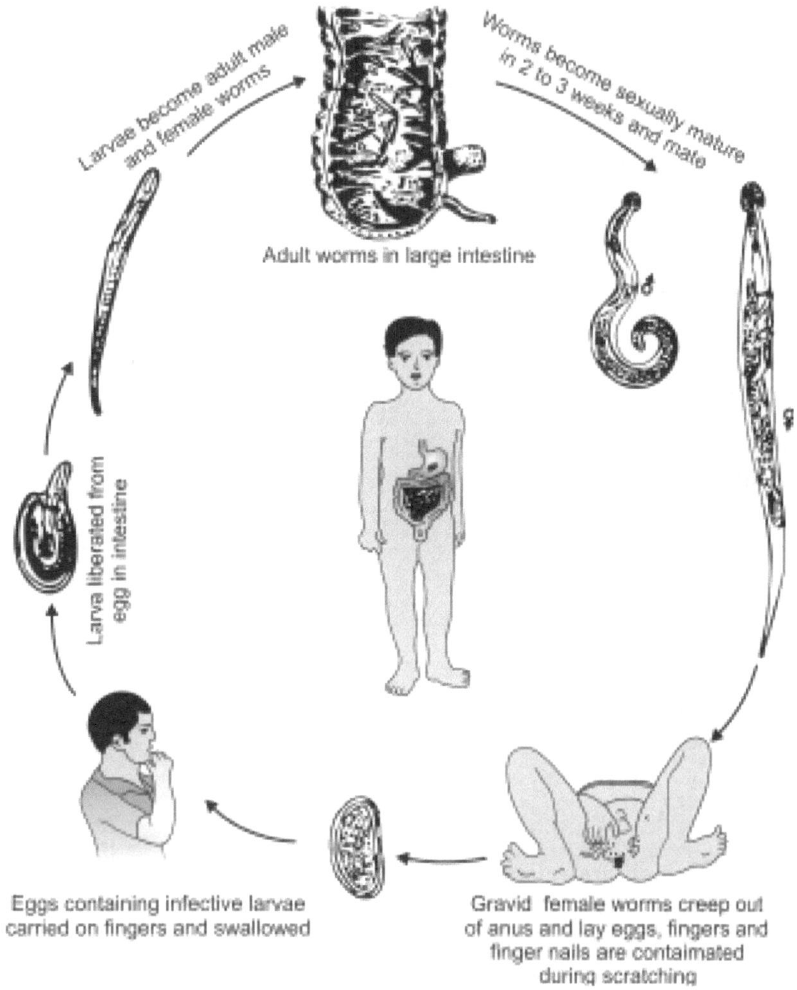

Fig. 6.21: Life cycle of threadworm

7

Nutrition

SCIENCE OF FOOD

Nutrition is a science of food, which influences the health of the individual, the community and nation. It is a requisite for body growth, body and mind development and maintenance of health.

Diet

Diet is menu, which a person consumes.

Public Health Importance

- Prevents infection
- Provides immunity
- Regulate fertility
- Protects the health of mother and child

Nutritional Epidemiology

This includes many facets of nutrition like:

- Community nutrition
- Community malnutrition
- Nutrition survey
- Diet survey
- Nutritional surveillance
- Growth monitoring
- Nutritional rehabilitation
- Nutritional policy

Other departments, which are related with health and nutrition are:

- Agriculture
- Education
- Demography
- Rural development
- Social welfare

Therapeutic Diet

It is the diet prescribed during illness or during the treatment.

Classification of Food Stuffs

Foodstuffs are classified into ten categories for the purpose of understanding and study. It also helps us to identify common characteristics of food stuff (Table 7.1).

Source of Nutrients

We get our energy, vitamins and minerals from regular use of foods. During advice, they are important as a part of diet treatment. They are specific in primary health care activities.

Table 7.1: Classification of food stuff

Food stuff category	*Examples*
1. Cereals and millets	
Cereals	Rice, wheat, maize
Millets	*Jowar*, *bazra*, *ragi*
2. Pulses	Bengal gram, red gram, soya bean, green gram, *urad*
3. Vegetables	
Green leaves	*Palak*, *amaranth* and *methi*
Roots, tubers	Potato, carrot, onion, radish, sweet potato
Other vegetables	Brinjal, tomato, cauliflower
4. Nuts and oilseeds	Groundnut, coconut, Mustard seed
5. Fruits	Banana, grapes, mango, guava
6. Animal food	milk, egg, fish
7. Fats and oils	Edible oil, vanaspathi, *ghee*, Butter
8. Sugars and Jaggery	*Shakkar*, *Gud*
9. Condiments and spices	Chilly, cardamom, ginger, cinnamon, jeera, pepper, *Methi*
10. Miscellaneous	Coffee, tea, soft drinks, cocoa

They can be tabulated as in Table 7.2.

Table 7.2: Nutrients and their source (food example)

Nutrient	*Food example*
Energy	Cereal, pulse, fat, oil
Protein	Pulses, meat
Fat	*Ghee*, vegetable oil
Carbohydrate	Cereals, sugar
Fibre	Vegetables, fruits
Calcium	*Ragi*, milk, greens
Iron	*Ragi*, green leafy vegetables
Vitamin A	Carrot, papaya, liver oil
Vitamin B complex	Less polished rice, milk, egg
Vitamin C	Sprouted grams, lime, orange
Vitamin D	Sunlight, milk

Food Value

The nutritive values of food stuff are required for *therapeutic diet* and for daily advice. They are tabulated for 100 grams of food as in Table 7.3.

Table 7.3: Nutritive values for 100 grams of food

Food	*Protein*	*Fat*	*Carbohydrate*	*Calories*
Cereal	9.9	2.3	71.0	344
Pulses	22.6	2.0	58.4	342
Green Leaves	3.8	0.6	6.0	45
Roots, tubers	1.2	0.2	16.0	70
Other vegetables	2.2	0.3	6.3	36
Nuts, oilseeds	15.2	46.6	20.4	578
Fruits	1.1	0.4	7.6	79
Meat	21.0	4.9	0.8	131
Oil	0.0	100.0	0.0	900
Jaggery	0.4	0.1	95.0	383
Spice (*masala*)	9.8	6.6	40.6	261
Milk	3.6	5.8	4.7	85
Curd	3.1	4.0	3.0	60

Nutritive Value of Selected Foods

Vitamin A:

- Cod liver oil – 18000 microgram vitamin A per 100 gram
- Egg – 140 µg of vitamin A per 100 gram
- Carrot – 1167 µg of vitamin A per 100 gram
- Spinach – 607 µg of vitamin A per 100 gram

Vitamin D:

- Butter – 1.5 µg of vitamin D per 100 gram
- Shark liver oil – 100 µg of vitamin D per 100 gram

Thiamine (Vit B_1):

- Raw rice – 0.21 mg per 100 gram
- Gingelli seed – 1.01 mg per 100 gram
- Groundnut – 0.90 mg per 100 gram

Riboflavin (Vit B_2):

- Sheep liver – 1.70 mg per 1000 gram
- Egg – 0.40 mg per 100 gram

Vitamin C

- *Amla* – 600 mg per 100 gram
- Guava – 212 mg per 100 gram
- Cabbage – 124 mg per 100 gram

Nutritive Value of Milk (Table 7.4)

Table 7.4: Nutritive value of milk (per 100 gm)

Nutrient	*Cow's milk (Calories)*	*Human milk (Calories)*
Fat (g)	4.1	3.4
Protein (g)	3.2	1.1
Lactose (g)	4.4	7.4
Calcium (mg)	120	28
Iron (mg)	0.2	Nil
Vitamin C (mg)	2	3
Energy	67	65

Public Health Importance of Food Stuffs

Cereal

Combination of cereals and pulses in food is better because cereals alone are deficient in amino acid lysine. This aspect is called *limiting amino acid.* Parboiling the rice helps to retain nutrients. It is a process where paddy is soaked in hot water at 70°C for 3 hours. Later, drying and steaming are followed, milled and kept for use.

Pulses

Germinated pulse is rich in vitamins. Kesari dhal is associated with lathyrism.

Vegetables

They are low calorie foods. They form bulky foods. They are high fibre diets.

Nuts and Oil Seeds

Balanced food formulations like MPF, Bala ahar, and malt foods are available.

Animal Foods

They are source of food toxins and tapeworm infections.

Milk and Egg

They are reference protein.

NUTRIENTS

Nutrients are grouped under:
- Proximate principles
- Vitamins
- Minerals

Proximate Principles

These include protein, fat and carbohydrates.

Protein

Human body contains 20 per cent protein. They are mainly nitrogenous compounds.

Functions of protein:
- Tissue repair
- Osmotic pressure maintained
- Produces antibodies

Requirement of protein	–	One gram per kg body weight is the requirement.
Source	–	Pulses, milk, meat, egg and fish.

Fat

Major intake of fat is usually by invisible fat and its measurement is difficult. Fat yields high calories (1 gram yields 9 calories). Vegetable fat is preferred because it contains unsaturated fatty acids.

Functions of fat:
- Gives high calorie
- Gives support to body cavities
- Acts as local hormones

Requirement of fat	–	Thirty per cent of total calories are obtained by fat.
Source of fat	–	Groundnut oil, coconut oil, *ghee*, butter and cheese
Hydrogenation	–	It is conversion of oil to semisolid form in the presence of catalyst, for example, vanaspati
Oil refining	–	Refining is removal of rancid material of oil or wax, for example, rice bran oil.
Public health importance	–	Fat is connected with obesity, skin changes like roughening, heart disease and cancer of some organs.

Carbohydrates

Starch, sugar and cellulose are three main sources of carbohydrates. The human body has always a store of "glycogen" which is called "carbohydrate reserve" which helps in body needs like fasting.

Carbohydrates in vegetables, fruit and whole grains form major components of dietary fibre. Dietary fibre encourages bowl movement.

Vitamins

They are organic compounds and essential to the human body. Very small quantity is sufficient for its function. They are grouped under two categories:
- Fat-soluble vitamins – Vitamins A, D, E and K
- Water-soluble vitamins – Vitamins B and C

Vitamin A

It is important for vision, glands, skin and bones.
Sources: Spinach, greens, papaya, mango, liver, egg, butter and meat

Requirement:
- Adult—600 microgram of retinol
- Child—400 microgram of retinol

Public health importance:
- Night blindness
- Bitot's spot
- Keratomalacia (softening of eye)

Vitamin prophylaxis: Two lakh units in oil orally every 6 months from 9th month to prevent preventable blindness.

Vitamin D

Sources: Sunlight, foods like liver, butter and cheese.

Requirement:
- Adult—100 IU
- Child—200 IU

Public health importance:
- Rickets in children
- Osteomalacia in adults

Vitamin K

Sources: Green leaves and cow's milk.

Requirement:
Adult—0.03 mg/kg

Public health importance:
Help in the control of bleeding

Vitamin B Complex

Vitamins B_1, B_6 and B_{12} are important among B complex group of vitamins.

Vitamin B_1: It is called thiamine. It helps in carbohydrate metabolism.

Sources: Raw rice, wheat, groundnut and milk

Requirement:
0.5 mg per 1000 calories of energy

Public health importance:
Deficiency produces neuritis and beriberi

Vitamin B_6: It is called pyridoxine. It helps in metabolism of carbohydrate, protein and fat.

Sources: Milk, liver and meat.

Requirement:
2 mg per day

Public health importance:
Deficiency produces neuritis

Vitamin B_{12}: It is also called cyanocobalamine.

Sources: Milk, egg, liver and meat

Requirement:
- Adult—1 microgram
- Child—0.2 microgram

Public health importance:
Deficiency produces megaloblastic anaemia.

Vitamin C

This is important in tissue oxidation and found useful in producing body protection against infection.

Source: Fresh fruits

Requirement: 60 mg per day

Public health importance:
Deficiency produces scurvy.

Minerals

Many minerals like calcium, phosphorus, iron and iodine are required for body functions. Since they are required in small quantity, minerals are called *trace elements.* Examples of trace elements are iron, iodine and fluorine.

Calcium

Bone formation, teeth formation, muscle activity, heart activity, nerve activity are regulated by calcium.

Sources: Milk, egg and fish

Requirement: 500 mg per day

Public health importance:
Hypocalcaemia

Iron

It is required for haemoglobin formation, brain development.

Sources: Green leaves, jaggery, liver and meat

Requirement: Adult 0.9 mg per day

Public health importance:
Anaemia.

Iodine

It is required for thyroid hormone preparation.
Sources: Sea fish, cod liver oil and salt.

Requirement: 150 μg per day.

Public health importance:
- Goitre
- Cretinism.

Fluorine

It is required for the formation of bone and teeth

Sources: Water, sea fish and tea.

Requirement: In drinking water, the acceptable level is 0.5 to 0.8 mg per litre.

Public health importance:
- Caries
- Dental fluorosis
- Skeletal fluorosis.

DAILY REQUIREMENT OF NUTRIENTS

For the promotion, protection and maintenance of health, nutrients are required. Recommended daily intake or allowances are known for most of the nutrients.

Calories

- Indian reference men
  - 20 to 39 years
  - 60 kg weight
  - 8-hour work
- Indian reference women
  - 20 to 39 years
  - 50 kg weight
  - 8-hour work

Supply of Calories by Proximate Principles

- Protein – 4 calories per gram
- Fat – 9 calories per gram
- Carbohydrate – 4 calories per gram

Requirement:
- Adult male—2500 calories
- Adult female—1900 calories

Requirement of Proximate Principles

Protein
Man—60 gram per day
Woman—50 gram per day

Fat:
Man/woman—20 gram per day

Carbohydrate:
Man—460 gram
Woman—410 gram

Requirement of Vitamins and Minerals

- Vitamin A—600 μg retinol
- Vitamin D—100 IU
- Vitamin B_1—1.4 mg
- Vitamin B_6—2 mg
- Vitamin B_{12}—1 μg
- Vitamin C—60 mg
- Calcium—500 mg
- Iron—0.9 mg

Balanced Diet

A diet is the type of food which man consumes everyday for his living.

A balanced diet is a diet, which contains sufficient calories, proximate principles, sufficient vitamins and minerals for maintaining a person's health (Tables 7.5 to 7.9).

Table 7.5: Balanced diet for adult man

	Sedentary	*Moderate work*	*Heavy work*
Cereals	460	520	670
Pulses	40	50	60
Leafy veg	40	40	40
Other veg	60	70	80
Roots, tubers	50	60	80
Milk	150	200	250
Oil, fat	40	45	65
Sugar, jaggery	30	35	55

Table 7.6: Balanced diet for adult woman

	Sedentary	*Moderate work*	*Heavy work*
Cereals	410	440	575
Pulses	40	45	50
Leafy veg	100	100	150
Other veg	40	40	100
Roots, tubers	50	50	60
Milk	100	150	200
Oil, fat	20	25	40
Sugar, jaggery	20	20	40

Table 7.7: Balanced diet for children

	1-3 yr child	*4-6 yr child*	*10-12 yr boy*	*10-12 yr girl*
Cereals	175	270	420	380
Pulses	35	35	45	45
Leafy veg	40	50	50	50
Other veg	20	30	50	50
Roots, tubers	10	20	30	30
Milk	300	250	250	250
Oil, fat	15	25	40	35
Sugar, jaggery	30	40	45	45

Table 7.8: Additional allowance during pregnancy

Food item	*Quantity*	*Calories*
Cereals	35 gram	118
Pulses	15 gram	52
Milk	100 gram	83
Sugar	10 gram	40
	Total	293 calories

Table 7.9: Additional allowance during lactation

Food item	*Quantity*	*Calories*
Cereals	60 gram	203
Pulses	30 gram	105
Milk	100 gram	83
Fat	10 gram	90
Sugar	10 gram	40
	Total	521 calories

Non-vegetarians' Substitution

30 grams of pulses

(Any one with 5 g oil) = 30 g meat
= 30 g fish
= 1 egg

60 grams of pulses

(Any one with 10 g oil) = 50 g meat
= 50 g fish
= 2 eggs

NUTRITIONAL REQUIREMENT OF SPECIAL GROUPS

Infants

Newborn and infants are best benefited by exclusive breast-feeding. Breast milk is the ideal infant food. Since exclusive breast-feeding is suggested up to 4 to 6 months, the requirement of breast milk is suggested as under:

- 0 to 3 months — 800 to 850 ml per day
- 3 to 6 months — 1100 to 1200 ml per day

Table 7.10 shows caloric and protein requirement of infant.

Table 7.10: Caloric and protein requirement of infant

Age	*Calories*	*Protein*
0 to 3 months	120/kg	2.3 g/kg
3 to 5 months	115/kg	1.8 g/kg
6 to 8 months	110/kg	1.8 g/kg
9 to 11 months	105/kg	1.5 g/kg
12 to 24 months	112/kg	1.5 g/kg

Weaning

From 4th month or 6th month onwards, gradual withdrawal of breast milk and introduction of supplementary food is called *weaning*. Common weaning foods are:

- Cow's milk
- *Dhal* water
- Fruit juice
- Mashed potato
- Soft-cooked rice
- Soft-cooked vegetable
- Soft-cooked egg

If weaning is delayed, it affects growth and development of a child.

By one year, the child should be able to eat cereal, pulse and vegetables.

India has low cost weaning foods based on locally available cereal, legume and oilseed.

Weaning is good, if weight gain of infant is as under:

- 4th month — double the birth weight
- 12th month — treble the birth weight

(If birth weight is 3 kg, then it should be 6 kg at 4th month and 9 kg at 12th month).

Pregnancy

An Indian reference woman is 20 to 39 years of age and weighs 50 kg.

Calorie requirement for a pregnant woman is 1900 plus an additional 300 calories per day.

Apart from one g per kg body weight, the pregnant woman requires an additional 15 g of protein per day.

Special mention must be made of IFA intake.

Lactation

Lactating woman requires additional calories as under:

About 550 calories per day during first 6 months of lactation is required. Thereafter, she needs 400 calories per day. This is apart from her requirement of 2000 calories per day.

Up to 6 months of lactation, lactating mother requires 25 g of additional protein per day apart from her daily requirement of 1 g per day per kg body weight.

Adequate intake of other nutrients is made available through balanced diet.

Lactating mother requires about 80 mg vitamin C per day during lactating period.

Preschool Child

One to 5-year child is called preschool child. Physical and mental growth is rapid in this age group; and, hence calorie requirement will be more.

Below 3-year child requires about 1240 calories per day (on an average).

Above 3-year child requires about 1690 calories per day (on an average).

Similarly, below 3-year child requires 1.83 g per kg + 22 grams of protein as additional allowance per day.

Above 3 years of age, child requires 1.52 g/kg protein + 30 grams of protein as additional allowance per day.

If 8 to 10 per cent of energy comes from protein, child maintains good health.

School Going Child

School going child requires about 2000 to 2400 calories per day and 1.5 g/kg protein with an additional allowance of 30 to 40 gram per day.

Since 1960, as per the Government of India recommendations, a mid-day meal is provided to a school child, which can provide 1/3rd of daily requirement of calories, protein and other nutrients.

A model menu for school going child can be as in Table 7.11.

Table 7.11: Model menu for school going child

Food	*Allowed*
Cereals, millets	75 gram per day per child
Pulses	30 gram per day per child
Oil	8 gram per day per child
Leafy vegetables	30 gram per day per child
Non-leafy vegetables	30 gram per day per child

School going child nutrition should also lay emphasis on the following:

- Eating habit
- Nutrition awareness
- Encouraging local food.

NUTRITIONAL ASSESSMENT

It is done on one person or for the family.

Individual Assessment (Table 7.12)

Table 7.12: Individual assessment by using nutritional assessment schedule

Name	*Age*	*Sex*	*Address*

Date of assessment

Clinical examination for deficiency signs

Appearance	Healthy or ill
Hair	Normal or abnormal
Face	Normal or moon face
Eyes has	Normal or abnormal (red eye or the eye Bitot's spot)
Lips	Normal or crack in mouth angle
Tongue	Normal or pale
Teeth	Normal or caries
Gums	Normal or bleeding
Thyroid and parotid	Normal or enlarged
Glands	Normal or enlarged
Skin	Normal or dry or scaly
Nails	Normal or abnormal
Oedema (swelling)	Normal or swollen legs
Rickets	Present or absent
Other changes	Normal or enlarged
Liver muscle wasting	Yes or no
Weight	Height
For children below 6 years	Head circumference Chest circumference Midupper arm circumference

Blood test for Hb%

Stool examination for parasites

Blood smear for malaria

Family Assessment

- Clinical examination of all members
- Height and weight for all
- Head circumference, chest circumference and skin fold for children
- Blood test for Hb% for all
- Diet survey is done by 7 days information on food intake to calculate per head consumption of calories and per capita consumption of nutrients. It is done by
  - Weighing raw food used by the family
  - Weighing cooked food used by the family
  - Oral questionnaire method by asking
  - Stock inventory in case of hostels

CULTURAL FACTORS IN NUTRITION

Hunger, malnutrition and religious factors are associated with food that we eat.

Major Factors Affecting Nutritional Status

There are some major factors that contribute to nutritional status of people. They are grouped under following categories.

Food Habits

Rice is the main diet in south India. Wheat is the main diet in north India.

Food Customs

Papaya is avoided in pregnancy on the belief that it causes abortion. Similarly, nursing mother is not given banana, *ghee*, green leaves on some belief.

Food Belief

People believe that certain foods are hot and certain are cold.

Food Fads

Likes and dislikes of food by people are called food fads.

Cooking Practices

Some traditional methods are found associated with loss of nutrients.

Child Rearing Practices

Feeding practice in infants and children determines child health.

Other Culture

Men eating first, alcoholism among people make the nutritional status of the family poor.

NUTRITION EDUCATION

It is a type of health education given to individual, family and community for the development of responsible attitude towards better nutrition and better health.

While creating awareness on nutrition, the following contents are to be kept in mind:

- Child care
  - Exclusive breast feeding
  - Weaning at after 6 months
  - Type of weaning foods
  - Clean utensil use
  - Growth monitoring
- Pregnant women care
  - Nutrition of pregnant women
- Lactating mothers' care
  - Nutrition of lactating mother
- Food hygiene
- Balanced diet

MALNUTRITION

It is a current nutritional health problem in public health. There are three main malnutrition conditions that need attention in the country. They are:

- LBW (low birth weight)
- PEM (protein-energy malnutrition)
- Iodine deficiency

Low Birth Weight (LBW)

When newborn has birth weight of less than 2500 gram, it is called LBW. It is calculated by:

$$\frac{\text{Live birth with weight of below 2.5 kg}}{\text{Total live birth}} \times 100$$

It is about 26 per cent in India.

Causes of LBW

- Twins
- Acute infection
- Hypertension in pregnancy
- Severe anaemia in mother
- PET
- No birth spacing
- Illiteracy

Prevention of LBW

- Identification of high-risk pregnancy
- Good RCH care
- Good nutritional care of mothers
- Control of anaemia in mothers
- Control of infection
- Early detection and treatment of medical disorders
- Family planning
- Women education

Protein-energy Malnutrition (PEM)

Diseases and deaths are common due to malnutrition. Since protein deficiency and calorie deficiency are there, it is called PEM. Clinically, there are two types. They are:

- Marasmus (Fig. 7.1)
- Kwashiorkor (Fig. 7.2)

They are clinically differentiated as in Table 7.13.

Table 7.13: Clinical difference between marasmus and kwashiorkor

Marasmus	*Kwashiorkor*
• Muscle wasting +	• No muscle wasting
• Fat is absent in skin	• Fat is retained
• No oedema	• Oedema +
• Quite child	• Irritable child
• Good appetite	• Poor appetite
• No skin change	• Skin change +
• No hair change	• Hair change +

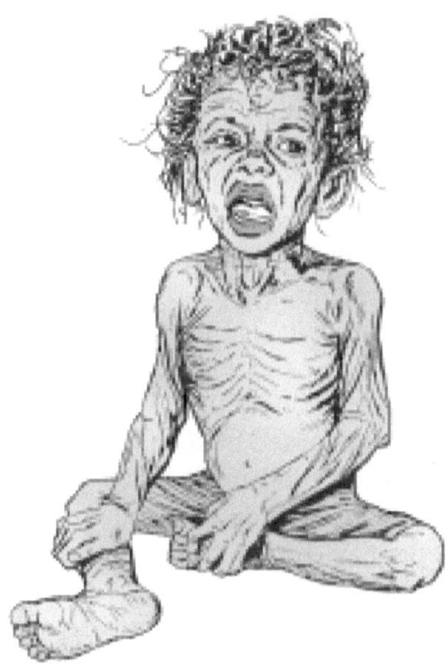

Fig. 7.1: Marasmus child

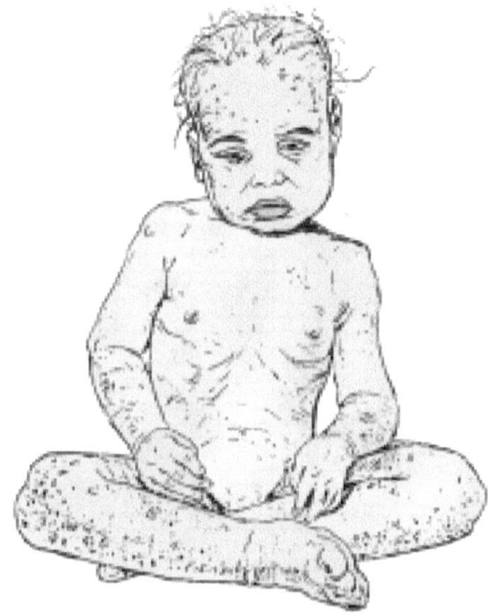

Fig. 7.2: Kwashiorkor child

Recording the child's body weight and charting in growth chart estimate the degree of malnutrition (Fig. 7.3).

Accordingly, we have the following degree of malnutrition:

- Normal — when the weight lies within the road to health in the chart
- Mild malnutrition — when grade I and grade II present
- Severe malnutrition — when grade III and grade IV present

Prevention

- Nutrition education and supplementary nutrition to pregnant and lactating women
- Promotion of breast-feeding
- Improvement of family diet
- Home economics
- Family planning
- High protein diet to children
- Good immunisation coverage in children
- Food fortification
- Treatment of infection and diarrhoea
- Deworming children

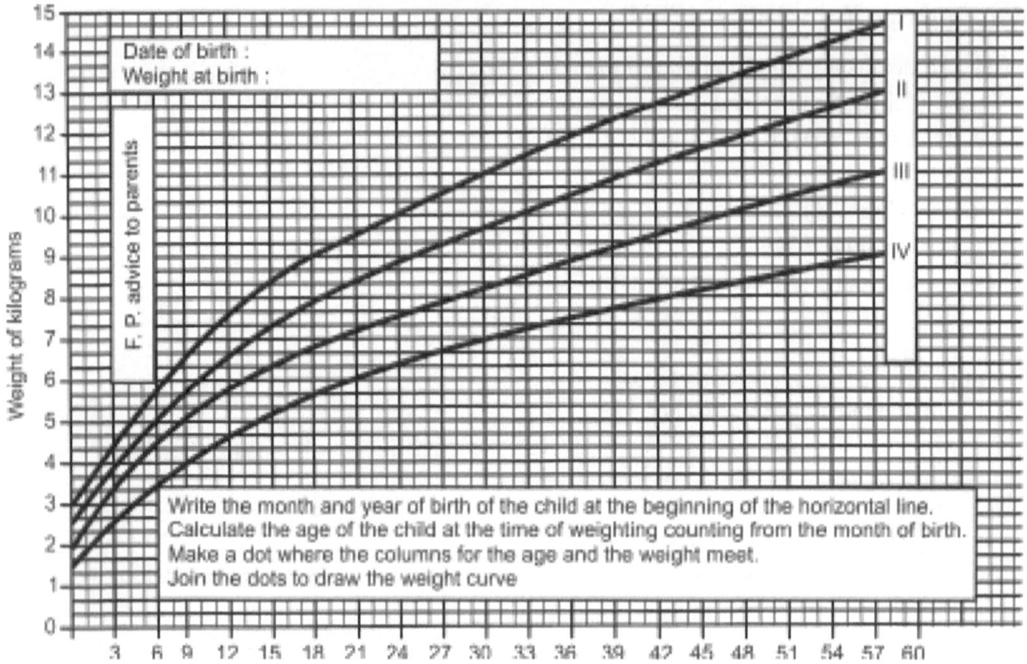

Fig. 7.3: Growth chart

Iodine Deficiency

Iodine deficiency is another major nutritional health problem in India (Fig. 7.4). It is leading to serious health problems and also social health problem.

Public Health Problem

About 150 million people are living in goitre endemic areas in India. It has produced the following disorders in the country:

- Goitre (Fig. 7.5)
- Low intelligence
- Delayed milestone
- Muscle weakness
- Abortion
- Hearing defect
- Speech defect

For the control and prevention, the steps taken are:

- Supply of iodised salt
- Health education on IDDCP
- Mass communication

THERAPEUTIC NUTRITION

Special care must be given to severe malnutrition children. They include grade III and grade IV who are given special food, which is called *therapeutic nutrition*. In other words, at-risk child is taken care with special attention.

The food provided as therapeutic nutrition may be different from supplementary nutrition. It can be given in semi liquid form, which can be easily ingested and digested by a child. The preparation aspect of such food must be easy. Therapeutic nutrition aims at providing 600 calories and 20 gram protein per day. Total 4 feeds should be given for this purpose.

Home management of severe malnourished child is very important, because mother should be educated for special care and proper feeding at home.

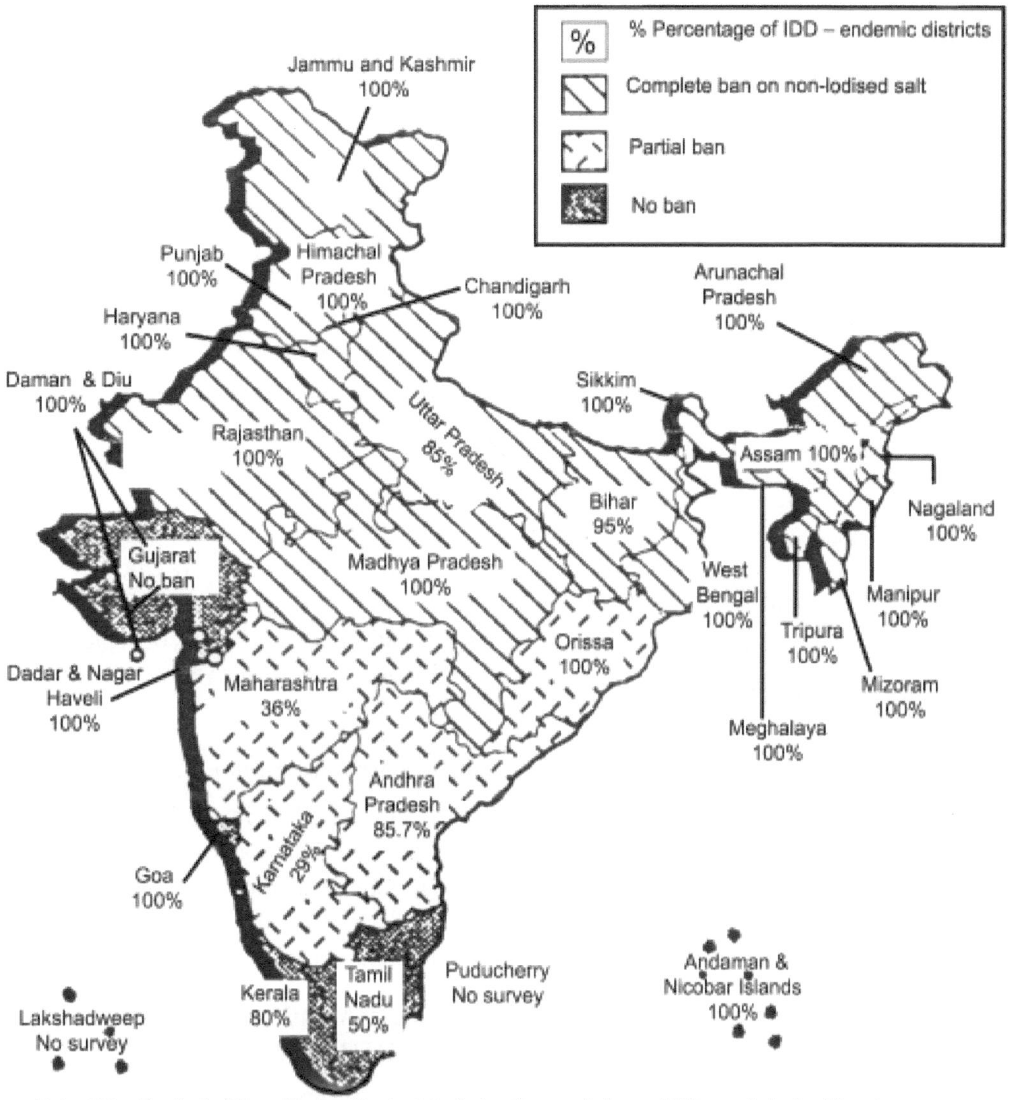

Note: Uttar Pradesh, Bihar, Madya Pradesh includes the newly formed Uttaranchal, Jharkhand and Chhatisgarh respectively

Fig. 7.4: IDD map of India

Therapeutic Diet

Instruction for Weight Reducing Diet

Foods to avoid:

- Whole milk, cream, butter, oil, *ghee*, fried food, honey
- Sugar, sweets
- Ovaltine, Horlicks, cocoa, cheese
- Banana, mango, grapes, potato
- Alcohol
- Dried fruits

Foods given freely:

- All vegetables, lime juice, pepper water
- Skimmed milk
- All fruits

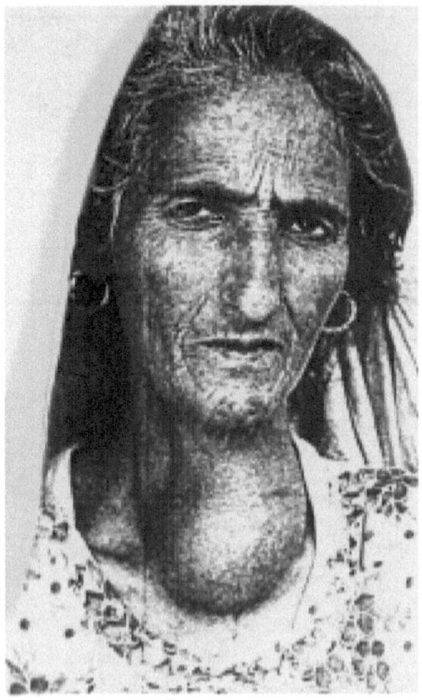

Fig. 7.5: Endow goitre in a women

Instruction for Low Fat Diet

Foods to avoid:

- Meat, liver, kidney, brain
- Whole milk, cream, butter, *ghee*
- Vanaspati
- Eggs
- Alcohol
- Sweets

Foods given freely:

- All vegetables and lime juice
- Skimmed milk
- Groundnut milk

Instructions for Bland Diet

Food permitted: Milk, bread, cooked vegetables, fruit juice, cooked *dhal*, rice *kanji* and tender coconut.

Food not permitted: Atta, high fibre vegetable, meat, all *masala.*

Instructions for Diabetic Patient

Free food: Leafy vegetable, tomato, cucumber, radish, lime, clear soup, black coffee, black tea, *lassi*, sour *chutney*, pickle, pepper and *zeera* water.

Food to avoid: Potato, *arvi*, mango, grapes, banana, alcohol and wine.

Food prohibited: Glucose, sugar, honey and all sweets.

Instructions for Cirrhosis of Liver

- Restrict fat and salt
- Give food in small quantity and frequently
- Make food palatable by adding fruit juice
- Diet must be bland
- Increase or decrease of sugar and rice help in increasing or decreasing calorie
- Vitamin and protein are supplemented
- Avoid fried food, cream, oil, spices and alcohol
- Plenty of fruit juice and vegetable soup are advocated

Instructions for Renal Stone

- If stone is uric acid; avoid meat, *dhal*, oatmeal, dried pea, beans and spinach.
- If stone is oxalic acid; avoid green plantain, spinach, *arvi*, potato, beetroot, almond, cashew nut and grapes.

HOME MANAGEMENT OF MALNUTRITION

Following factors are kept in mind for a good home management of malnutrition.

- Poverty
- Incorrect family food habit
- Parental ignorance regarding proper feeding and diet

An infant is best managed with only breast-feeding because it is clean, safe, contains all necessary nutrients and there is no cost. If possible, it can be continued as long as possible. It is dangerous to use a bottle and nipple for feeding because it cannot be cleaned and can be a source for child infection.

- Group A: Bread, rice, wheat, potato, sugar and jaggery (Fig 7.6).

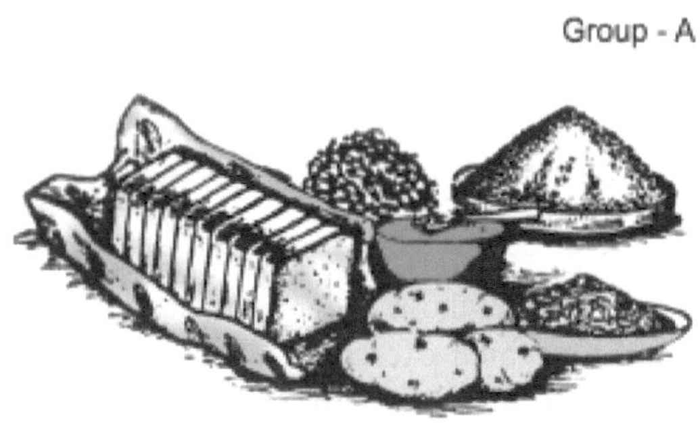

Fig. 7.6: Bread, rice, wheat, potato, sugar and jaggery

- Group B: Meat, fish, egg, milk, groundnut, *dhal* and beans (Fig. 7.7).

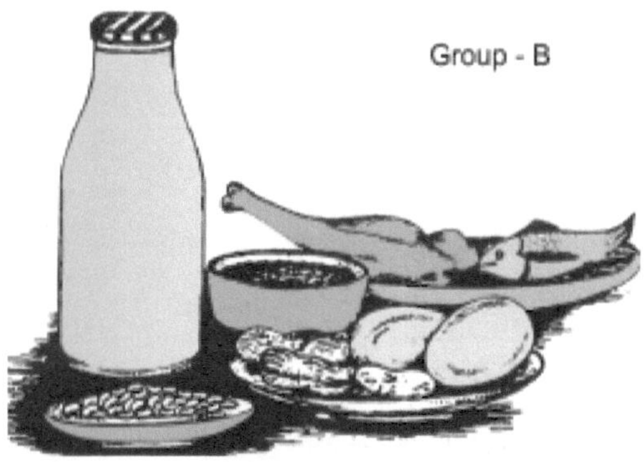

Fig. 7.7: Meat, fish, egg, milk, groundnut, dhal and beans

- Group C: Orange, banana, lime, papaya, mango and guava (Fig. 7.8).

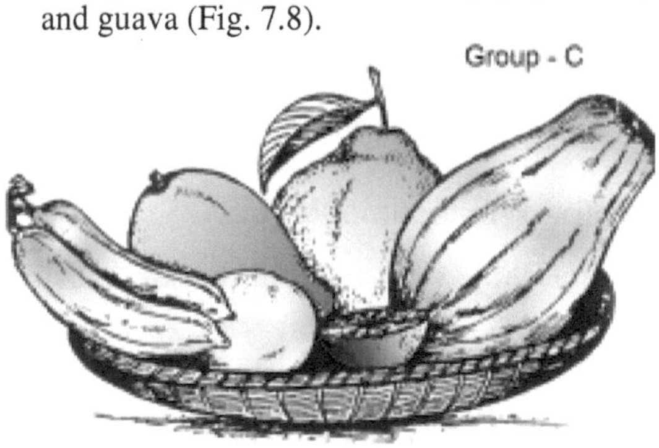

Fig. 7.8: Orange, banana, lime, papaya, mango and guava

- Group D: Pea, capsicum, carrot, Ladies fingers (Okra), brinjal, tomato, bittergourd, cauliflower, *palak* and *methi* (Fig 7.9).

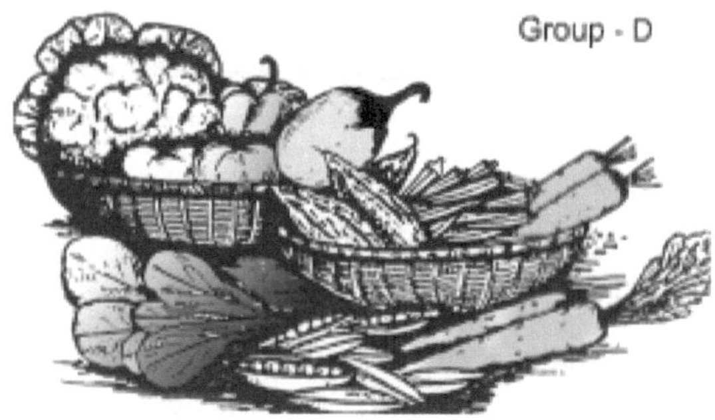

Fig. 7.9: Pea, capsicum, carrot, ladies fingers, brinjal, tomato, bittergourd, cauliflower, *palak* and *methi*

- Group E: *Ghee*, oil and butter (Fig 7.10).

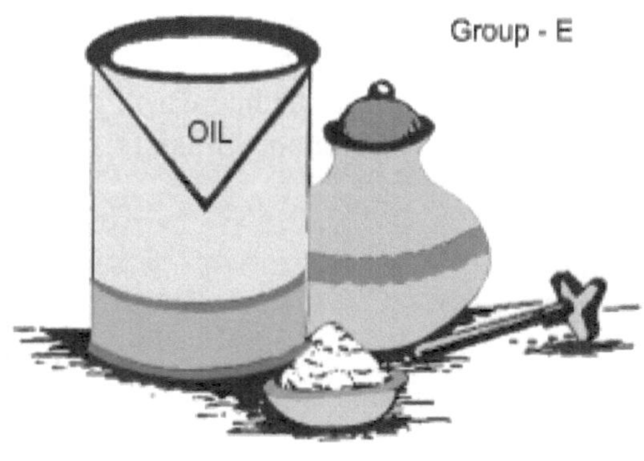

Fig. 7.10: Ghee, oil and butter

About 4 to 6 months onwards, weaning foods are advocated. First weaning food can be cow's milk. Later, ripe banana, well-cooked mashed rice, cooked potato and spices are avoided to children.

New food, when started, is to be given by spoon and later gradually increased in quantity. Supplementary food should be added gradually over a period of time rather than all at once.

Clean hands and clean utensil and freshly prepared food are necessary to prevent infection.

At 6th month, baby should be given *dhal* and greens. Food is grouped into five groups called group A, B, C, D and E. One or more from these groups are to be selected for the suggested food provision and food care for the child.

8

Environmental Health

INTRODUCTION

Our surrounding is environment. Physical items like water, air, light, radiation and workplace surrounding us, house we live in thrown out wastes and the food we eat, all these constitute *physical environment.*

Germs and disease-causing agents around us constitute *biological environment.*

Our tradition, custom and society around us constitute *social environment.*

Cleanliness of our surrounding which goes to form physical environment consists of the following:

- Water
- Solid waste
- Liquid waste
- Human excreta
- Residential environment (house)
- Air and ventilation
- Workplace called industry and trade
- Public gathering
- School surrounding
- Food sanitation
- Climate
- Health care waste

ENVIRONMENTAL SANITATION

Definition

"It is science of cleanliness of our surrounding."

"It is science of controlling man's physical environment which bring about disease, defect and death."

Environmental sanitation is called *environmental health.*

WHO's Definition of Environmental Sanitation

"The control of all those factors in man's physical environment which exercise or may exercise a deleterious effect in his physical development, health and survival."

Environmental health is to be protected by many areas. They are:

- Public health
- Epidemiology
- Public health engineering
- Town planning
- Sociologist
- Economist
- Health inspectors

WATER

In our life, safe drinking water which is readily available throughout the year and which is free of contamination brings about total and positive health.

Water is responsible for socioeconomic development of our country.

Under primary health care, water is the main basic element.

Safe and Wholesome Water

- Water should not contain disease-causing pathogens.
- Water should not contain harmful chemicals.
- Should have acceptable colour and taste.
- It should be potable or useable.

Requirement

- Drinking purpose — 2 litre per day per man
- Household purpose — 200 litre per day per man

Uses of Water (Table 8.1)

Table 8.1: Different uses of water

House	*Public place*	*Industry*	*Agriculture*	*Others*
Drinking	Swimming pool	Small scale	Farm	Electricity
Cooking	Fire protection	Large scale	Land	Waste clean
Clothe wash		Food	Wetland	
Regular bath		Iron	Horticulture	
Toilet cleaning		Steel		
Gardening		Ice		

Sources of Water (Fig 8.1)

Rain Water

It forms the main source for agriculture. The water from rain is pure in the beginning. When it starts running on the surface, it gets polluted.

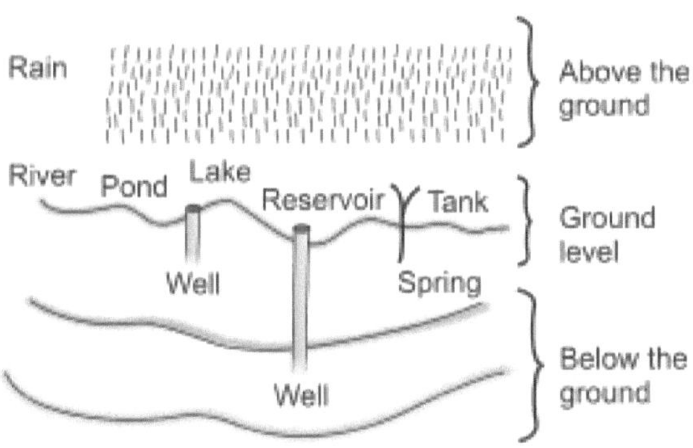

Fig. 8.1: Sources of water

Surface Water

We have reservoirs, rivers, tanks, ponds and lakes as surface water. These get impurities by human activities and human culture. River water is better because it gets purified during its flow on the ground surface.

Groundwater

Well water is the common water source in India as ground water. Different types of wells seen are:

- *Katcha* dug well — is simple dug well
- *Pucca* dug well — brick or stonewall is present
- Tube well — borewell by public health engineering department
- Step well — steps are present to get down to water
- Artisan well — water rises by pressure

Tube wells are sanitary because any means do not contaminate the water.

Step wells are responsible for spreading guinea worm infection.

Wells

In public health two types of wells are described. One is *shallow well* and the other is *deep well* (Table 8.2). These definitions are based on first impervious layer either above or below the water source. Deep wells are good and healthy from public health point of view (Fig. 8.2).

Table 8.2: Differences between shallow and deep well

Shallow well	*Deep well*
• Water is drawn from above the first impervious layer	• Water is drawn from below the first impervious layer
• Not hard	• Hard
• Contaminated	• Not contaminated
• Not available always	• Gives constant supply

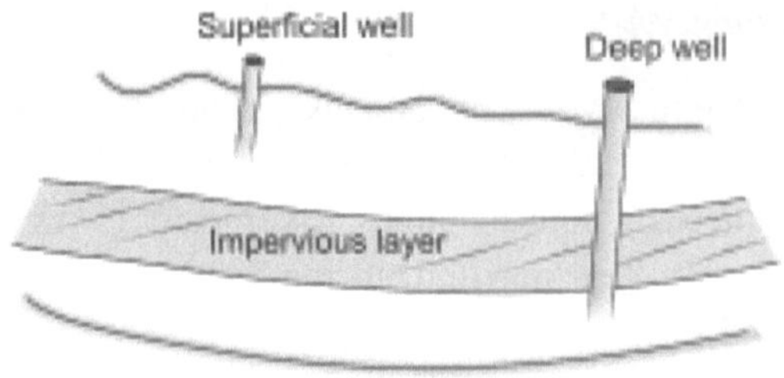

Fig. 8.2: Shallow well and deep well

Sanitary Well

There is a need for the well which is to be located in a good place, has wall constructed by bricks and does not allow water contamination. Such a well is called *sanitary well* (Fig. 8.3).

It is recommended that a sanitary well should have the following (Fig 8.4):

- Constructed at a higher level than ground level
- Walls are of brick and cement
- Has parapet wall

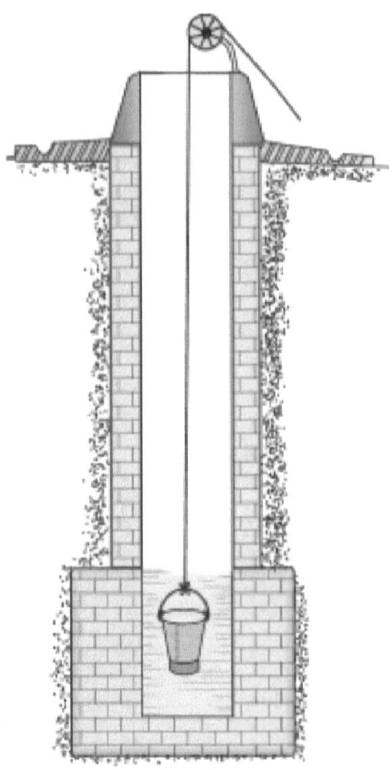

Fig. 8.3: Sanitary well

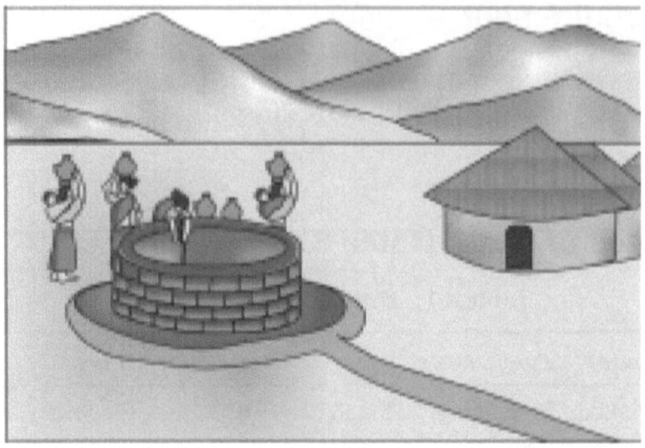

Fig. 8.4: A protected well in a village

- Has platform
- Has a drain
- It is better if it has a cover above

Tube Well

They are called borewells. Health Inspectors should advice public to follow certain instructions:

- Not to use the borewell 24 hours continuously
- To give rest at least for 8 hours in the night
- If water collected from tube well shows sand particle, people should stop collecting water and give time for water to collect in the water layer of the ground.
- If above instructions are not followed, it develops *critical velocity* (i.e. sand also comes with water by pressure because of less water) and borewell gets damaged.

Water-borne Diseases

By Pathogens

- Jaundice
- Polio
- Diarrhoea
- Typhoid
- Cholera
- Amoebic dysentery
- Roundworm
- Threadworm
- Guinea worm

By Chemicals

Low level of fluoride causes caries. The minimum level of fluoride recommended is 1 mg/litre.

By Soft Water

Heart diseases are known to occur by continuous consumption of soft water.

Conservation of Sources of Water

Water source and water catchments area should be protected. Every effort should be made to site the obstruction point above the source of pollution. Protection zone should be demarcated. Waste, effluent, fertilisers, etc. should not be allowed.

Wastage of water must be restricted thereby water source is made available for all the time in a year.

Minimum safe distance should be kept for stable, latrine and human contamination activities.

Conservation of water includes:

- Source protection
- Catchments area protection
- Groundwater protection

At Collection Point

Well, river, tank or any water collection point should be kept clean. Strict cleanliness must be maintained. Restriction on human activities removes the fear of water contamination.

Care at collection is necessary because people waste 20 litres of water when they collect 2 litres for their use.

At Storage Point

Care is exercised to avoid dust, impurities, vegetables, etc. at storage. Periodic cleaning of con-tainer, overhead tank or even big reservoir is a suggested guideline in conservation of water. Simple chlorination adds to the quality of water.

At Distribution

This refers to tap water or well water in most of the cases. Following care is needed and health education for water care awareness helps a lot:

- Not to spill water unnecessarily
- Collection of only required quantity
- No animal bath at the distribution point
- No transport cleaning or utensil cleaning at distribution point
- Waste water at collection is allowed to drain away from point of distribution
- Good maintenance is required.

Quality of Water

Standards are laid down to ensure safe water supply in the community. These standards are highlighted below.

Acceptability of Water

1. Water must be free from any turbidity. The taste, colour and odour should be acceptable by the community.
2. Levels of certain chemicals are standardised for their level in the safe water. The upper limits of these chemicals are as under:
   - Chlorides — up to 600 mg/L
   - Water must be moderately hard (calcium level up to 300 mg/L)
   - Ammonia content should be 1 mg/L
   - Total solids should be up to 600 mg/L

Disease-causing Pathogens

They should not be present.

Coliform organism test: It is done by PCT (Presumptive Coliform Test) in microbiology department and standard criteria are fixed to say the potability of water (Table 8.3).

Table 8.3: Coliform organism test

Standard criteria	*Coliform count/ 100 ml*	*Condition of water*
Class I	Zero	Excellent
Class II	1 to 2	Satisfactory
Class III	3 to 10	Suspicious
Class IV	Above 10	Unsatisfactory

Common coliforms found in water are:

- *Escherichia coli*
- Klebsiella
- Faecal *Streptococci*
- *Clostridium perfringens*

Chemicals

Chemicals, which indicate water pollution, are called chemical *indicators of water pollution.* They are:

- Arsenic — should be absent
- Cyanide — should be absent
- Fluoride — 1.5 mg/L
- Lead — should be zero
- Nitrogen in the form of NO_3 which is stable compound, if found above 50 ppm (mg/L) it indicates remote pollution or old pollution.
- Nitrogen in the form of NO_2, which is unstable, actually should be zero. But provisional guideline is given up to 3 mg/L. It indicates recent water pollution.

Radioactive Materials

No radioactive materials should be present in drinking water.

Sanitary Inspection of Water Supply

- Community survey is done to map out community source and their current status.
- On-the-spot inspection of water supply system is conducted.
- Sanitary inspector report forms are used for report making.
- Health inspector should inform local community in advance of the visit.
- Basic data are collected.
- Minimum annual frequency of sanitary inspection is given in Table 8.4.

Table 8.4: Minimum annual frequency of sanitary inspection

Dug well without pump	6 per year
Dug well with pump	4 per year
Dug well shallow	4 per year
Piped supply of well water	1 per year
Piped supply of river water	12 per year

Water Sampling (Collection of Water Sample)

Two litres of water in clean pharmacy bottle (Winchester' suart bottle) is collected, sealed and sent for physical and chemical analysis.

Sterilised bottles are used to collect 200 ml of water and are sent in transport box (Fig. 8.5).

If the sample is from tap, the tap is sterilised and midstream is collected. In case of well, river, etc. water is collected from little inside the water. Periodical collection of sample of water is necessary for good water surveillance system.

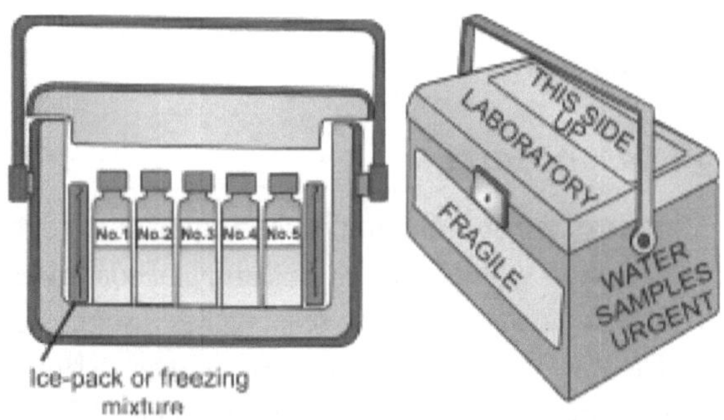

Fig. 8.5: Transport box (Cross-section and outside look)

Tap Water

Collection of water from a tap (sampling of tap water for public health examination).

Steps:

- Step 1 — clean the tap (Fig. 8.6)
- Step 2 — open the tap (Fig. 8.7)
- Step 3 — sterilise the tap (Fig. 8.8)
- Step 4 — open the tap (Fig. 8.9)
- Step 5 — collect the water (Fig. 8.10)
- Step 6 — allow air space (Fig. 8.11)
- Step 7 — close and seal (Fig. 8.12)

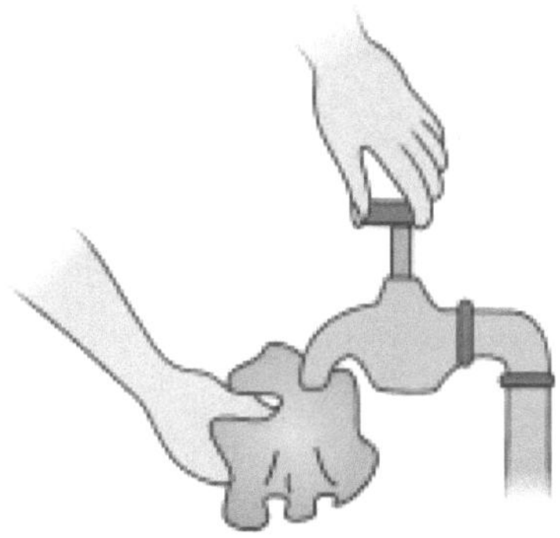

Fig. 8.6: Clean the tap

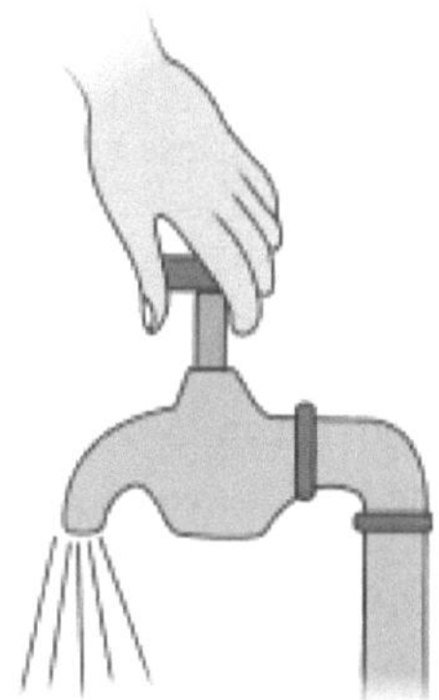

Fig. 8.9: Open the tap

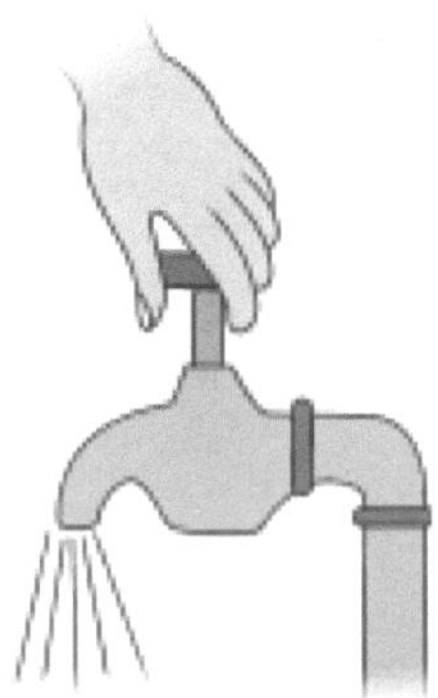

Fig. 8.7: Open the tap

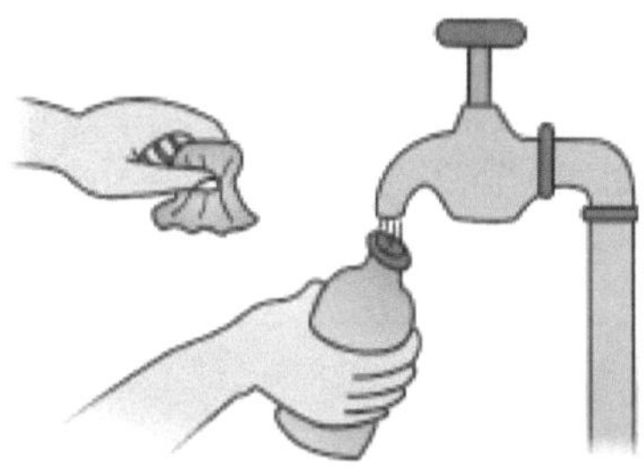

Fig. 8.10: Collect the water

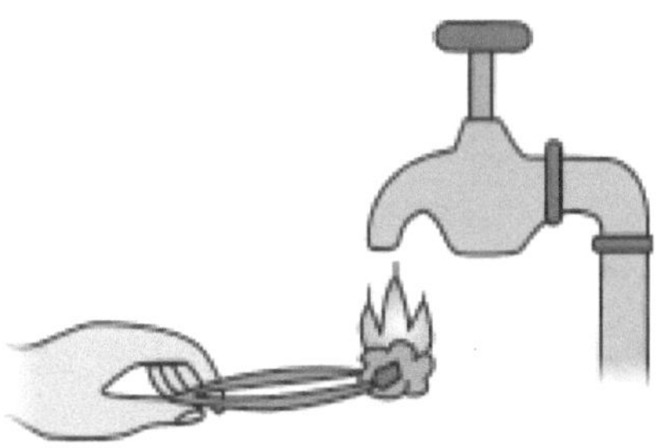

Fig. 8.8: Sterilise the tap

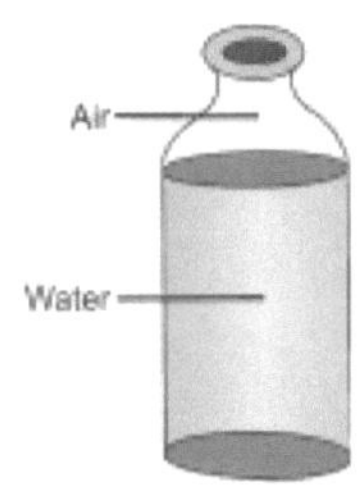

Fig. 8.11: Allow air space

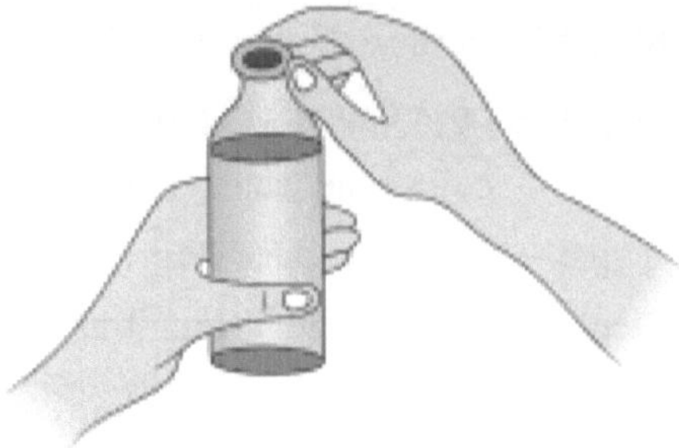

Fig. 8.12: Close and seal

Well Water

Collection of water from a well (sampling of well water for public health examination) (Table 8.5).

Steps:

a. Step 1—attach the bottle to the string (Fig. 8.13)
b. Step 2—lower the bottle. Should not touch the wall of well (Fig. 8.14)
c. Step 3—fill with water (Fig. 8.15)
   - Without hitting
   - Without disturbing any sediment

Table 8.5: Population and sample per month

Population	*Sample per month*
5000	One per month
5000 to 10000	One per 5000 per month
Above one lakh	1 per 10000 per month plus 10 extra samples

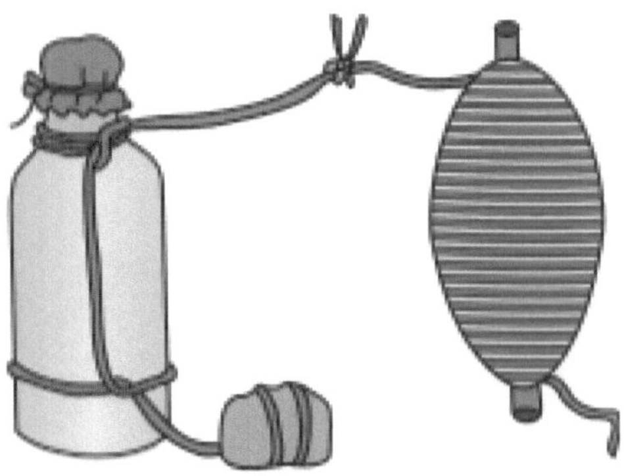

Fig. 8.13: String to the bottle

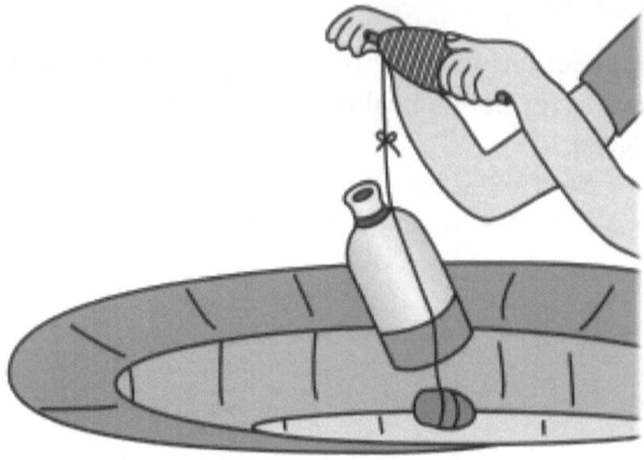

Fig. 8.14: Lower the bottle

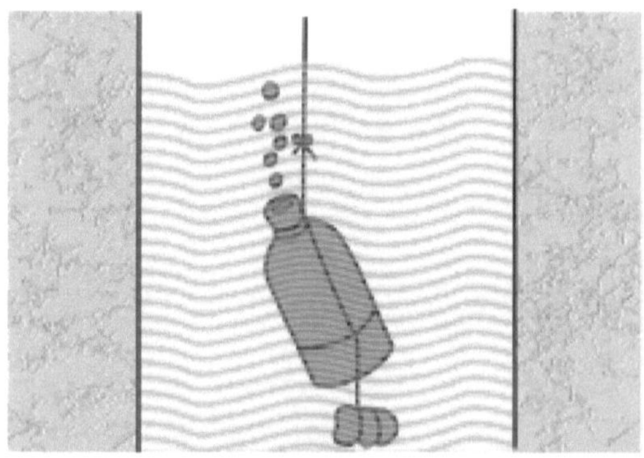

Fig. 8.15: Fill with water

Table 8.6 shows sample form.

Table 8.6: Sample form—information

Name of the office__________	Locality__________
	Site collected_______
	Place_____________
	Source____________
	Residual chlorine____
	Date of sampling____ Time of sampling___
Sender_______________	Dt. of previous collection____
Sample No.___________	

Public Health Aspect of Very Hard Water

- Waste of soap and water
- Scaling of boilers
- Cooking time is more
- Clothes get spoiled
- Not useful to industry
- Water pipe gets destroyed

It is advocated that boiling and base exchange process can reduce hardness of water for better public health use.

Swimming Pools

In urban areas, the Health Inspector working in a corporation jurisdiction has to inspect and take care to see that the following diseases do not occur among swimmers.

- Fungal infection
- Skin infection
- Eye and ear infection
- Respiratory infection
- Accidents

Compulsory rules are applied for 15 per cent water change everyday and chlorination for 1-PPM residual chlorine is advocated.

Health education is given to the public; not to spit in water, not to urinate in water and to take clean bath before coming for swimming.

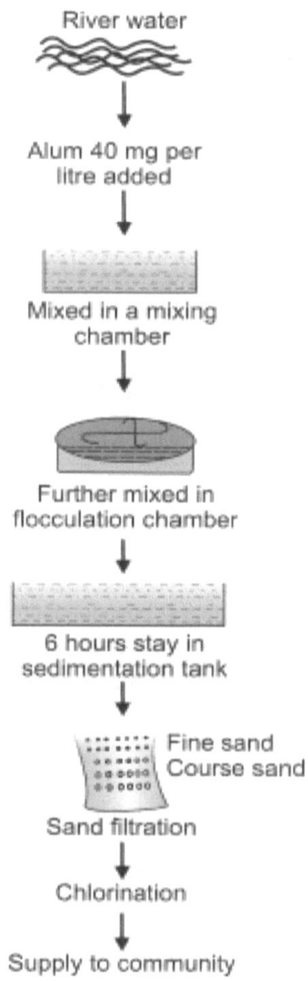

Fig. 8.16: Rapid sand filtration

Purification of Water in Urban Area

Rapid Sand Filtration

At present, rapid sand filtration is widely used as a measure of purification of water in urban community water supply (Fig. 8.16).

Steps of Purification (Table 8.7)

Usual steps of purification of water for urban supply include:

- Storage to remove suspended impurities
- Filtration through sand for purification
- Addition of bleaching powder to kill pathogens

Step I: River water is taken to a tank (mixing chamber) and on the way Alum (Aluminium sulphate) is added at the rate of 40 mg/L. The alum is a coagulant *(note that alum is not going to purify water but helps the dust to settle down).*

Step II: Then water from mixing chamber is allowed to flocculation chamber where it mixes well for 30 minutes by mechanical stirring through motors.

Step III: From flocculation chamber water is allowed to settle in a sedimentation tank.

Step IV: Later water is allowed to pass through sand bed. This stage is actual water purification. During the process of filtration, dirt collected brings some obstruction. To remove this obstruction, *backwash* is done.

Step V: Chlorine in the form of bleaching powder is added and later sent to the storage tank for storage. Further, it is distributed through pumping stations.

Table 8.7: Difference between rapid sand filtration and slow sand filtration

Rapid sand filtration	*Slow sand filtration*
• Small space needed	• Large space needed
• About 200 million gallons/acre/hour	• About 2 million gallons/acre/day
• Sand size 0.6 mm	• Sand size 0.3 mm
• Alum added	• No alum
• Backwash for cleaning	• By manual scarping clean
• A skilled operation	• An unskilled operation
• Loss of head 8 feet	• Loss of head 4 feet
• Removes turbidity	• Removes turbidity
• Removes colour	• Removes colour
• Bacterial removal is 98 per cent	• Bacteria removal is 100 per cent
• There is no vital layer formation	• Vital layer is formed and cleans

Chlorination

When water acts with bleaching powder, there is liberation of hydrogen ion and hypochlorite ion, which act as disinfectants.

$$H_2O + Cl_2 \text{ (of } CaOCl_2) \longrightarrow HCl + HOCl$$

$$HOCl \longrightarrow H + OCl$$

Types of Chlorination

- Prechlorination – Done before sand filtration
- Postchlorination – Done after sand filtration
- Combined chlorination – Both pre- and postchlorination done
- Super chlorination – Large quantities of bleaching powder added
- Breakpoint chlorination – When no pathogens are there and free chlorine starts appearing

Principles of Chlorination

- Water must be clean or it is made clean.
- Chlorine demand is found out by Horrock's test or by rough formula.
- Contact period must be one hour.
- Free chlorine should be 0.5 ppm at 1 hour.

Purification of Water in Rural Areas

Sanitary Well Purification

Concepts and principles: It is a properly well-located, well-constructed, protected against contamination for the supply of safe water (Fig. 8.17).

Minimum requirements of a sanitary well:

- Located 15 metres away from stable and latrine
- Brick or stone lining used for the wall

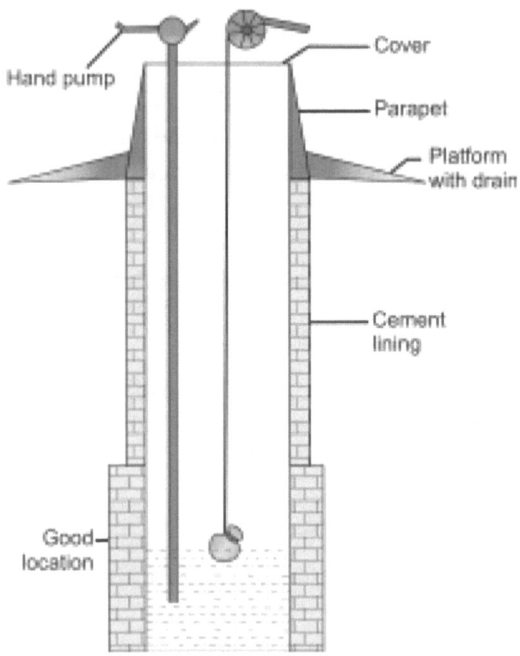

Fig. 8.17: Minimum requirement of a sanitary well

- Two to three feet high parapet above the ground should be erected
- Should have concrete platform
- *Pucca* drain for spilled water
- Top is covered
- Hand pump is preferred.

Steps of Disinfections of a Well

Open wells should be disinfected once a week. Ponds, tanks, other sources are done only during epidemic, if they are found contaminated.

Step I

Volume of water is found out by measuring water depth and diameter of well and using the following formulae.

Formula I

$$\frac{3.14 \times (d^2) \times (h)}{4} \times 1000 = \text{litres (multiply by 5 for gallons)}$$

where, d = diameter of the well in metres
h = height of the water in the well in metres

Formula II

$$D^2 \times (W) \times (5) = \text{gallons of water}$$

where, D = Diameter of the well in feet
W = Depth of the water in the well in feet

Step II

Find the bleaching powder demand.

- By 2.5 g/1000 litres or 1 ounce (one matchbox full)/1000 gallons
- By doing the Horrock's test

Horrock's apparatus: This consists of the following (Fig. 8.18):

- Six white enamel cups (200 ml capacity)
- One black enamel cup with a mark on inside

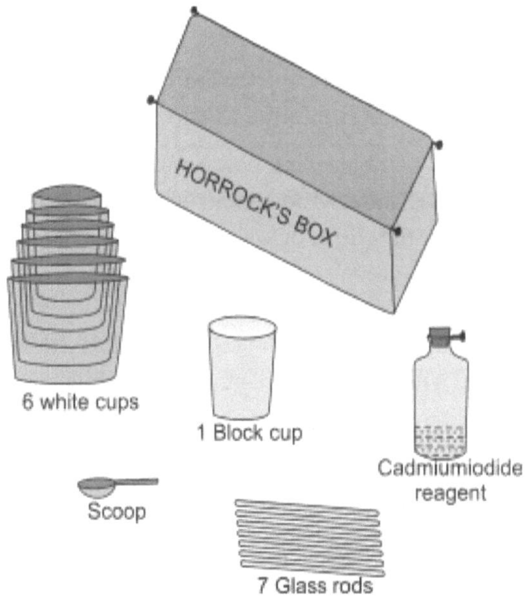

Fig. 8.18: Horrock's apparatus

- One scoop (spoon like) with capacity 2 g
- Glass stirrers
- One pipette
- Two droppers
- Starch iodine indicator.

Doing the Horrock's test: One scoop bleaching powder is taken, prepared into a paste in the beginning, and later making a homogeneous solution by adding further water up to the mark of the black cup (it is stock solution prepared in black cup).

- White cups are filled with sample of water up to the mark and are numbered from 1 to 6.
- To these white, stock solution is added as — One drop to the first cup, 2 drops to the second, etc. till 6 drops to the sixth cup.
- They are stirred with separate glass rods provided.
- Half an hour contact period is given for the action to take place.

Now, to each of these 6 cups, 3 drops of starch iodide indicator added, one by one.

Now they are observed for any colour change.

Result: Suppose 5th cup onward blue colour has appeared, then it is inferred as under:

5 × 2 = 10 g of bleaching powder is required
to disinfect 100 gallons of water
(or 500 litres of water)

Note: Suppose no colour has appeared in any of the six cups, then the whole experiment is to be repeated with giving 7 to 12 numbers to white cups.

Step III

Required bleaching powder is taken in a bucket, solution is prepared by adding water, making into a homogeneous solution, allowing for 10 minutes. Clear upper solution is taken in another bucket for use.

Step IV

The supernatant solution of bleaching powder is taken in a bucket. With the help of a rope, it is immersed into water and mixed well by jerky movement.

Step V

It is allowed overnight for action to take place (it is one hour if water is required).

Step VI

After one hour or after the overnight, well water is taken; orthotolidine test is done to find out the free residual chlorine level.

Step VII

If the free chlorine or residual chlorine level is below 0.5 ppm, the chlorination procedure is to be repeated once again.

Methods of Well Disinfections

Chlorine Tablets

If chlorine tablets are provided for well disinfections, then follow the following procedure:
- Chlorine tablet given will be 0.5 g each.
- Mix the required amount of chlorine tablets in a bucket three fourths full of water. One tablet is sufficient for 20 litres of water.
- Fix the rope or chain to the bucket handle and lower the bucket containing the solution in the well.
- Shake the bucket to ensure proper mixing, taking care that the bottom of the well is not disturbed.
- Allow 30 minutes or 1 hour as contact period.

Earthen Pot Method

If an Earthen pot is to be used, then follow the following procedure:
- Take an Earthen pot.
- In the bottom of the pot make 7 holes, each 0.6 cm diameter.
- Fill the lower part of the pot with small stones and cover these with a layer of gravel (Fig. 8.19).

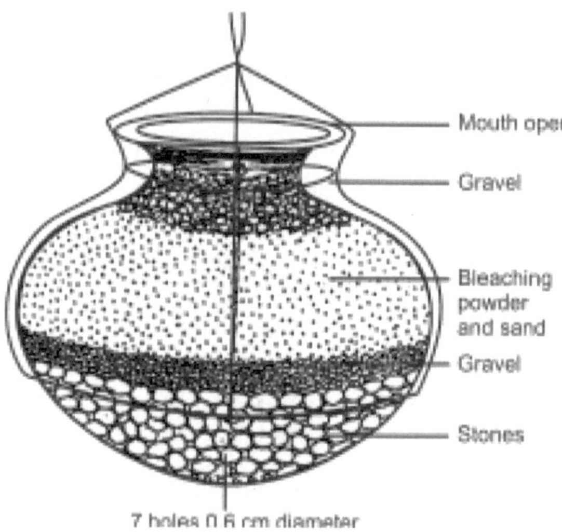

Fig. 8.19: Earthen pot method of well disinfections

- Over this, place a mixture of the following:
  - 1.5 kg bleaching powder
  - 3 kg course sand
  - 75 grams of sodium hexametaphosphate
- Pack the rest of the pot with gravel up to the top.
- Leave the mouth of the pot open.
- Suspend the pot in the well one metre below water level.

One pot is enough to chlorine a well-containing 9000 to 13000 litres of water and serving about 20 to 30 people per day. The packing in the earthen pot has to be changed once a week.

This method is suitable for individual house well. It is necessary to educate the public on the following aspects:

- To be careful while lowering buckets to avoid breaking the pot
- To prevent children from deliberately cutting the rope
- Suspending the pot.

Double Pot Method

In case of a double pot provided, follow the following procedure to disinfect the well:

It is an improvement by NEERI Nagpur, where bleaching powder and sand are mixed, a hole in upper aspect of inner pot and a hole in the lower aspect of outer pot are made. Similar to Earthen pot, it allows slow release of bleaching powder for disinfections of the well, when it is immersed in the well by a rope and left there (Fig. 8.20).

It is useful for a house well to disinfect about 5000 litre of water a day for the people of the house.

Other Methods

Other methods of disinfections of water on a small scale:

- Boiling for 10 minutes and keeping in same container.
- Chlorine tablets 0.5 g per 20 litres and use after half an hour later.

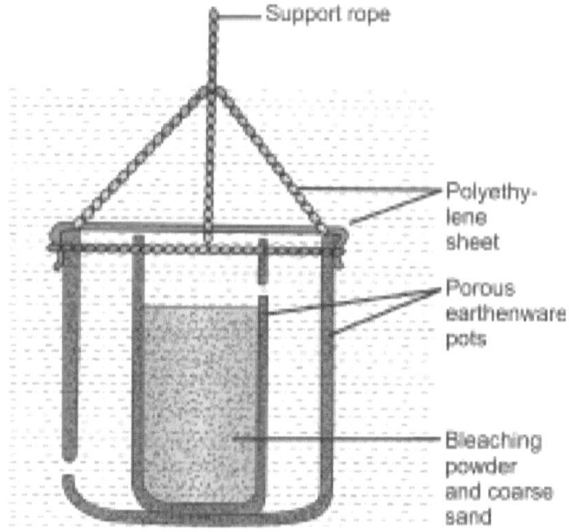

Fig. 8.20: Double pot for well disinfection

- Potassium permanganate ($KMnO_4$) is a good disinfectant. But because of colour change of water, the public do not accept it.

Water filters: They are commonly used at homes. They are of three types:

- Pasteur Chamber land filter
- Berkefeld filter
- Katadyn filter

The most essential part of the filter is the candle (Fig. 8.21).

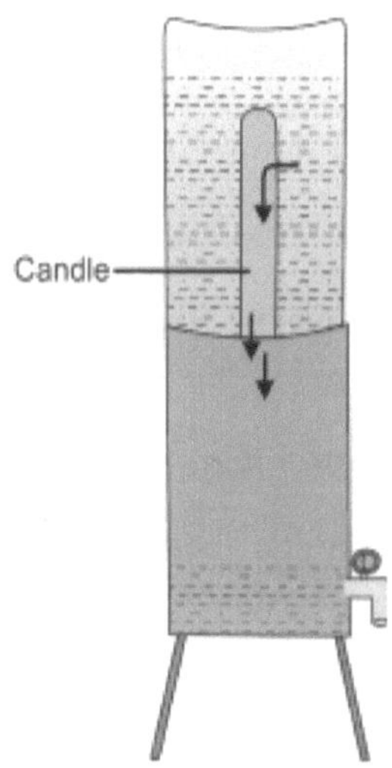

Fig. 8.21: Water filter

The candle in the water filter filters the bacteria, but not the virus. Hence, water filters are not useful in prevention of viral diseases like jaundice and polio.

Borewells: They are sanitary wells. They need maintenance, which has been mentioned in the early part of this chapter under water conservation.

Interpretation of Water Analysis in Public Health Laboratory

The State Public Health Laboratory and District PH Laboratories in every district examine the water sample sent for report.

Interpretation of water analysis should include:
- Source of water
- Physical quality, good or not good
- Chemical character, satisfactory or not satisfactory
- Bacteriological character, fit for drinking or not

The above interpretations are done based on water quality criteria and standards laid down in Public Health Laboratory set up.

WASTE DISPOSAL

Solid Waste

Waste includes paper, plastic, wood, metal, old container, glass, old bricks, old pipes and plant leaves and other thrown-out household material.

On an average 2 kg of waste per person gets accumulated.

Health hazards are fly breeding, rat breeding, water pollution and soil pollution.

Source of Generation

Depending upon the source of generation, it can be grouped as:
- House waste
- Street waste
- Market waste
- Industry waste
- Stable waste.

Storage

It is suggested that they are stored in dustbin, use me bins.

Collection

Corporation collects house-to-house waste in urban areas. In rural areas, it is dumped in the backyard everyday.

Sanitary Method of Disposal of Solid Waste (Fig. 8.22)

Landfill

An area is selected, or a trench is dug to put solid waste and cover with mud. When it is buried in the soil, decomposition occurs and even disease-producing germs are killed.

Burning

It is hygienic method and is called *incineration.*

Composting

Animal waste and solid household waste can be hygienically disposed of by composting. An advantage of this method is that the resulting compost serves as useful fertiliser.

Health inspectors' responsibilities are:
- Find out which families in your area would like to construct a compost pit and inform the area health worker.
- Assist the family in constructing a compost pit as under:
  - The pit should be near the house but away from the water source.
  - Dig a pit 4 metres by 3 metres by 1.25 metres or 3 metres by 2 metres by 1 metre.

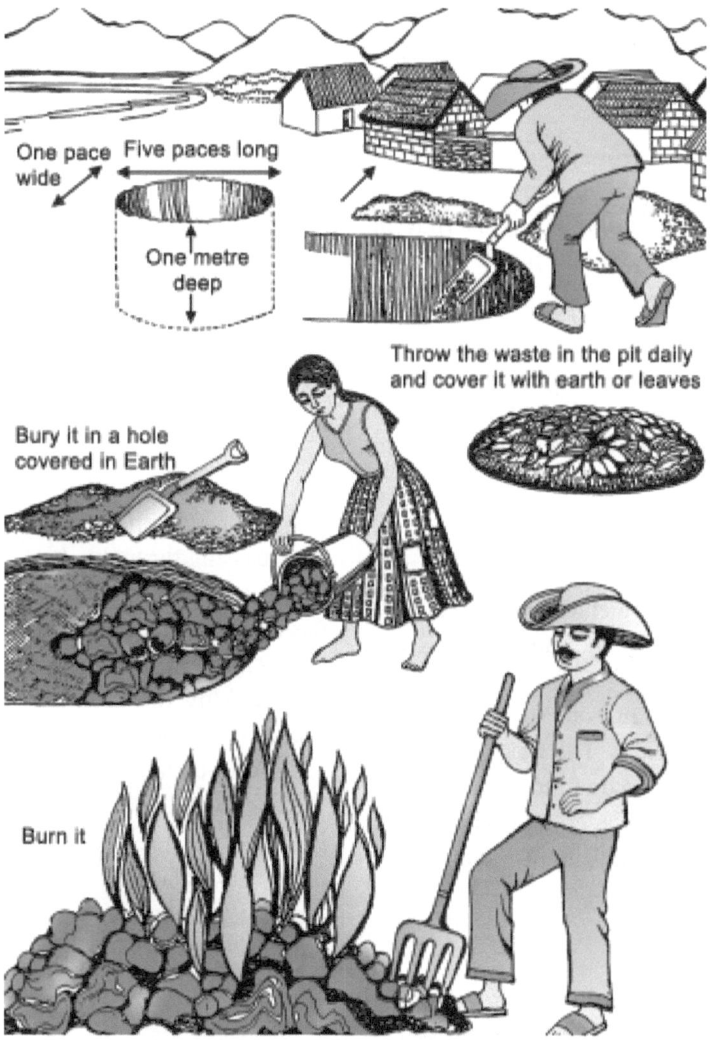

Fig. 8.22: Simple methods of waste disposal

- Instruct the family to fill the pit with layers of refuse and cow dung in the ratio of 3 to 1 volume until the whole content of the pit reaches 30 cm above ground level. The uppermost layer should consist of soil.
- Leave the pit for 6 months after which the compost can be used as fertiliser.
- When the pit is full, dig another pit.

In cities, hot fermentation process called *Bangalore method of composting* is done where solid waste and night soil are alternatively put and buried to get decomposed.

Public awareness on the following is advocated:

- Indiscriminate collections of refuse lead to fly breeding, attract rats and dogs, are unsightly and cause unpleasant odours.

- Refuse should not be dumped in drains as the drains become choked and produce stagnant water collections, which lead to mosquito breeding.
- Refuse should be properly disposed of by composting, burying or burning.
- The advantage of composting is that the compost serves as a good fertiliser.

Biogasification

Cow dung is collected and by simple process biogas is produced which is economic, viable and made available for public use for cooking and electricity.

Liquid Waste

Soakage Pits

Soakage pits provide a hygienic method of disposal of waste water (Fig. 8.23). They are cheap and easy to construct.

A soakage pit is a dug out space filled with stones or over burnt bricks. The waste water from the house is led through a drain to the soakage pit and seeps gradually into the ground. This reduces the danger of polluting wells in the vicinity.

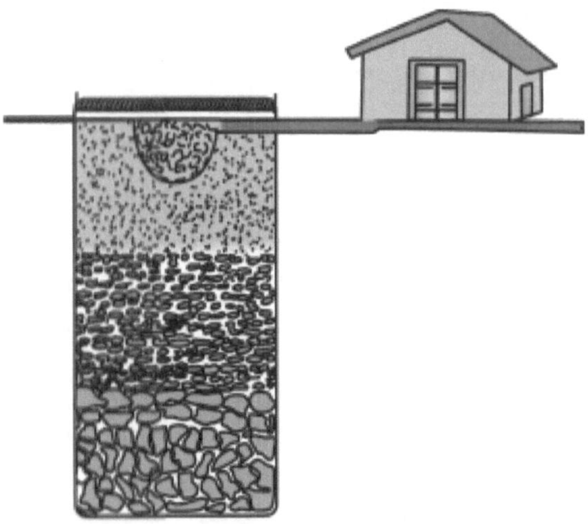

Fig. 8.23: Soakage pit

Construction of Soakage Pit

It is constructed as under:

- Dig a pit 2 metres deep and 1.5 metres square or 1.5 metres in diameter.
- Divide it vertically into three equal portions.
- The lowest portion is filled with stones or preferably over burnt bricks of 3/4th size.
- The middle portion is filled with bricks of ½ size, and the uppermost portion with bricks of 1/4th size, which is covered by a layer of earth.

The opening is protected by a parapet 10 cm high to prevent rainwater from entering the pit.

The house drain should join the soakage pit through a pipe opening into the middle of the pit after passing through a basket filled with straw or leaves which serves as filter. The contents of this basket are periodically removed and replaced by fresh dry straw or leaves.

Blocking the drain during the rainy season should disconnect the soakage pit

After a certain period, the soakage pit becomes "sewage sick" and will start overflowing. The pit has to be emptied, and the stones or bricks washed, dried and replaced.

Soakage pits cannot be used in waterlogged areas.

Kitchen Garden

If the household is small, the amount of waste water is limited and can easily be disposed of by leading it into a kitchen garden. In such a garden, vegetables and fruits can be grown which the family could use to improve their nutrition.

Health inspectors' responsibilities are:

- Find out the interested families who would like to have a kitchen garden.
- Assist that family in constructing a kitchen garden and supervise its construction.
- See that the family keeps the drain leading from the house to the kitchen garden clean so that water flows freely.

- Seek the advice of the Horticulturist as to which fruits and vegetables are suitable for starting and maintaining a kitchen garden.

Hygienic Methods of Disposal of Liquid Waste

- Water collections around the houses are a health hazard as they lead to mosquito breeding
- Collections of waste water give rise to unpleasant odours
- Waste water can be safely disposed of by constructing:
  - Soakage pits
  - Kitchen gardens

In urban areas, sewerage system is adopted for collecting and transporting liquid waste from dwelling places.

The water carriage system contains:

- House drain pipe
- Public sewer pipe
- Traps and manholes in the sewer pipes.

Night Soil

Sewage is liquid waste-containing human excreta.

Health hazards of unsanitary disposal of sewage are:

- Fly nuisance
- Soil pollution
- Water pollution
- Food contamination.

Faecal-borne diseases due to unsanitary disposal of sewage are (Fig. 8.24):

- Typhoid
- Diarrhoea
- Dysentery
- Cholera
- Hookworm
- Roundworm
- Jaundice.

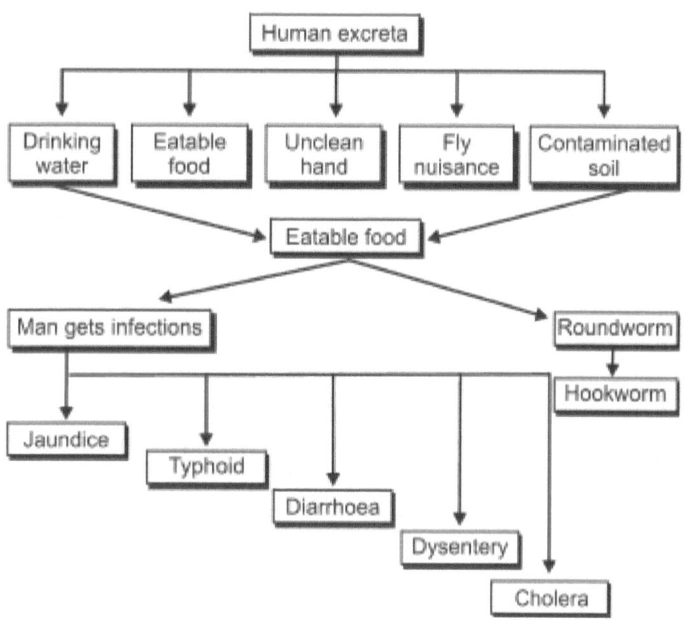

Fig. 8.24: Diseases by human excreta

Sanitary Latrine

Unhygienic disposal of human excreta leads to disease transmission through:

- Flies settling on food
- Drinking polluted water
- Eating contaminated raw vegetables
- Walking barefoot.

Sanitary latrine is also called RCA latrine.

Precautions should be taken to see that RCA latrine is located 15 metres away from the water source in the area. It has the following components:

- Squatting plate 3' × 3'
- A pan with 17 inches length
- Trap to hold water
- Connecting pipe between pan and dug well
- Dug well with 30 inches diameter and 12 feet depth.

In rural areas, the proper disposal of human excreta by the use of sanitary latrines is primary responsibility of the house owner. In cities, trust board or town planning authorities do not approve the licence without the presence of sanitary latrine in a house.

In remote areas, there are people who cannot afford to construct a latrine and who use open field should be advised to dig a small pit with a "*khurpi*" for defaecation. After use, the pit should be covered with earth.

The parts of sanitary latrine (RCA latrine) are depicted in Figure 8.25.

Health inspectors' responsibilities are:

- Find out which houses do not have the latrine and use open field defaecation.
- Motivate them to have at least a sanitary latrine.
- Assist the household in procuring from the Block Development Officer the material for constructing the latrine (Fig. 8.26).

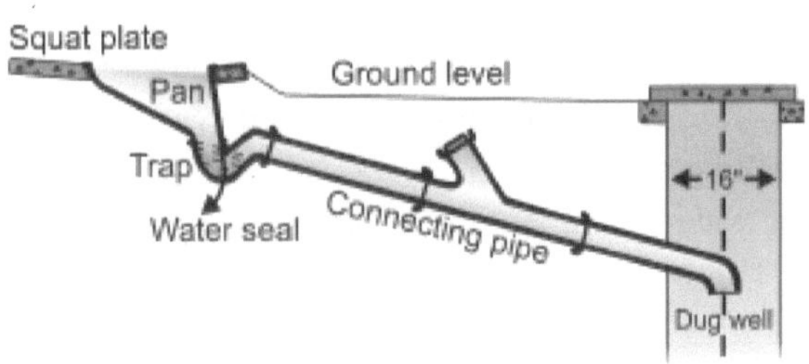

Fig. 8.25: RCA latrine

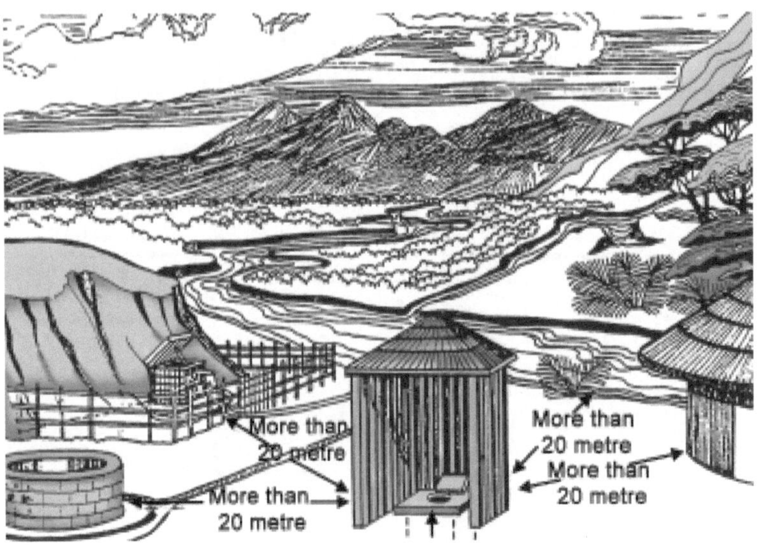

Fig. 8.26: Sanitary community latrine

- Carry out instructions given to you by the authorities or the BDO or City Health Officer
- Ensure the latrine is properly used and maintained.

Septic Tank

It is a watertight tank into which sewage from the house is allowed (Fig 8.27). It is good for a small family.

Solid content of sewage is made harmless by anaerobic digestion. The liquid form of sewage (effluent) is percolated through subsoil and is digested by aerobic digestion.

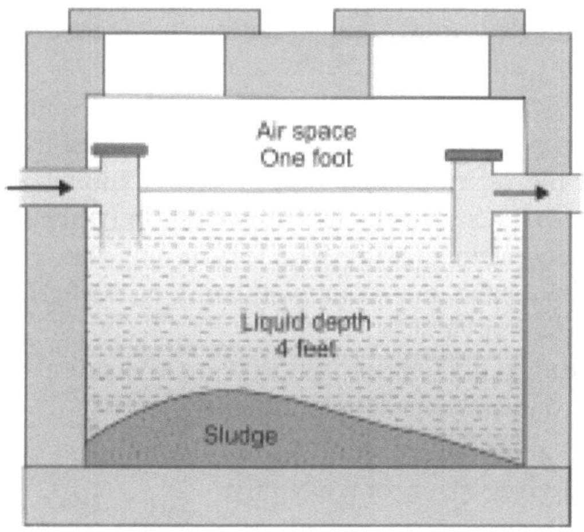

Fig. 8.27: Septic tank

HEALTH HAZARDS

Health Hazards due to Improper Management of Waste Material

By Solid Waste

- Fly breeding
- Rat menace
- Dog menace
- Intolerable smell
- Drains get blocked
- Produce stagnant water and mosquito breeding.

By Liquid Waste

- Mosquito breeding
- Bad smell.

By Sewage

- Soil pollution
- Water pollution
- Food contamination
- Fly nuisance
- Diseases like typhoid, diarrhoea, dysentery, cholera, hookworm, roundworm and jaundice.

Protective Devices

Protective devices for the prevention of diseases due to solid waste and liquid waste:

- Facemask
- Hand gloves
- Hand operating appliances to collect and transport waste
- Goggle
- Pump shoe
- Rubber gown for workers working in sewerages.

Universal Precaution

Universal precaution for the protection against hazards due to wastes:

- Always wash hands before eating (hand hygiene)
- Change and wash clothes if they are soiled and contaminated
- Avoid areas where air is polluted with waste matter
- Food hygiene
- Personal hygiene.

Sewage Treatment Methods

Based on the principles of aerobic digestion and anaerobic digestion, sewage purification is done by sewage treatment plants (Fig. 8.28).

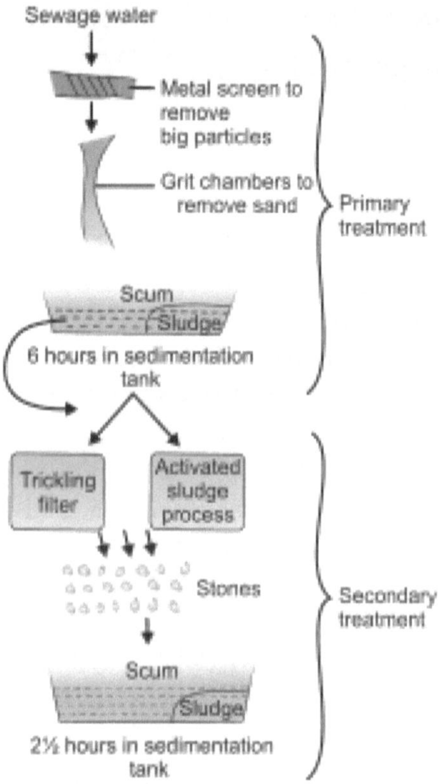

Fig. 8.28: Sewage treatment plant

- By metal screen rods provided in the sewage treatment plant, wood, dead animals and garbage, etc. are removed.
- By grit chamber, sand and gravel are removed.
- By primary sedimentation for 6 hours, sludge settles and undergoes anaerobic digestion.
- Scum floats are taken for:
  - Trickling filter (sprinkling by revolving device)
  - Activated sludge process (aerobic bacteria added and allowed for 6 hours)
- Later, the sewage is passed through crushed stone and allowed to sediment in secondary sedimentation tank for 2 ½ hours
- Sludge undergoes anaerobic digestion and effluent undergoes aerobic digestion
- The effluent is tested for *suspended solids*, which should be below 30 mg/L (30 ppm)
- The biological oxygen demand (BOD) for 5 days should be less than 20 mg/L (20 ppm) and can be land disposed or stream dilution allowed.
- Sewage farming allows growing fodder grass, potato, and fruit trees.

RESIDENTIAL ENVIRONMENT

Housing

General Principles of Healthy Housing

Housing includes physical structure of house, its surrounding and home facility available for good health. New word "human settlement" is used for healthy housing.

According to the WHO, definition of residential environment is "physical structure that man uses and the environs of the structure including all necessary services, facilities, equipment and devices needed or desired for the physical and mental health and social well-being of the family and the individual".

Basic principles adopted in a residential environment or healthy housing are:

- It gives shelter.
- It gives space for the family.
- It is accessible to school, shop, temple, mosque, church.
- It gives space for the family for religious activities.
- It is a capital investment.

Home Sanitation

A clean home leads to good health and the absence of disease.

Characteristics

The characteristics of a healthy home are as follows:

- It is built with a tin, wooden or cement roof.
- The floors and walls are smooth and can be easily cleaned.

- The house is well-ventilated.
- There is sufficient natural light and sunshine.
- It has a sanitary latrine.
- The waste water leads to a soakage pit or a kitchen garden.
- If the house does not have its own well, there are hygienic arrangements for water storage.
- There is a compost pit or a place for burying or burning refuse.
- Poultry and livestock are kept in a separate place away from the living place.
- The kitchen is free from smoke.
- Food and grains are stored properly so that insects and vermin cannot reach them.
- There is no overcrowding.

The house should be cleaned regularly and whitewashed or pasted with cow dung periodically

Storing and drawing drinking water: It is the responsibility of family to see that the drinking water is stored and kept clean (Fig. 8.29).

Smokeless chulha: The smoke nuisance is avoided by the use of smokeless *chulha* (Fig. 8.30).

Smoky kitchens are not comfortable to work and are hazardous. Irritation of the eye, infection of the eye, wall damage and wall discolouring, etc. will occur.

This is avoided by allowing the smoke to outside the house through chimney. The *chulha* is built by mud and straw. The size will be:

(75 cm) × (40 cm) × (20 cm)

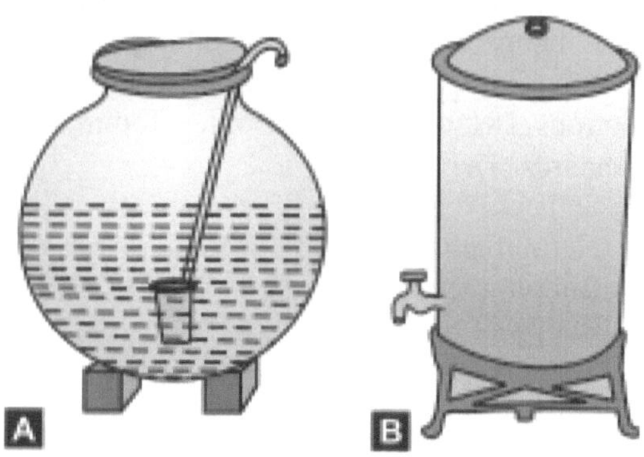

Figs 8.29A and B: Storing and drawing drinking water

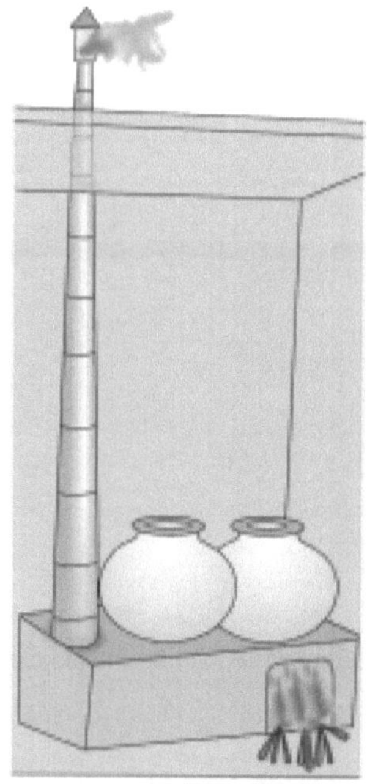

Fig. 8.30: Smokeless chulha

Clay pipe of 10 cm diameter kept one over the other and tapering to 8.75 cm gives the shape of chimney. The chimney will be projected outside the house. By fixing a cowl (hat-like cover) at the end of the chimney, rainwater entry is prevented.

Food Hygiene at Home

Food will be in short supply and its proper storage is important to protect it from being eaten by rats and from being contaminated by flies and other insects (Fig. 8.31).

- It must be stored in a good ventilated place.
- Food should be covered, thereby it is not accessible to flies or rats.
- Raw foods, like fruit and vegetables, are washed well before eating.
- Cooked food should not be stored for a long time because disease-producing germs will multiply in them and cause disease like diarrhoea and vomiting.
- Food grains should be kept in such a way that it is not accessible to rats.

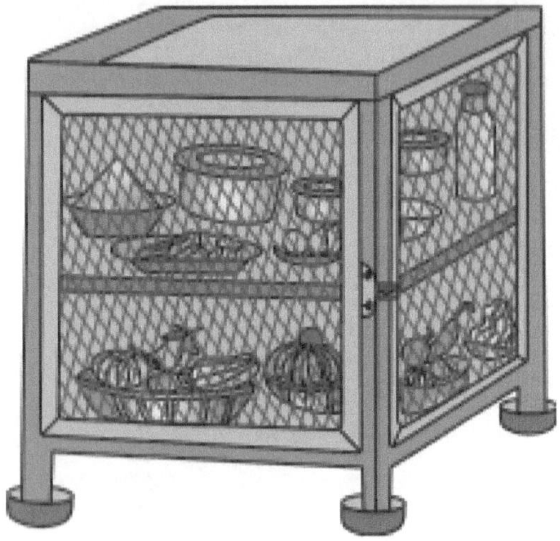

Fig. 8.31: Food kept in safe place

Specifications for Healthy Housing

Health inspectors' inspection for the following specifications for healthy housing.

Site

- Elevated
- No breeding place
- No traffic.

Foundation

- On a hard, dry and safe foundation
- No subsoil water.

Material

- Good quality sand
- Good quality bricks
- Good quality cement
- Good quality iron.

Construction

- Should be as per approved plan
- As per town-planning criteria
- As per municipality obligation.

Walls

- Strong
- 9" thick
- White-washed.

Floor

- *Pucca* concrete
- Damp proof
- Plinth preferred is 3 feet (height of floor from the ground is called plinth).

Rooms

- According to space per person recommended
- Minimum 2 rooms suggested.

Ventilation (ventilators)

- Should have cross-ventilation.

Lighting

- Day light factor should be 1 per cent.
- Sufficient light for work, studies and household duties.

Facilities

- Kitchen facility
- Bath facility
- Water source
- RCA latrine.

Codes/Regulations and Legislations Pertaining to Scrutiny of Building

As per power to regulate building, houses, mansions, bungalows, commercial buildings, entertainment buildings, etc. Municipalities Act 1964, sections 181 to 192 are adopted for minimum standards. They are:

- Setback
- Non-inflammable roof
- Building level
- Rat proof building
- No misrepresentations
- Completion certificate by Corporation or Municipality before occupation

The codes pertaining to drainage and water works, etc. vide Municipality Act 1964, sections 193 to 207 are adopted for minimum standards like:

- Drainage for the house
- Privies
- Alternations and repair license
- Work from licensed plumber and water supply contractor.

Regulations pertaining to public health safety and conveniences as per the Municipality Act 1964, sections 213 to 223 are adopted for minimum standards like:

- Dangerous building
- Pavement
- Road cutting
- Dog and pig menace.

AIR AND VENTILATION

Concepts and Importance of Adequate Ventilation

Ventilation is good air movement. Bad and hot air driven out and fresh and cold air is taken in is called ventilation. Purity, tolerable temperature and tolerable humidity are characteristics of good ventilation.

It is acceptable to have 300 cubic feet of air space and a floor space of 100 square feet per person. It is found adequate for good ventilation.

Ill Effects of Inadequate Ventilation

It affects functioning of special senses like smell and hearing

Polluted air can cause sickness

Ill-ventilated room can cause discomfort. This discomfort is due to physical changes in the air by high temperature, high humidity and poor air movement.

Types of Ventilation

Natural Ventilation

- By wind movement
- By diffusion through small space
- Airflow from high-density area to low-density area.

Mechanical Ventilation

- Exhaust fans (Air is pushed out)
- Non-exhaust fans (Plenum) (Air is taken in)
- Air conditioning.

Indicators of Air Pollution

Man by his activities makes the air polluted and in turn suffers from effects of air pollution.

Air gets polluted with gases, suspended particles, smoke and pathogens. Common sources of air pollution are automobiles, factories, domestic coal burning and nuclear energy programmes.

Air Pollutants

Common air pollutants are:

- Carbon monoxide (CO)
- Sulphur dioxide (SO_2)
- Lead (Pb)
- Hydrocarbons
- Hydrogen sulphides (H_2S)
- Cadmium
- Ozone (O_3)
- Polynuclear aromatic hydrocarbons (PAH)
- Dust particles from factory

Best indicators of air pollution are indicated below with permissible values (Table 8.8).

The National Air Quality Monitoring Programme by Central Pollution Control Board (CPCB) has given the following indicator to say that there is air pollution.

For example, suspended particulate matter (SPM).

Measures to Reduce Air Pollution

- By good enclosure, good ventilation and air cleaning. This is called containment measure.
- More use of electricity, natural gas and central heating can reduce air pollution.

Table 8.8: Indicators of air pollution

Indicators	*Permissible values*
SO_2 content in the air	500 microgram/m^3 in 10 minutes
Smoke measurement of the air	
Dust measurement of the air	
Haziness of atmosphere	

- Through law making in the country like:
  - Clean Air Act
  - Air (Prevention and Control of Pollution) Act
- Disinfections of air by mechanical ventilation, UV radiation of air, triethylene glycol vapour use and application of oil to floors are suggested.

INDUSTRY AND TRADE

In early days, occupational health was concentrating on factories and mines; hence the word "Industry and Trade" has come. But modern concept includes all types of occupation.

Aims

In industry and trade, the aims are for the promotion and maintenance of well-being of workers, prevention of disabilities, death and protection of workers from accidents.

Ergonomics

It is a recognised area for fitting the job to the worker.

Hazards during occupation are grouped under five major categories. They are:

1. Physical hazards
2. Chemical hazards
3. Mechanical hazards
4. Biological hazards
5. Psychological hazards

Industrial Hygiene

The term *industrial hygiene* means that principles and practice of modern medicine and hygiene to the special problems of health and disease as they are met with in India.

Trade

They are mainly animal matter require to be supervised by the Health Inspector as due to nuisance of smell and trade waste which are injurious to health.

Offensive Trade

It is a source of nuisance from public health point of view.

Regulations

Under the Municipalities Act, following trades are regulated:

- Animal skin dressing, it is called tanning
- Blood boiling or blood drying as seen in sugar factory, blood albumin preparation, Turkey red pigment manufacturing, etc.
- Bone boiling as in phosphatic manure for tea garden, gelatin, glue, fat, knives, handles, etc.
- Brick and lime kilns (brick and lime burning)
- Fat and tallow melting as in soap manufacturing
- Gut scraping as in making sausage skin, catgut, etc.
- Keeping animals like cows, buffalos, pigs, goats, hens, ducks, etc.
- Oil mills
- Paper making
- Rice mills
- Sugar factories
- Smoke nuisance as in rubber industry
- Slaughtering of animals where unhygienic slaughter houses are nuisance and menace to public health.

Pneumoconiosis

They are dusty trades. Pneumoconiosis is lung condition produced by chronic inhalation of dusts for a longer time. Common ones are:

- Anthracosis — coal dust
- Asbestosis — asbestos

- Byssinosis — cotton
- Silicosis — stone dust
- Siderosis — iron dust
- Tobaccosis — tobacco

Occupational Poisons

Lead: Paint, smelting metal, glass industry, lead pipes and rubber compounds are common industries that cause lead poisoning.

Workers' Health Protection

Following measures are undertaken for the health protection of workers in Industry and Trades.

Location

It must be away from residential areas and schools. Hard soil is preferred for the establishment of industries. There must not be water logging in the site area. No industry is permitted on the banks of river.

Ventilation

Good ventilation reduces the chance of infections from person to person. Ventilation brings about physical and mental efficiency of the workers. It is needed to control dust and fumes.

Water Supply

Basic requirement is drinking water supply to workers. Sufficient water for cleaning and industry maintenance is advocated. Drinking water fountains are preferred in industry.

Sanitation

Sufficient number of urinals and latrines are provided separately for men and women. Minimum recommended are:

- One sanitary convenience for every 25 workers (male and female separately)
- Provision for garbage disposal and waste disposal should be present.

Lighting

To avoid eye fatigue, to reduce accidents, to increase production and for accuracy in finished products, good lighting is very essential. Poor lighting causes permanent impairment of vision. There must be natural lighting and sufficient artificial light in every industry. Even corridor and passages must be illuminated.

Control of Dust and Other Hazardous Substances

- Industrial building is constructed with a view to check dust collection and easy disposal.
- Good cleanliness, washing and maintenance will not allow dust congregation.
- Minimum of 5 square feet per person ventilation is allowed for dust control.
- Hand mixing is replaced by mechanical arrangements.
- Use of less toxic chemicals in industry.
- Water spray minimises dust problem.
- If dust producing machine is kept in an enclosed room, it can prevent dust problem.
- Harmful process and offensive process must be done in a separate building.
- Trapping the dust by exhaust ventilation is recommended.
- Mask-wearing reduces dust inhalation.

In summary, best-suited methods for the control of dust and other hazardous material are:

- Avoid contact with chemicals
- Avoid respiring with barriers

Occupational Risk Factors and Safety Measures

They are enumerated below:

- High temperature produces fatigue, accident, hot spots, radiant heat and heat stagnation.
- Poor illumination in working area
- Continuous noise and vibration
- Radiation
- Direct touch of chemicals can cause eczema, ulcer, cancer, burns

- Dust inhaling causes pneumoconiosis
- Toxic effect of lead by contact and inhalation
- Anthrax, fungal infections and brucella infection with animal products
- Tear in the skin, cut in the skin, hand cut, and vision loss by carelessness or improper training in machineries
- Emotion and tension at work

Safety Measures for Occupational Risk Factors

- Proper temperature maintenance
- Good lighting
- Good maintenance of machines
- Lead sheet wearing by people connected with radiation (e.g., X-ray technician)
- Use of mechanised tool to handle harmful chemicals
- Mask use in dusty occupation
- Personal protection and personal hygiene to control lead poisoning
- Care by personal hygiene and personal protection in handling animals and animal products
- Alertness at work and good training in the job when they are expected to use machine
- Good employee and employer relationship for better and positive mental make up

Legislative Provisions

To safeguard the health and welfare of workers in Industry and Trade, we have Factory Laws. They are:

- The Factory Act
- The ESI Act
- The Mines Act
- The Minimum Wage Act
- The Maternity Benefit Act
- The Plantation Act
- The Municipalities Act

The Factory Act 1948

It is applicable to industries and trade where more than 20 people are working. In electrically operated industries, it is applicable if more than 10 workers are working.

- Factories should maintain cleanliness, lighting, ventilation, and elimination of dusts for safety of workers.
- Young persons below the age of 14 years should not be appointed.
- Weekly working hour must be 48 hours. Every day it should be 9 hours and a break of half an hour.
- Every worker is allowed leave 1 day for 20 working days.
- Any injury or accident in the factory should be notified.

Employees State Insurance Act (ESI Act) 1948

It is a measure of social security and health insurance for workers in an industry or trade. Since 01-01-1997, it covers all types of factories and all types of employees.

Benefits to Employees

Medical benefits: Free medical care and free treatment to all workers and for certain diseases like tuberculosis, cancer, paralysis, cataract, etc. it allows 309 days of benefit.

Sickness benefits: In sickness, benefit of leave with 7/12th of wage is given. For other sickness on certification, the worker will get 91 days of benefit.

Maternity benefits: For delivery 12 weeks and for sickness during pregnancy 6 weeks are available for pregnant women.

Dependents' benefits: Pension at the rate of 40 per cent to the widow or unmarried child, in case of accident or death of the worker.

Funeral benefit: Rs.1000 is provided for the funerals.

Disablement benefits: Monthly payment of Rs.10 by the worker, become insurable and the family members will get free treatment in case of their disability or retirement from occupation.

Rehabilitation benefits

Public Gathering

Sanitation of public gathering or Fair and Festival is highlighted in Appendix VI.

School Environment

School health is highlighted in Chapter 21.

Food Sanitation

Food sanitation is highlighted in Chapter 7 and also at the beginning of this chapter.

CLIMATOLOGY

General Effects of Climate on Health

Climate is the condition of the weather at any place over a period of time taking into consideration temperature, rainfall, atmospheric pressure, humidity, fog, mist, etc.

Effects of Climate on Health

High Temperature

It causes:
- Heat stroke (this can cause death)
- Heat exhaustion (salt and water loss)
- Heat cramps (muscle cramps)
- Heat syncope (BP falls)
- Heat pyrexia (high body temperature).

Low Temperature

It causes:
- Cold injury (hypothermia)
- Numbness of hand
- Numbness of feet
- Trench foot (severe cold injury)
- Frostbite (severe cold injury)

Rainfall

It is associated with:
- Low metabolic activity
- Cold and viral infection
- Allergic manifestations

Atmospheric Pressure

High altitude:
- Cannot survive above 25000 ft high
- Acute mountain sickness
- Pulmonary oedema.

Low altitude:
Compression syndrome called Caisson disease.

Humidity

- Low humidity causes dryness and predisposes to sore throat and cough.

Fog and Mist

- Motor accident
- Plane accident

Prevention of Cold Climate Effects

- Good woollen clothing
- Gloves, socks
- Important to dress suitably for cold areas
- Cold injury part is warmed in hot water
- Hot fluid intake

Prevention of Hot Climate Effects

- Person is encouraged to drink sufficient water.
- There is no need to take extra salt in Indian climate.
- Person working in hot climate should rest in between.
- If dizziness's or headache occurs, person should be taken to a shelter or to a cold place.
- Loose cotton white cloth should be worn.
- Cooling glass (goggle), head cover or hat use at work is advised.
- Good ventilation and air conditioning suggested.

MANAGEMENT OF HEALTH CARE WASTE

Public Health Importance

Health care waste is major source of infection of hospital patients, hospital staff and public. Since health care waste is from the sick, it is always contaminated and carries bacteria, virus, fungus and other disease-causing pathogens.

Therefore, it is vital to regulate health care waste management through scientific and sanitary way of handling. It is necessary to check the spread of infection and injury from the sick to the normal.

Health care waste is also called "Hospital waste". Proper and sanitary disposal of health care waste protects environmental health and thereby the health of the community.

Disease Transmission

Diseases transmitted due to improper hospital waste management:
- HIV infection
- Hepatitis B infection
- Hepatitis C infection
- Acute bacterial infections
- Chronic bacterial infections
- Epidemic of SARS
- Epidemic of anthrax

Hazards due to improper hospital waste management:
- Burns on the skin
- Corrosion of skin, eye
- Body toxicity
- Inhalation of dust or aerosol of disposal of expired drugs
- Headache and vomiting by radioactive waste collection and transport.

Definition

"Any health care waste generated during patients' examination, diagnosis, treatment and operation which include the following list of items."
- Human body part
- Animal waste
- Microbiology waste
- Biochemistry waste
- Needles, syringes, scalpel, blade and glass
- Discarded medicine and drug
- Solid waste like cotton, dressing, linen, bedding, tubing, catheter and IV set
- Liquid waste at cleaning and disposal
- Thrown out chemicals and disinfectants.

Classification of Health Care Waste (Table 8.9)

CONCEPTS IN WASTE MANAGEMENT

Point of Generation

Generation of waste depends on type of hospital. Government hospital, Hi-tech hospital, private hospital, private nursing home, private clinics,

Table 8.9: Classification of health care waste

Category examples	*Examples*
Infectious waste	Cultures, swabs, tissues and patient's stool
Pathological waste	Blood, body fluid, foetus
Sharps	Needles, infusion set, scalpel, knife, blade, broken glass
Pharmaceutical waste	Bottles, boxes, expired drugs
Genotoxic waste	Cytotoxic drugs and chemicals
Chemical waste	Lab reagents, film developer, expired disinfectants, expired solvents
Waste with high heavy metals	Batteries, broken thermometer, BP gauges
Pressurised containers	Gas cylinder, gas cartridge, aerosol cans
Radioactive waste	Unused liquids of radiology department

orthopaedic hospitals and trauma centres, each have their own statistics in the generation of hospital waste.

Four kg per patient and 40 tonne per city is an average figure available.

Usual hospital waste contains paper, plastics, rags, metals, infectious waste, dressing, linen, glass, and food waste and hospital sweepings.

Usual proportion of hospital waste is shown in Table 8.10.

Segregation

Routine procedure is to segregate the biomedical waste and accordingly we have 10 different types of waste categories. They are:

- Human anatomical waste (From OT)
- Animal waste (From animal house)
- Microbiology and biotechnology waste (Labs of Departments)
- Sharp waste (Injection room, OT)
- Discarded medicines and cytotoxic drugs
- Solid waste (Plaster, dressing)
- Solid waste from disposables (IV set, syringe)
- Liquid waste (By washing, disinfections)
- Ash (Incinerated)
- Chemicals (Reagents).

Table 8.10: Proportion of hospital waste

Category	*Percentage*
Infectious waste	8.0
Pathological waste	7.0
Sharps	1.0
Pharmaceutical waste	1.5
Chemical waste	1.5
Heavy metal waste	0.4
Pressurised container waste	0.3
Radioactive waste	0.3
Other general waste	80.0
Total	100.0

Sanitary Landfill

There should not be any open dumping. Environmental isolation is planned, site is selected, and it should be controlled by the efficient organisation.

Incineration

Before incineration, the following are excluded or segregated: Chemical, silver, photography, heavy metals, plastics and glass (Fig 8.32).

Medical Waste Sterilisation Unit (Central Sterilisation Unit)

The central sterilisation unit (CSU) or the medical waste sterilisation unit (MWSU) is a self-contained unit, readily portable and easy to install and commission, totally sterilises the waste by heating to 155°C in a pressure vessel for 15 minutes (Fig. 8.33).

Universal Precautions to Prevent HBV/HIV

- Entry to outsiders is restricted
- Door is written with symbol BIOHAZARD, no admission (Fig. 8.34)
- Workers should wear working white coats
- Gloves should be worn at all work

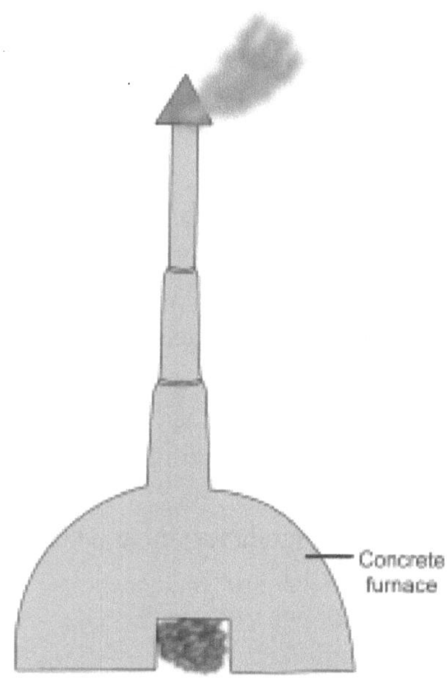

Fig. 8.32: Diagram of furnace for incineration

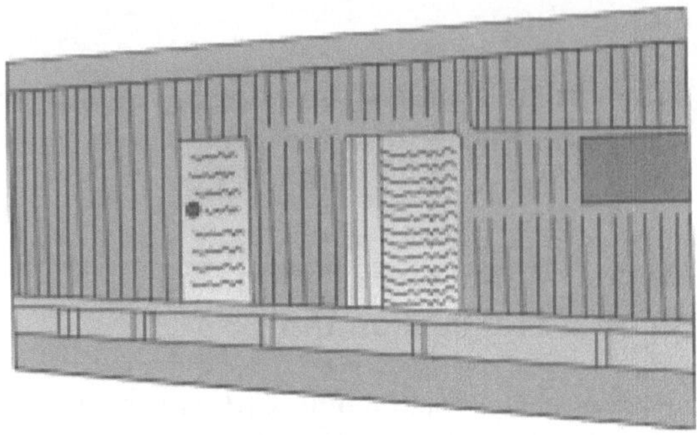

Fig. 8.33: Medical waste sterilisation unit

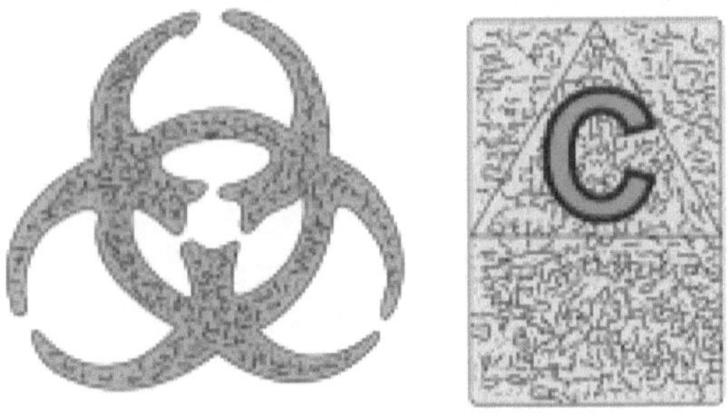

A B

Figs 8.34A and B: Symbols of BIOHAZARD at use

- Work surface should be disinfected
- Care at use of needles and instruments
- Do not recap used needles and do not remove needles from syringes
- Avoid mouth pipetting
- No air blow is done
- All should go to discard pan
- Avoid splashes, spills, aerosols and droplets
- Frequent hand wash done
- Touching mouth, nose and eyes is avoided
- Eating, drinking, smoking or storing food is prohibited
- Inspect cut or scratches in hand before work
- Always wear lab gown
- Seal all specimen positively
- Take precaution for needle prick injury
- Read instructions before any act.

Methods of Waste Management

Different types of waste and the recommended methods of health care management are described in Appendix XX.

There are three hierarchies suggested in waste management. They are:

- Reduction is done by incineration process. Recycling is allowed only to certain categories of material. Now plastic recycling is stopped. Permitted recycling is allowed for reducing the load of waste.
- Final disposal by deep burial is advocated
- Sanitary landfill and incineration are made routine in waste management

Occupational Hazards of Waste Handlers

By Waste and Sharps

HIV, hepatitis B, hepatitis C, acute and chronic infections

By Chemicals

Intoxication, burns and injury

Genotoxic Waste

Drug reaction and reproductive organ exposure to tissue damage

Radioactive Waste

Headache, vomiting and reproductive organ exposure to tissue damage

Importance of Monitoring and Recording

The Ministry of Environment and Forests notification, on 20th July 1998 has made emphasis on the monitoring and recording of Biomedical Waste (Management and Handling) Rules 1998. Vide item no.10 annual report submission and vide rule 11.0, maintenance of records say as under:

"Every operator shall submit report to the authority in form II by 31st January every year which include information about the categories and quantities of biomedical wastes handled during the preceding year. The prescribed authority shall send this information in a compiled form to the Central Pollution Control Board by 31st March every year."

"When any accident occurs at any institution or facility or any other site where biomedial waste is handled or during transportation of such waste, the authorised person shall report the accident in Form III to the prescribed authorities forthwith."

"Maintenance of records every authorised person shall maintain records related to the generation, collection, reception, storage, transportation, treatment, disposal and/or any form of handling of biomedical waste in accordance with these rules and any guidelines issued."

"All records shall be subject to inspection and verification by the prescribed authority at any time".

Colour Coding for Biomedical Waste (For Waste Category Mentioned)

- Yellow (1, 2, 3 and 6) – Plastic bag
- Red (3, 6 and 7) – Disinfected container/plastic bag
- Blue/white (4 and 7) – Plastic bag/puncture proof container
- Black (5, 9 and 10) – Plastic bag

9

Personal Hygiene

PERSONAL HEALTH

Hygiene is derived from the word Hygiea who is the Goddess of Health. Personal hygiene is also called *personal health.*

Definition

Personal hygiene deals with practices of cleanliness, which help in maintaining and promoting the physical, mental, social and spiritual health.

Habits and Customs Affecting Personal Hygiene

Indian culture has many time-tested habits and customs, which are closely linked with rituals. These rituals may be religious or magic by origin. *Examples*:

- Twigs of oil neem is used as toothbrush
- Pan leaf is eaten with lime
- Oil bath at home is a custom
- Taking bath after menstruation, after visit to burial ground, etc.
- Traditional barber does haircut and shaving who may not use sterilised instruments
- Smoking hubble-bubble is a social custom, which can spread tuberculosis
- People walk barefoot in open field and get hookworm infection.

The above examples give an idea as to how habits and customs affect personal hygiene (Fig. 9.1).

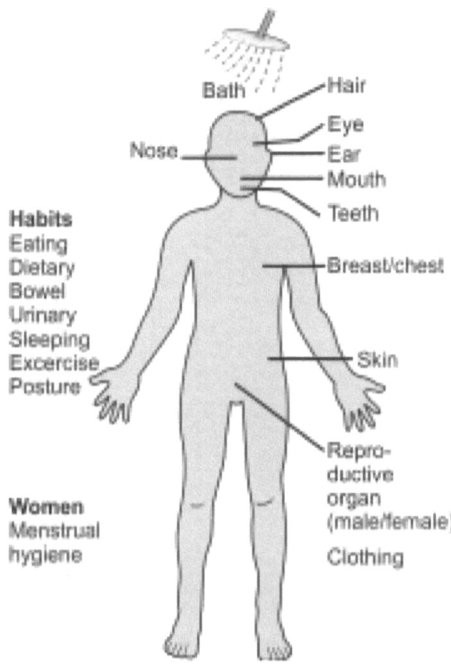

Fig. 9.1: Parts connected with personal hygiene

Care of the Body

Skin cleaning is important because we produce sweat. Sweat is thrown out waste from our body. Regular bath and good clothing is required for skin cleanliness.

Bath with soap nut powder, soap is a common habit. Bathing cleans and increases blood circulation, gives muscle tone and improves appetite. Bath can be of the following types:

- Cold bath When water is 33 to 35°C
- Warm bath When water is 35 to 36°C
- Hot bath When water is 36 to 43°C

Traditional families have oil bath which gives coolness and softness to the skin.

Ritual bath is taken after menstruation, after childbirth, after haircut and after attending to a funeral. Bath in the swimming pool gives opportunity for an exercise.

Since food and water is contaminated with dirty hand, care of the hand is important in personal hygiene. Handwash before eating, handwash after attending toilet, and after visiting the latrine are advocated.

Combing the hair is required for a better personal hygiene. This is a useful measure in head louse infestation.

Habits

Urine is waste excretion and should not be controlled at the cost of civilised life. Similarly, good bowel habit prevents constipation. High fibre diet helps in good bowel habit. Education on personal hygiene is given to women for cleaning from the vagina to rectum to prevent chance of infection of urethra and vagina from rectum.

Good dietary habits are required for good health. Knowledge of balanced diet, roughage use, avoiding junk foods is suggested under personal hygiene.

Regular exercise is a must for personal health. Household activities, socially useful productive work and rituals give opportunities for exercise.

Good posture in standing, walking and sitting are necessary for positive health.

The amount of sleep needed varies with age, occupation and habit. Usually, 8 hours of sleep is found sufficient for good body function and good mind function.

Clothing

Cloth protects our body from heat, cold, insect bite, etc. Cotton cloth is useful in tropics. Woollen cloths are useful in winter. Synthetic cloths produce skin allergy.

Menstrual Hygiene

Menstruation is a physiological process in women. Washing and cleaning of groin and vulva is required. Sanitary napkin (or a clean cloth) should be used and changed regularly and disposed of hygienically. Menses is not an illness.

Care of Special Sensory Organs

Eyes

If a refractory error is there (either short sight or long sight), it should be got corrected. Chemicals should not be used for eye beauty. Common stick should not be used for kajal. Minimum light is required while reading. At work, protective goggles must be used.

Ears

Repeated removal of earwax is not necessary. Finger, stick, etc. should not be put into the ears.

Nose

Mouth breathing is common in enlarged tonsils. Hence, treatment of enlarged tonsils is advised. Hair in the nostrils should not be plucked. A handkerchief should be used while sneezing.

Oral Hygiene

Oral hygiene means good teeth, good gums, and good buccal cavity. Good chewing helps in secretion of saliva and helps in digestion.

Mouth

After every meal, cleaning or rinsing of mouth is a good personal hygiene. Hot food, spicy food, tobacco, etc. cause irritation. If mouth hygiene is not attended to, it leads to gum infection and loss of teeth. Bad breath indicates poor mouth hygiene.

Teeth

After eating sweets or any sticky substances, mouthwash helps in preventing caries. Regular brushing of teeth helps in avoiding tooth problem.

Other Aspects of Personal Hygiene

- Footwear helps to avoid hookworm infection in the open field
- Observing purdha and avoiding sunrays cause respiratory infection like tuberculosis
- If a person is alcoholic, he will not maintain good personal hygiene
- Hygiene in tattooing, and circumcision help in preventing skin infection, AIDS, tetanus and scabies.

Public Bath

Personal hygiene in the form of avoiding spitting, not urinating in public bath, etc. reduces some infections. This is also called "Swimming pool sanitation".

CONCLUSION

Personal hygiene by good habit and culture helps in maintaining personal health of an individual.

10

Basic Epidemiology

EPIDEMIOLOGY

Definition

There are two noted definitions. They are:

- By Epidemiologist Mac Mahan (1960), "Epidemiology is the study of the distribution and determinants of disease frequency in man."
- By Epidemiologist John M Last (1988), "The study of the distribution and determinants of health-related states or health-related events in specified populations, and the application of this study to the control of health problems."

Epidemiology of infectious diseases is the fundamental part to be known by the Health Inspectors. It deals with public health problem, pattern of disease in the community, occurrence of new diseases and epidemics.

Selected Definitions

Infection

Entry of bacteria, virus or other pathogens to our body and produce body response.

Contamination

When bacteria, virus or pathogen mixes with non-living material like clothe, articles, etc. of man.

Infestation

Infection on the surface of our body like scabies, body louse, skin infection, etc.

Agent

Usually, bacteria, viruses or other pathogens that produce infection.

Host

This refers to man who gets disease.

Environment

Our surrounding which influence the diseases.

Infectious Diseases

Which quickly spread like measles, hepatitis, SARS, anthrax, dengue, etc.

Contagious Disease

It is by contact like scabies, fungal infection, STD, etc.

Communicable Disease

When a disease is passed on from man, animal, or environment to another man.

Endemic

If a disease is always present in one area, for example, typhoid, common cold, etc.

Epidemic

Sudden unexpected more number of cases in a community is called epidemic, for example, dengue fever, cholera and SARS.

Zoonoses

When man gets diseases that are present in vertebrate animals, for example, plague, anthrax and KFD.

Epizootic

When epidemic occurs in animals, for example, anthrax epidemic in sheep, rabies epidemic in dogs and JE in pigs.

Incubation Period

It is the time taken from entry of pathogens till signs and symptoms are manifested, for example, IP of cholera—5 days and IP of chickenpox—14 days.

Disease Distribution

This deals with the pattern of disease in a community. How it is distributed is recorded under the following points:

- *Time*: Which part of a year a disease is more is known
- *Place*: Which place in the world or a nation, it is more is known
- *Person*: Who are affected more? Man, woman, children, old people, low socio-economic people, etc.

Disease Determinants

Epidemiologists study many risk factors, which are known to be associated with diseases, for example,

- Overcrowding leads to many ARI cases, many scabies
- Using a common stick to apply *kajal* help in spread of eye infection.

Disease Measurement

- By measuring deaths occurring due to diseases
  - Crude death rate
  - Specific death rate
  - Case fatality rate
- By measuring sickness and disability.

Prevalence of a Disease

$$\frac{\text{Number of old cases + new cases at a given point of time or during one year}}{\text{Mid - year population}} \times 100$$

Incidence

$$\frac{\text{Number of new cases at a given point of time or during one year}}{\text{Population exposed}} \times 100$$

Types of Epidemiological Studies Conducted

- Cross-sectional study done at one point
- Longitudinal study done over a period of one year.

Risk Estimation in Diseases

Usually, risk is obtained by the following formula:

$$\text{Relative risk} = \frac{\text{Incidence among exposed}}{\text{Incidence among unexposed}} \times 100$$

The above value is a ratio obtained by dividing incidence among exposed with incidence among unexposed.

EXPERIMENTAL EPIDEMIOLOGY

This is done by conducting experiments with animals or conducting field trial with human beings.

Uses of Epidemiology

- Helps in identification of pathology in the community
- Explains the pattern of disease in the community
- Helps to find out risk factors of a disease
- Helps in screening of disease
- Helps in survey of a community for a community diagnosis
- Identifies seasonal variation of a disease
- Helps in taking up control measures or preventive measures in the community

Spectrum of Health and Illness

Since health and disease are interrelated and overlap each other, we come across a range of people with their health ranging from positive health to negative health (Fig. 10.1).

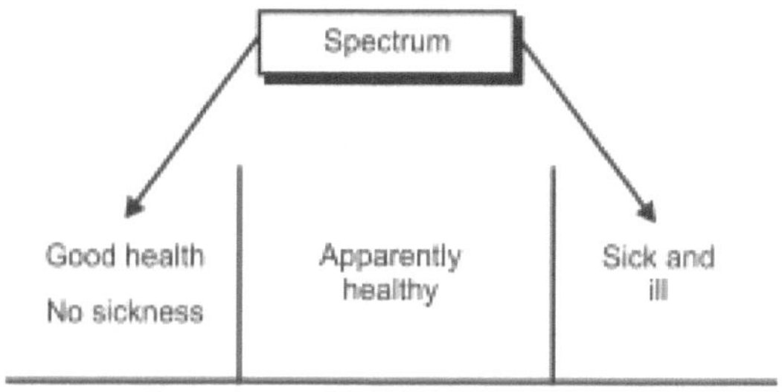

Fig. 10.1: Spectrum of health and illness

Factors Influencing Health and Illness

They are also called determinants of disease and health. They are:

- Genetic make up which runs in the family
- Lifestyle of person
- Our surrounding called environment
- Economic status of the person or the family
- Literacy status of the person or the family
- Occupation of the person or the family
- Availability of health services

Human life in his environment is also termed as ecology of health.

Web of Causation

All possible causes and influencing factors are interrelated and interwoven to form *web of causation of a disease.* This includes all possible causes, all possible risk factors and all possible influencing factors in a disease (Figs 10.2 and 10.3).

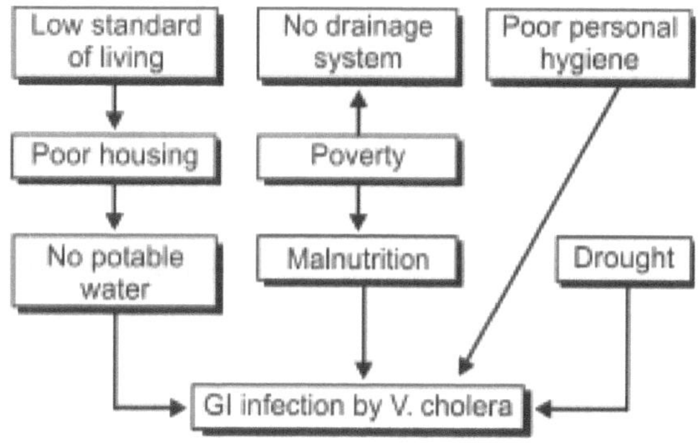

Fig. 10.2: Web of causation of cholera

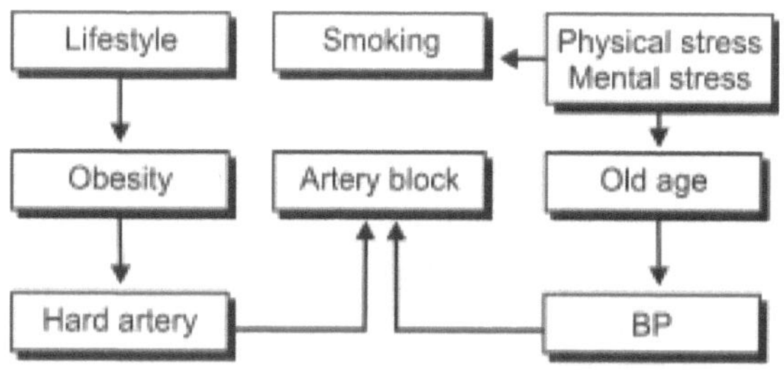

Fig. 10.3: Web of causation of heart attack

Epidemiological Triad

The causes of diseases are grouped under three heads. Hence, the name *triad of epidemiology.* They are depicted in Figure 10.4.

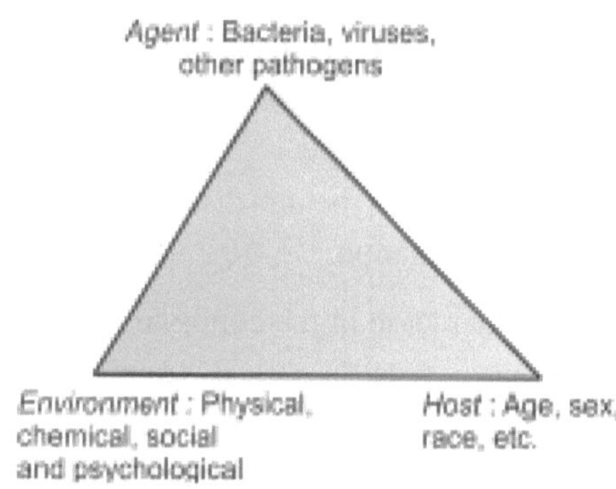

Fig. 10.4: Triad of epidemiology

Disease Iceberg

In a community, we see a small portion of ill health and many illnesses are not seen at all. This is compared with an ice-immersed in water, which shows only an upper small portion (depicting small portion of sickness) and big submerged portion (unseen illness of the community). This phenomenon is called *iceberg of disease.*

11

Dynamics of Disease Transmission

DISEASE TRANSMISSION CHAIN

In the dynamics of disease transmission, usually the following links are highlighted (Figs 11.1 to 11.4).

- Reservoir of infection
- Mode of transmission of infection
- Host or the man who gets infection

Reservoir of Infection

Reservoir is a man, animal or non-living things where pathogens survive, reproduce and transmit to new host.

- Non-living things are soil, paper, cloth, etc.
- Animal reservoirs are dogs, monkeys, pigs, etc.
- Human reservoir is a person who harbours pathogen. He is called a case when he is having a disease, or has health disorder and who is under investigation.

First human case in the community is called a **primary case.** When a case is seen as first case during the survey in the locality; it is called an **index case.** If a person does not show signs and symptoms but harbour pathogens, then he is called a **carrier.** Different kinds of carrier states are given below.

- *Healthy carrier*: When a person does not suffer, apparently healthy but harbours pathogen, he is called a healthy carrier.
- *Temporary carrier*: When a person is lodging pathogen for a short time is called temporary carrier (it is usually 3 to 7 days).

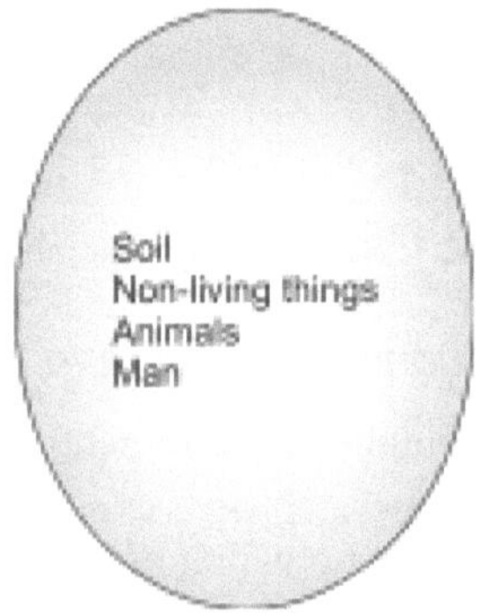

Fig. 11.1: First link of disease transmission chain

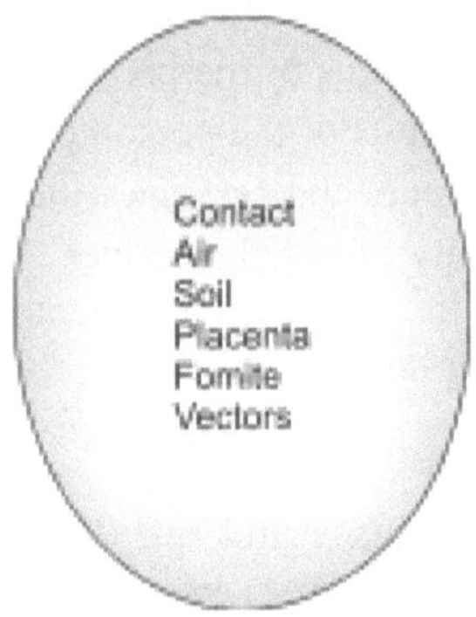

Fig. 11.2: Second link of disease transmission

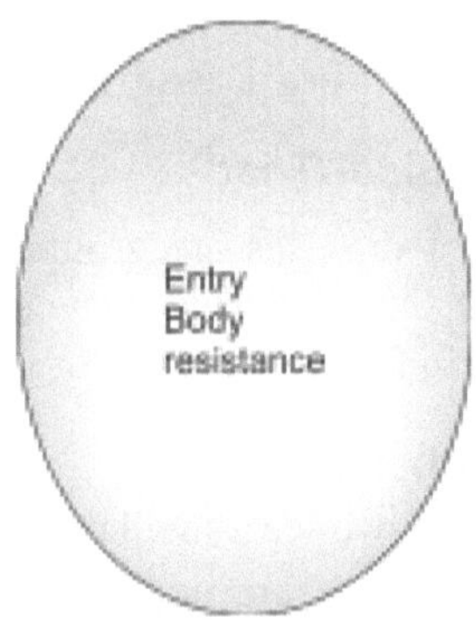

Fig. 11.3: Third link of disease transmission

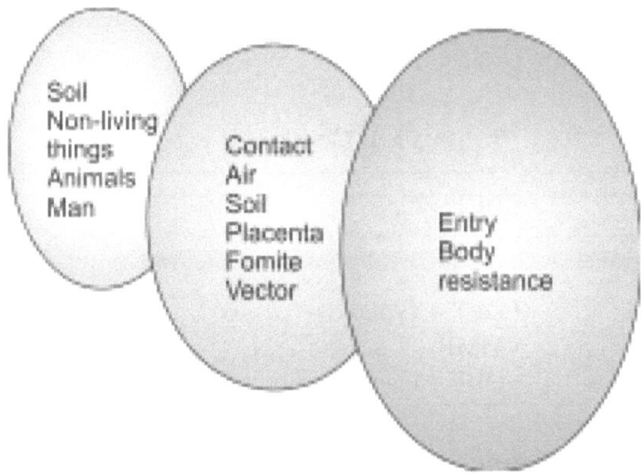

Fig. 11.4: Linked links of disease transmission

- *Chronic carrier*: When a person or patient is lodging pathogen for a longer time, he is called chronic carrier (it is usually over 3 months).

Mode of Transmission of Infection

There are many modes of disease transmission. They are:

- Direct—Scabies, STD
- Droplet—TB, whooping cough
- Soil—Tetanus, hookworm
- Placenta—Syphilis, rubella
- Water—Hepatitis, cholera
- Food—GE, typhoid
- Vector—Cyclops transmitting guinea worm, mosquitoes transmitting malaria
- Fomite—Typhoid, skin infection

Host

When man becomes susceptible, he gets the disease. Usually, through air, through food or through contact, pathogen enters and takes a few days for the development of signs and symptoms. This period is called *incubation period.*

SERIAL INTERVAL

It is the period of time gap between first case (primary case) and second case (secondary case). If more secondary cases are there, the infection is said to be spreading quickly. It is called *secondary attack rate.* The secondary attack rate (SAR) is calculated by:

$$\text{SAR} = \frac{\text{Number of contacts developing disease}}{\text{Total people exposed}} \times 100$$

SAR is specifically applicable to infectious diseases. SAR helps in identification of susceptible in case of chickenpox and measles. In a population, where vaccination is done, the attack rate among vaccinated can be found out. This is an added advantage in infectious disease epidemiology.

MAN'S IMMUNITY AGAINST DISEASE

There are two types of immunity:

- *Active immunity*:
  - It is obtained after an attack of infection
  - It is obtained after subclinical attack of infection
  - It is obtained after giving vaccine for a given disease.
- *Passive immunity*:
  - It is obtained by giving immunoglobulins
  - It is obtained by giving antiserum
  - A baby can get from mother through placenta.

In the dynamics of disease transmission, *herd immunity* is an important component, which determines disease occurrence in the community. Herd immunity gives body protection to whole population and a disease is not allowed to occur in a community. If this type of herd immunity is not there, an attack by a disease leads to many deaths and severe illness in the community. By collecting blood sample and sending for serology test, we can find out the existence of herd immunity.

Vaccines

It is prepared from pathogens, which are inactivated or killed. Even some of the vaccines are extracted from the cells of organism.

Recent vaccines are available in the following form:

- Recombinant vaccines
- Subunit vaccines

Common vaccines used in public health practice (Table 11.1).

Table 11.1: Common vaccines

Vaccine		*Nature*
OPV	Viral	Live-attenuated vaccine
Cholera	Bacterial	Killed vaccine
Diphtheria	Bacterial	Toxoid
Whooping cough	Bacterial	Killed vaccine
Tetanus	Bacterial	Toxoid
BCG	Bacterial	Live-attenuated
Typhoid oral	Bacterial	Live-attenuated
Measles	Viral	Live-attenuated
Meningitis	Bacterial	Killed
Rabies	Viral	Killed
JE	Viral	Killed

Common immunoglobulins used in public health practice (Table 11.2).

Table 11.2: Common immunoglobulins

Immunoglobulins	*Nature*
Tetanus	Human normal immunoglobulin
Rabies	Human normal immunoglobulin
Measles	Human normal immunoglobulin
Hepatitis A	Human normal immunoglobulin
Diphtheria	Human specific immunoglobulin

Common antisera used in public health practice (Table 11.3).

Table 11.3: Common antisera

Antisera	*Nature*
ADS	Bacterial non-human
ATS	Bacterial non-human
ARS	Viral non-human

Combined vaccines used in public health practice (Table 11.4)

Table 11.4: Combined vaccines

• DPT
• DT
• DP
• DPT + Typhoid
• MMR
• DPT + Inactivated polio

Cold Chain

Cold chain is maintained to keep vaccine fit for human use. It should have safety and potency. Cold chain is the centre for success of immunisation programme.

If temperature of ILR/DF/Fridge falls below +2°C or raised above + 8°C, it indicates a break in cold chain.

Thus, cold chain is a system of storing and transporting vaccines at recommended temperature from the point of manufacture to use point.

Equipment

- WIF (Walk in freezer)
  - For OPV, measles
  - For ice packs
  - Maintains – 20°C
  - At state level
- WIC (Walk in cooler)
  - At regional level use
  - Maintain + 2 to + 8°C
  - Store large quantity
  - Has alarm system
- DF (Deep freezer)
  - Under UIP
  - Maintain – 18 to – 20°C
  - For OPV, measles
  - For ice packs
  - 300 litre capacity for district level
- ILR (Ice-linked refrigerator)
  - MK 300 is for district level
  - MK 140 is for PHC level
  - Maintain + 2 to + 8°C

- Top for BCG, DPT, DT, TT
- Bottom for OPV, measles

Special note: No electrical cold chain equipment should be installed without a voltage stabiliser.

Cold Box

They are 5 litre and 20 litre capacities for 1500 dose and 6000 dose respectively (Figs 11.5 to 11.7). Temperature maintenance is 90 hours for 5 litres, 6 days for 20-litre box.

Vaccine Carrier

It is used for carrying 16 to 20 vials to subcentre for 1 day use.

Day Carrier

It is used for carrying 6 to 8 vials to immunisation session. Storage time is 6 hours.

General instructions:

- Record of storage temperature is kept
- Record of storage is maintained
- Action is taken when warranted
- FIFO (First in First Rule) is followed
- FEFO (First to Expire First to out) is followed

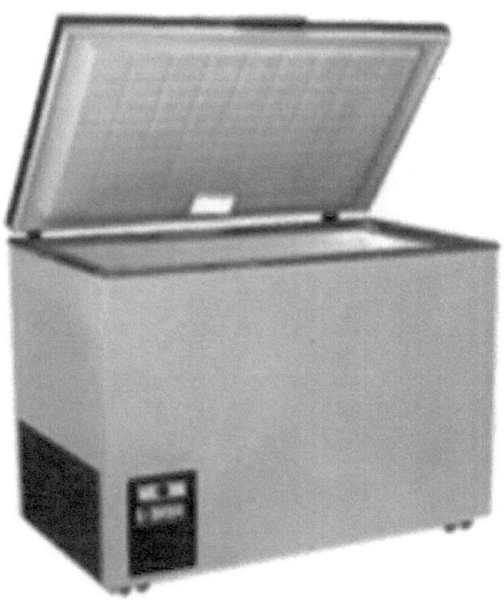

Fig. 11.5: Deep freezer (300 litre)

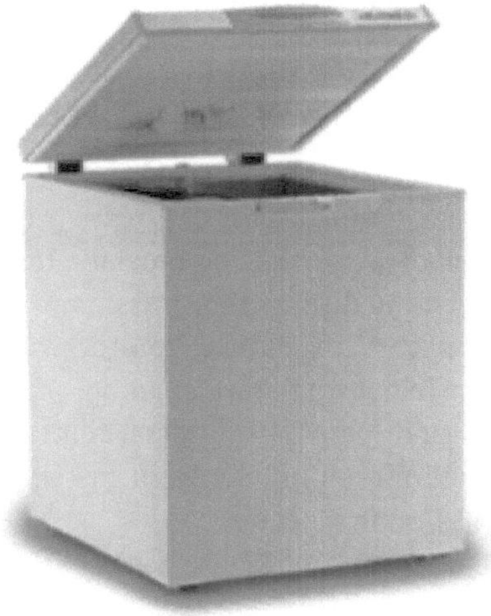

Fig. 11.6: Deep freezer (140 litre)

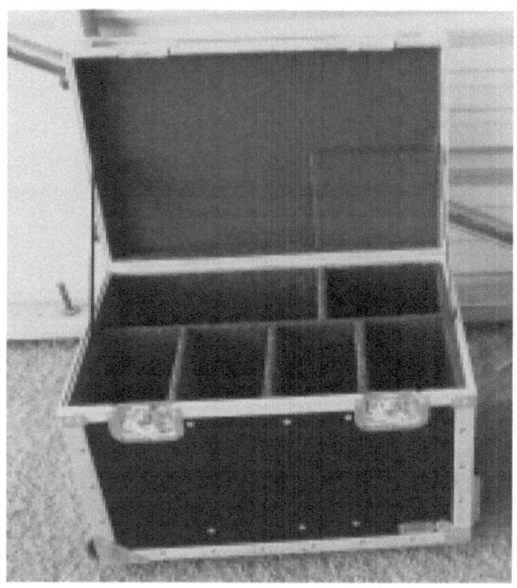

Fig. 11.7: Cold box (22 litre)

REACTION TO IMMUNISATION

Commonly local reactions like pain, swelling, redness, tenderness, and small nodule development are noticed. General reactions like fever and body ache are common. Giving paracetamol tablet at immunisation session will overcome this problem.

For any unusual reaction, MOH or Doctors concerned are referred.

Identification of the Weak Link of Disease Transmission

Weak link varies from disease to disease (Fig 11.8). Identification of weak link and breaking them will help in preventing disease transmission.

In the history of public health, we know removing the handle of the water pump, which was responsible for disease transmission, controlled the cholera epidemic (John Snow in his historical discovery at London).

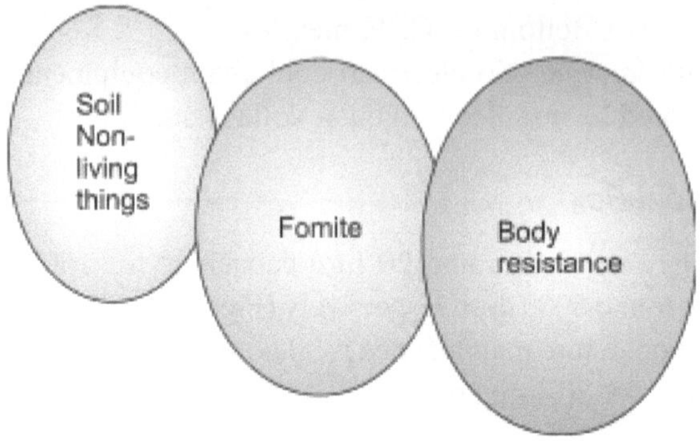

Fig. 11.8: Weak links in disease transmission

12

Concept of Disease Prevention and Control

INTRODUCTION

Knowledge of epidemiology of disease helps us in its control and prevention. Depending on available resources, measures are to be taken for the control and prevention. Sometimes, more than one method may have to be adopted. During policymaking and implementation, we require:

- Political acceptance
- Availability of funds
- Public acceptability for the method used
- Community participation
- Intersectoral coordination.

LEVELS AND MEASURES OF DISEASE PREVENTION AND CONTROL

Disease prevention is applied at three levels; and, hence, there are three measures available for the disease elimination from the community.

- *I level*: Tackling at source of infection which will be usually a reservoir (man or animal or nonliving thing)
- *II level*: Tackling at routes of transmission (air, water, food, contact, vectors, etc.)
- *III level*: Tackling at risk group in a community

I level

Tackling at Source

Health inspector is expected to follow the following procedures to control and prevent disease at source:

- Visit the family for first hand information. Taking MOH for case diagnosis in the field should follow this.
- When once the case is diagnosed by MOH, local authorities namely DH and FWO must be informed. This is called *notification.*
- Procedure laid down under investigation of an epidemic is followed.
- Isolation of suspected case till he is made noninfectious. Period of isolation is specified by the District Health Authorities (DHAs) as in Table 12.1.

Table 12.1: Period of isolation specified by the DHAs

Disease	*Period of isolation*
Cholera	Till negative culture after antibiotics
Jaundice (hepatitis A)	Three weeks from the start of illness
Measles	After rash, patient is isolated for minimum 3 days
Chickenpox	After rash, patient is isolated for 6 days
Polio	Child is isolated for 1½ months Adult is isolated for 15 days
TB	Till he is made AFB negative
Meningococcal meningitis	Till next day of completed antibiotic course

- With the help of MOH and LMO, specific treatments are got done to the cases.
- *Quarantine*: In case of cholera, plague, relapsing fever and yellow fever (yellow fever is not present in India) quarantine, i.e. limiting the freedom of movement is done as in Table 12.2.

Table 12.2: Quarantine

Disease	*Number of days quarantine*
Cholera	6 days
Plague	8 days
Relapsing fever	8 days for tick-borne relapsing fever
Yellow fever	6 days

II Level

Tackling at the Route of Transmission

Public health measures are taken to stop further spread in the following situations:

- Water purification and provision of protected water
- Food hygiene including personal hygiene
- Control of breeding of mosquitoes, flies, etc.
- Control of soil pollution
- Sanitary disposal of human excreta

III Level

Tackling at Risk Group

Following immunisation is done:

a. *Under UIP*
   - DPT
   - OPV
   - BCG
   - Measles

b. *Under special circumstances*
   - Cholera
   - Plague
   - Typhoid

OTHER MEASURES

Other measures in the control and prevention of diseases are as follows:

Surveillance

It is continuous scrutiny of occurrence and spread of diseases. For example,

- STD surveillance
- AIDS surveillance
- AFP surveillance

Advice to Travellers

Travellers are susceptible to the following diseases:

- Malaria
- Diarrhoea
- Dengue
- Influenza
- STD
- AIDS
- Typhoid
- Viral hepatitis.

Advice to travellers include the following:

- Food hygiene
- Use of protected water
- Use of mosquito curtain or repellents
- Avoid injections
- Get required vaccines before travel

Now, the health of travellers are guided through a discipline called **emporiatrics**

Disinfection

Disinfectants are chemicals that kill pathogens; if they inhibit growth, they are called antiseptic.

Types of Disinfection

They are as follow (Table 12.3):

- Concurrent, when done during treatment
- Terminal, when done after discharge or death
- Prophylactic, when done to prevent infection

Table 12.3: Types of disinfection

Disinfection	*Example*
Concurrent	Sputum is disinfected
Terminal	Ward disinfection after death of a patient
Prophylactic	Water chlorination and milk pasteurisation

Common Disinfectants

Common disinfectants used in day-to-day practice are given in Table 12.4

Table 12.4: Common disinfectants

Natural	*Physical*	*Chemical*
Sunlight	Boiling	Phenol
Drying in air	Autoclaving	Dettol Savlon Bleaching powder Sodium hypochlorite

13

Medical Entomology

Medical entomology deals with insects of public health importance. They transmit many diseases.

INSECTS

Insects have jointed appendages, segmented body and bilaterally symmetrical and body cavity consists of an open vascular system.

Modes of Transmission

Modes of transmission of diseases by insects are:

1. *Direct transmission*
   - Scabies
   - Myiasis by fly maggots
2. *Indirect transmission*
   - Mechanically, e.g. housefly
   - Biological
   - Propagative (plague by rat flea)
   - Cyclodevelopment (microfilaria in culex)
   - Cyclopropagative (malaria by anopheles).

Vector

Vector is an arthropod, which is responsible for biological transmission of diseases of public health importance (Table 13.1). For example, anopheles mosquito is vector of malaria.

Table 13.1: List of Arthropods (Insects)

Family	*Vector*
Insecta	Mosquitoes • Anopheles • Culex • Aedes • Monsonoides Housefly Sandfly Rat flea
Arachnida	Ticks • Hard tick • Soft tick Mite • Trombiculoid • Itch mite
Crustacea	Cyclops

HOUSEFLY

Morphology

The body is divisible into head, thorax and abdomen. It is mouse gray in colour. Head bears antennae, compound eyes and proboscis. Thorax has four stripes, wings, and legs. Abdomen also shows dark markings (Fig. 13.1).

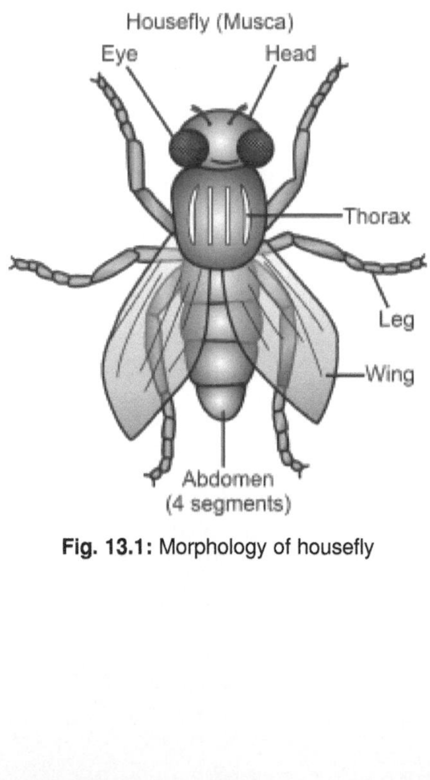

Fig. 13.1: Morphology of housefly

Life Cycle

Housefly has life history through four stages—egg, maggot, pupa and adult (Fig. 13.2).

Bionomics

Housefly breeds on horse manure, human excreta, garbage and decomposed fruits. Fly vomits frequently and defaecates continuously.

Public Health Importance

Housefly is often found abundantly around human and animal excreta, breeds and transmits diarrhoea, dysentery, typhoid, cholera, eye infection, trachoma, yaws, etc.

Control Measures

Environmental control: Store garbage in rustproof cans with lids. They are dispatched in a landfill. Pit privy, aqua privy, water seal latrine, subsoil drainage, septic tank help in the control of houseflies.

Insecticidal control:
- DDT 5%
- Methoxychlor 5%
- Lindane 0.5%
- Dieldrin (4 litres per 100 sq m) 1.25%
- Fenthion 2.5%

Bait

Dry bait: Sugar or corn meal containing 2.0% diazinon.

Liquid bait: 0.2% dichlorvos in 12.5% sugar water gives longer control.

Spray

Outdoor spray: 2.0% lindane

Indoor spray: 0.2% synergised pyrethrum

Fly cords: Impregnated with parathion installed at a rate of 10 metres of cord per 10 sqm.

Larvicide: 0.5% diazinon (56 litres per 100 sqm).

LOUSE

Morphology

Lice are wingless and are of three types—head louse, body louse and pubic louse (Figs 13.3 and 13.4).

Head louse and body louse have head, thorax and abdomen.

Head of a louse has antennae. Adapted mouthpart helps in sucking. Thorax has three pairs of legs. Abdomen has nine segments.

Life History

Lice have three stages namely, egg, nymph and adult (Fig. 13.5).

Bionomics

Lice are found on head, body and pubic hairy parts. Pubic louse has crab-like appearance. Their presence highlights personal hygiene of the individual.

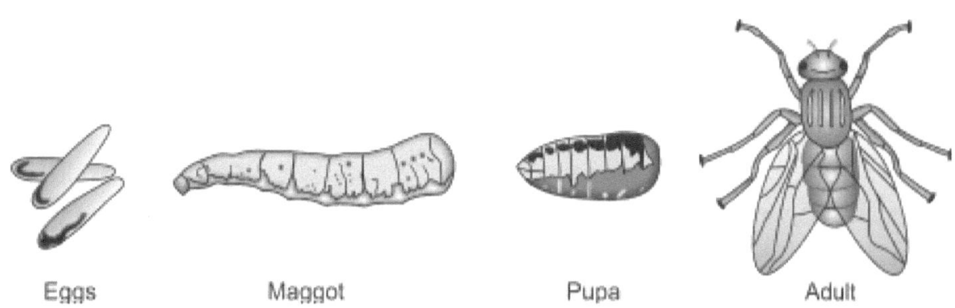

Fig. 13.2: Life cycle of housefly

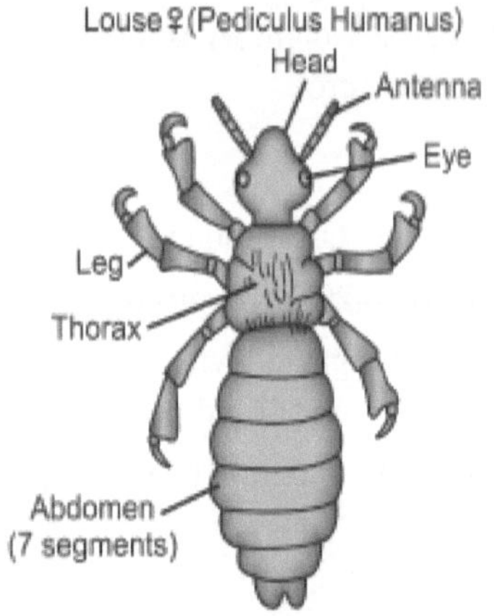

Fig. 13.3: Morphology of louse (Head louse or Body louse)

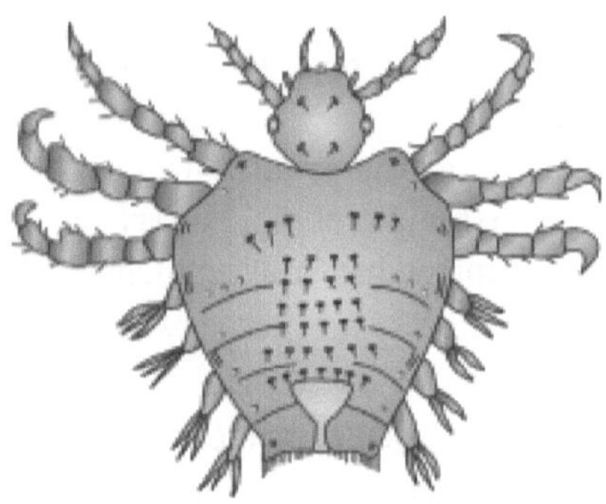

Fig. 13.4: Morphology of pubic louse

Public Health Importance

Head louse and body louse bite man severely. In some, there may not be any reaction. In others, it produces skin irritation and distress. Body louse transmits epidemic typhus, relapsing fever and trench fever.

Control Measures

Environmental control: Bath frequently with hot soapy water to limit infestation. To control body louse, launder clothing and press with hot iron. To control head louse and pubic louse, the hair is cut and destroyed to get rid of eggs, nymphs and adults.

Insecticidal control: Dust people with 10% DDT, 1% lindane, 1% malathion, 0.2% synergised pyrethrum (Fig. 13.6). Apply 50 grams of dust per person. If dust is inadvisable, then use 12% benzyl benzoate or 0.1% lindane liquid preparations.

Treatment: Repeat treatment in 7 days to kill late hatching lice to make sure of eradication. Contacts are found and are treated.

TICKS

Ticks are of two types:

a. Hard tick
b. Soft tick.

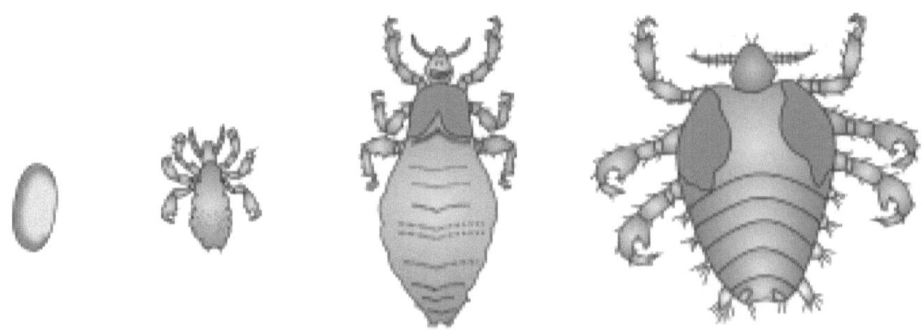

Fig. 13.5: Life history of lice

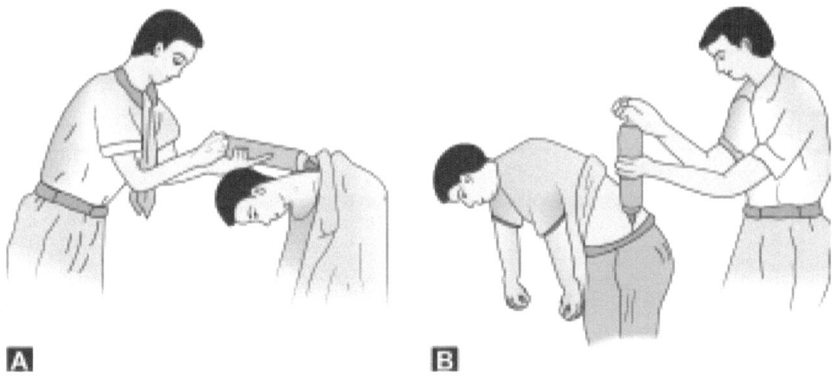

Fig. 13.6: Dusting in louse infestation

Morphology

Tick is oval in shape and one cannot make out head, body, thorax or abdomen. It has four pairs of legs. Scutum is covered on the dorsal surface of hard tick (fully covered in male and partially covered in female) (Fig 13.7).

Life History

Tick passes through the stages of egg, larva, nymph and adult (Fig. 13.8).

Bionomics

By mouthpart, tick attaches to the body of host. It sucks blood from the body of the host.

Major differences between the hard tick and soft tick are given in Table 13.2.

Public Health Importance

Ticks suck blood and cause skin inflammation and distress. Soft ticks transmit relapsing fever and hard ticks typhus, haemorrhagic fever like Kyasanur forest disease (KFD).

Control Measures

Environmental control: Reduce the number of cracks in ground, near the building and path. Reduce wild rodents.

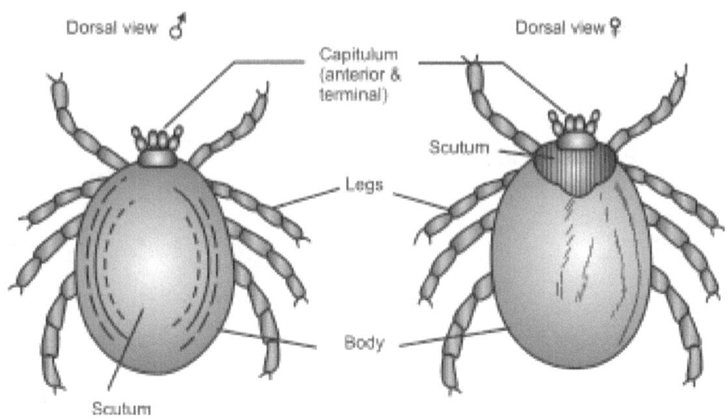

Fig. 13.7: Morphology of tick

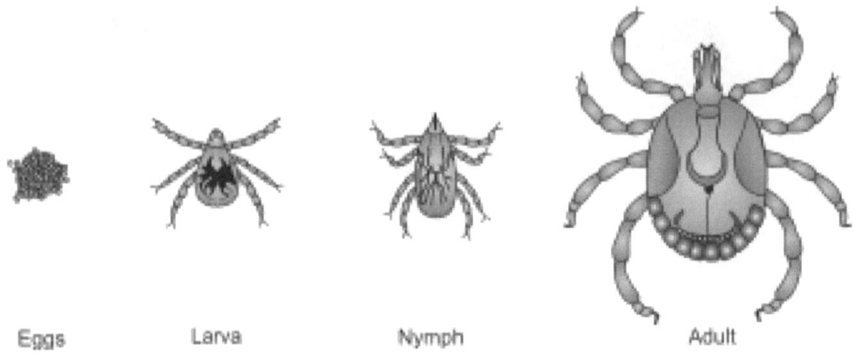

Fig. 13.8: Life cycle of tick

Table 13.2: Differences between hard and soft ticks

	Hard tick	*Soft tick*
Scutum	Present	Absent
Head	Anterior	Ventral
Nymph stage	One	Five
Habit	Frequently suck the blood (cannot starve)	Once in a way suck blood (can starve)

Insecticidal control:

a. On dogs—use
   - Carbaryl dust — 5%
   - Chlordane — 2%
   - DDT — 5%
   - Dieldrin — 0.5%
   - Lindane — 0.5%
   - Malathion — 5%
   - Trichlorphos — 1%

b. In houses—spray cracks with 0.5% diazinon or 3% fenthion.

c. Area control is done by 5% dust with DDT.

Use tick repellents like:
- Meta diethyl toluamide
- Dimethyl phthalate.

Apply repellents to clothing: Use protective clothing like close fitting trouser legs, shirts with sleeves and coats. Shirts should be tucked into top of trousers.

MITES

Morphology

Mites resemble ticks. They have four pairs of legs. Body is not demarcated like head, thorax and abdomen (Fig. 13.9). Trombiculoid and itch mites are two important mites.

Life History

Mite is complex in nature and is variable. Quite often it passes through four stages (Fig. 13.10).
- Egg
- 6-legged larva
- 8-legged nymph
- 8-legged adult mite.

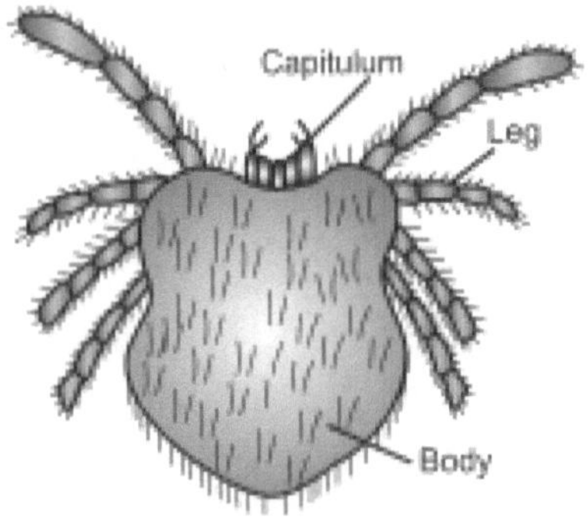

Fig. 13.9: Morphology of mite

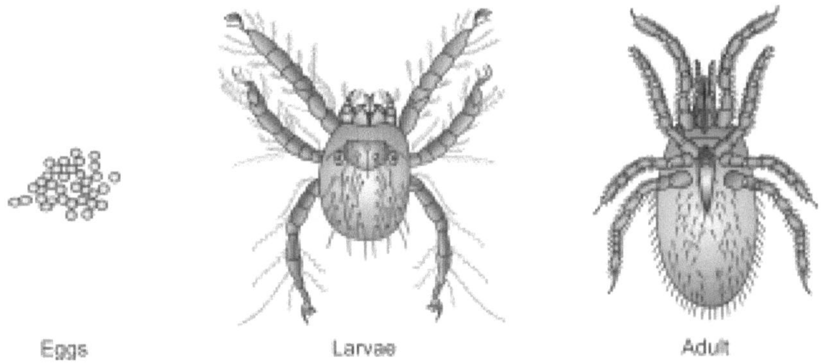

Fig. 13.10: Life history of mite

Bionomics

Larva attacks man and rodents. When they are blown with blood, they start moulting.

Public Health Importance

When they bite man, mites cause inflammation and severe distress. Scabies mites live in the skin. Other mites transmit scrub typhus, haemorrhagic fever and rickettisialpox.

Control Measures

Environmental control: Avoid contact with mite infested people, keep out of mite-infested areas. Prevent bats, birds and rodents from harbouring in or near the buildings. Keep vegetations closely trimmed. Destroy mite-infested foods. Wear impregnated protective clothing in mite-infested areas.

Insecticidal control:
- Chlordane—5% dust, 0.625% spray
- Dieldrine—5% dust, 0.625% spray

SANDFLY

Morphology

The body is divided into head, thorax and abdomen. They are dark brown in colour and smaller than mosquitoes. Antenna palpi and proboscis are present in the head. Thorax has three pairs of legs and a pair of wings. Wings are upright, lanceolate and hairy. Abdomen has ten segments (Fig. 13.11). Differences between mosquitoes and sand flies are shown in Table 13.3.

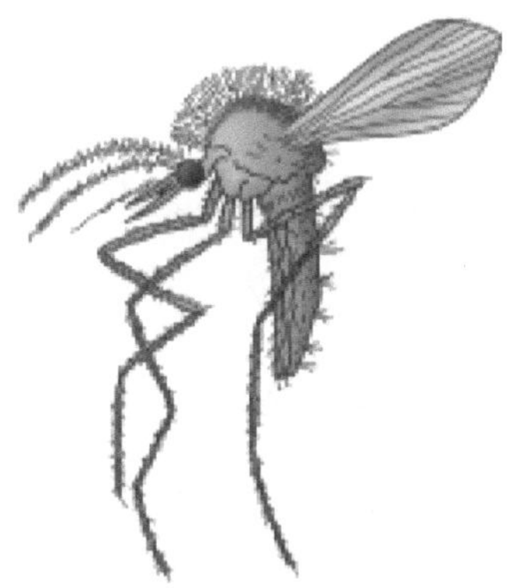

Fig. 13.11: Morphology of sandfly

Life History

Sandfly passes through the stages of egg, larva, pupa and adult (Fig. 13.12).

Bionomics

Sandfly is a nocturnal pest. It is found in dark room, trees and storeroom. They cannot fly long distances. They only hop about.

Table 13.3: Differences between mosquito and sandfly

	Sandfly	*Mosquito*
Size	Small	Large
Wings	Upright, lanceolate	Not lanceolate
Legs	Long	Not long
Hair	Plenty	Very less
Movement	Hops	Flies

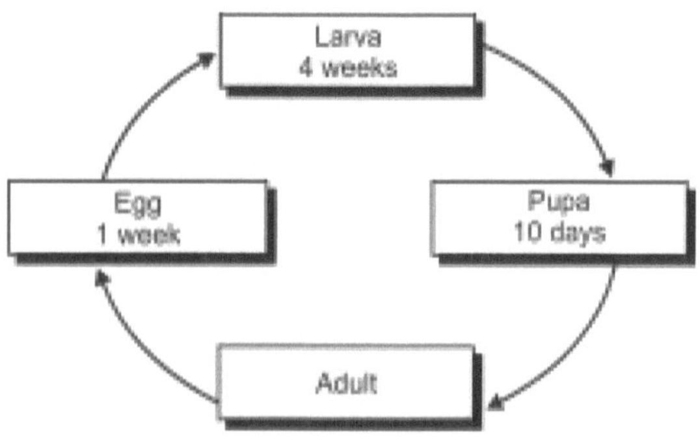

Fig. 13.12: Life cycle of sand fly

Public Health Importance

Sand fly transmits the following diseases:

- Kala-azar
- Sand fly fever
- Oriental sore

Control Measures

Environmental control: Removal of shrubs, vegetations, filling-up cracks in the wall, keeping animal sheds away from house.

Insecticidal control:

- DDT 2 gram per sqm.
- Lindane 0.25 gram per sqm.

RAT FLEA

Morphology

Rat fleas are bilaterally compressed, wingless with hard covering. The body is divisible into head, thorax and abdomen. Head has mouthparts. Thorax has three pairs of legs. Abdomen has ten segments (Fig 13.13).

Life Cycle

Rat flea passes through four stages of life cycle (Fig 13.14). They are:

- Egg
- Larva
- Pupa
- Adult

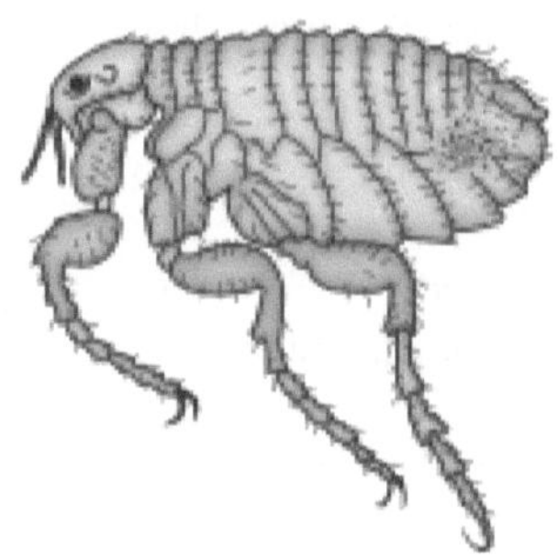

Fig: 13.13: Morphology of rat flea

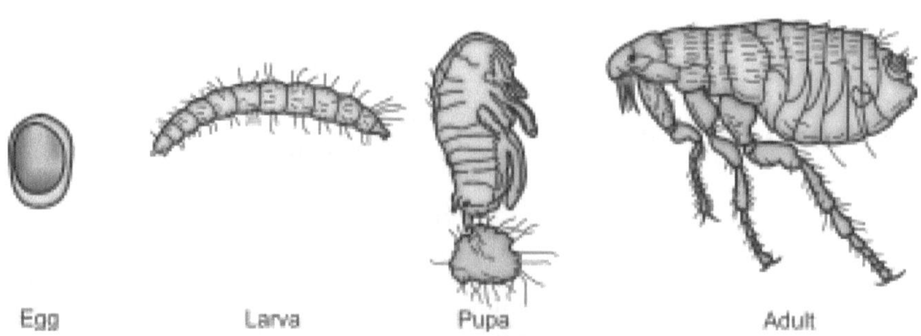

Fig. 13.14: Life cycle of rat flea

Bionomics

Rat fleas harbour on the body of mammals and birds. Usually, they are attached to one host and suck the blood from the same host.

Public Health Importance

Rat flea transmits organisms causing murine typhus.

Control Measures

Environmental control: If possible, vacuum clean floors and rugs weekly to pick-up fleas. Avoid unhygienic conditions, which attract rats. In severe infestations, keep premises free of pets.

Insecticidal control: Dust rat runs, burrows with:
- DDT — 10%
- Dieldrin — 1.5%
- Aldrin — 2.0%
- Malathion — 5%

Treat animals to keep flea off by 5% DDT; 10% methoxychlor; 1% lindane; 2% chlordane; 5% malathion.

Outdoor spray; 1% emulsion of chlordane, diazinon, lindane (4 litres per 100 sqm).

MOSQUITOES

They are major insects of public health importance. They are of four types:
- Anopheles
- Culex
- Aedes
- Mansonia

Morphology

Body is divisible into head, thorax and abdomen (Fig. 13.15).

Head has compound eye, proboscis, palpi and antennae. Thorax has a pair of wings and three pairs of legs. Abdomen has ten segments.

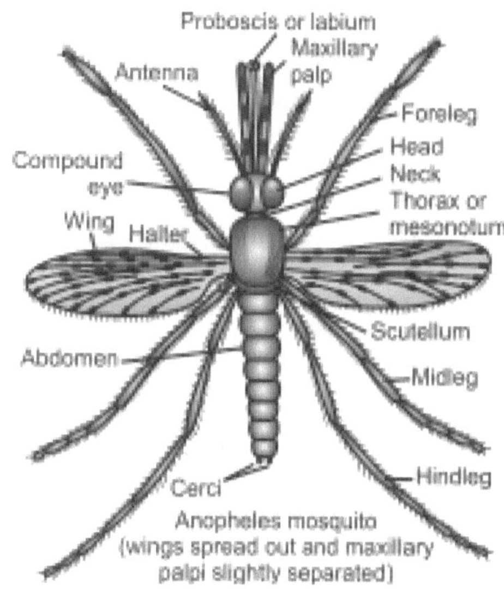

Fig. 13.15: Morphology of mosquito

Life History

Mosquitoes pass their life cycle in four stages (Fig. 13.16).
- Egg
- Larva
- Pupa
- Adult.

Culex, *Aedes* and *Mansonia* have common characteristics, which differentiate *anopheles* (Fig. 13.17, Table 13.4).

Bionomics

Mosquitoes are found everywhere. All types of mosquitoes feed on human blood. Male mosquitoes do not bite.

Female mosquitoes bite at night. They rest in darker places. *Anopheles* breed in clean water, *Culex* in dirty water, *Aedes* in collected water and *Mansonia* in water plants.

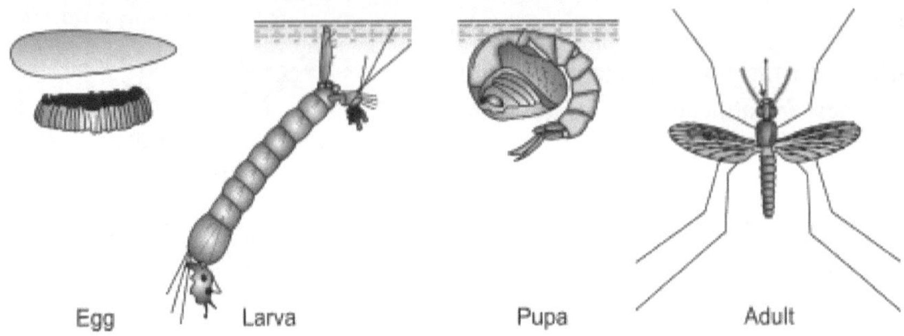

Fig. 13.16: Life history of mosquito

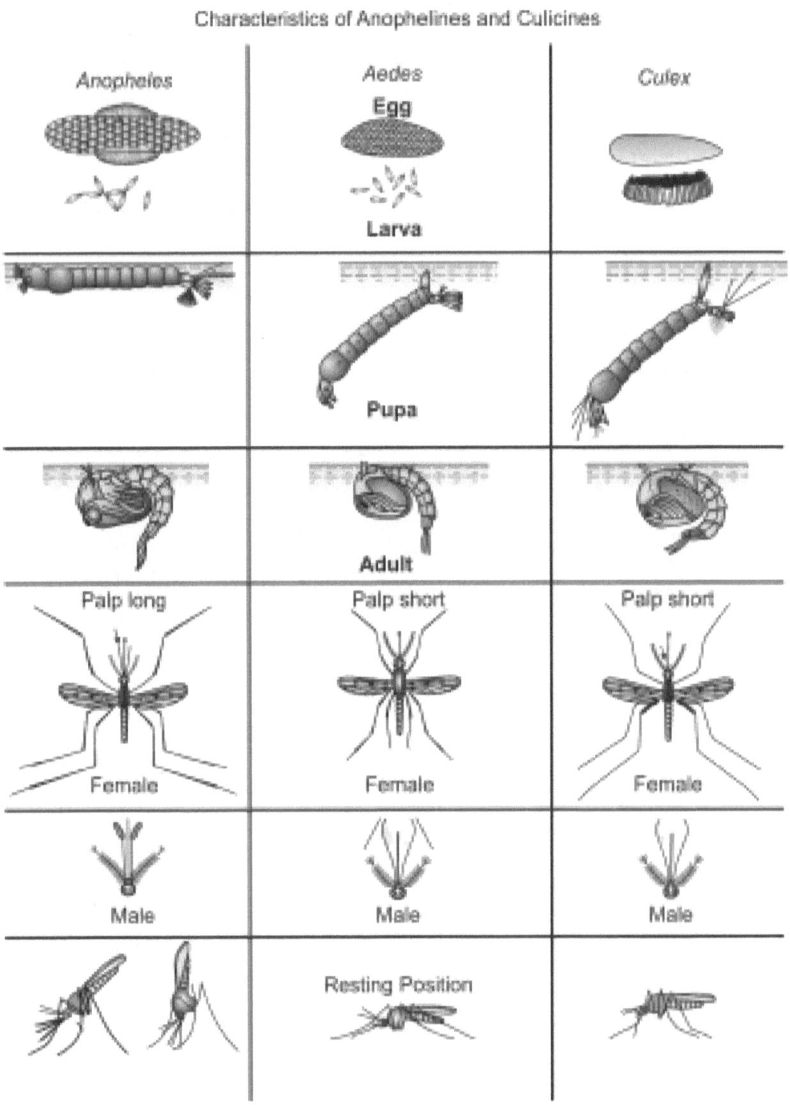

Fig. 13.17: Characteristics of mosquitoes

Table 13.4: Common characteristics of mosquitoes

	Anopheles	*Culex, Aedes and Mansonia*
Egg	Single, boat-shaped	Cluster, raft, oval-shaped
Larva	Float parallel	Float perpendicular
	No siphon tube	Siphon tube present
	Palmate hair present	No palmate hair
Pupa	Broad, short siphon tube	Long, narrow siphon tube
Adult	No hunch backs	Hunch back present
	Spotted wings	Not spotted wings
	Long palpi in male and female	Short palpi in female

Public Health Importance

Mosquitoes suck blood, cause skin inflammation; transmit malaria, filaria, dengue fever and yellow fever (not present in India), brain fever and haemorrhagic fever.

Control Measures

Environmental control: Clean up old tyre, tin can, bottle and junks. Screen water containers. Fill up low areas and drain other low areas. Maintain a clean shoreline free of weeds, which provide protection to larvae. Clean water plants. Install dams with automatic flushing device.

Insecticidal control:

a. Residual spray (4 litres per 100 sq m)
   - DDT — 5 %
   - Malathion — 5 %
   - Lindane — 1.25 %
   - Dieldrin — 1.25 %

b. Outdoor space spray
   - DDT — 0.4 Lb/acre
   - Lindane — 0.2 Lb/acre
   - Malathion — 0.5 Lb/acre
   - Fenthion — 0.1 Lb/acre
   - Dichlorvos — 0.25 Lb/acre

c. Indoor space spray
   - Synergised pyrethrum — 0.25 %
   - DDT — 3 %
   - Residual fumigants
   - Dichlorvos resin strips

- Larvicide
  i. Fuel oil — 100 litres/hectare
  ii. Chlordane spray — 1.25%/hectare
  iii. Fenthion — 5 litres/hectare
  iv. Paris green — 16 kg/hectare

d. Aeroplane disperse (fogging)
   - Parathion-methyl—10 litres/hectare
   - Repellents
   - Diethyl toluamide
   - Dimethyl phthalate

CYCLOPS

It is a water flea.

Morphology

Cyclops is 1 mm in length, pear-shaped body, has a forked tail, two pairs antennae, five pairs legs and a pigmented eye (Fig 13.18).

Life Cycle (Fig. 13.19)

Bionomics

Cyclops are found in fresh water ponds and step wells. They rest in shady areas. Infected cyclops are more in water bottom.

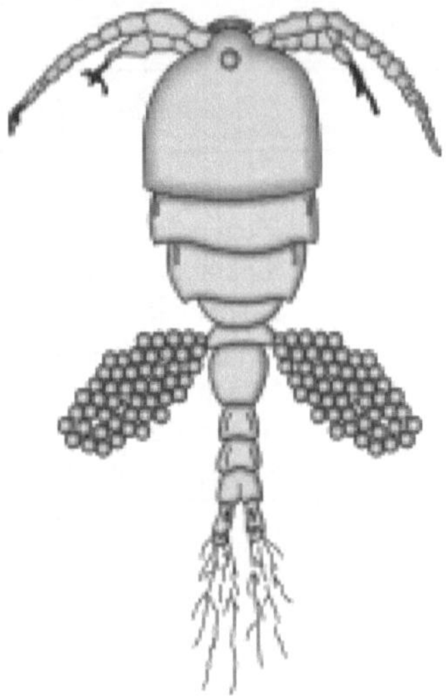

Fig. 13.18: Morphology of cyclops

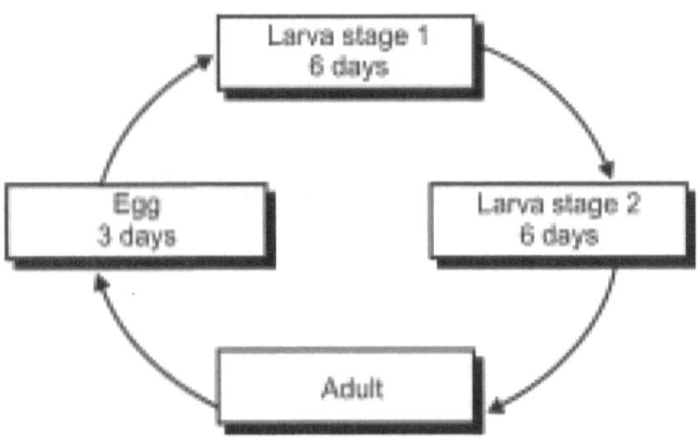

Fig. 13.19: Life history of cyclops

Public Health Importance

Cyclops transmits guinea worm infection in man.

Control Measures

Environmental control: People are not allowed to enter step well. Provision of sanitary well is ideal. Boiling and filtering help in protection from infection by cyclops.

Insecticidal control: DDT 5 ppm in water source is found effective.

Biological control: Fishes are tried which eat away cyclops.

IDENTIFICATION OF COMMON INSECTICIDES

1. *DDT:* White amorphous powder
   - Has mild unpleasant smell
   - Not soluble in water
   - Dissolves in organic solvents
   - It is a contact poison
   - Has residual action
2. *BHC*: A chocolate-coloured powder
   - Has musty smell
   - Produces irritation to eyes, nose and skin
   - It is a contact poison
   - Has residual action
3. *Malathion*: Brown liquid
   Has unpleasant smell
4. *Abate*: Brown viscous liquid
5. *Pyrethrum*: Extracted from a flower
6. *Paris green*: It is an emerald green powder.

Insecticide Equipment (Fig. 13.20)

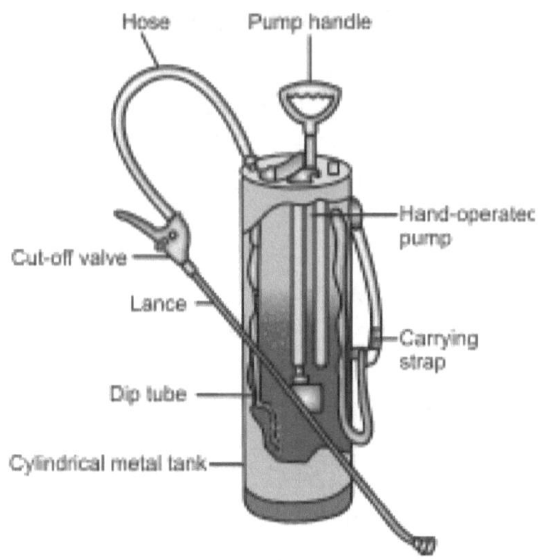

Fig. 13.20: Hand-operated compressor sprayer

ADDITIONAL INFORMATION ON MEDICAL ENTOMOLOGY

- *Integrated approach*: It is used for more than one method of vector control
- *Common malaria-spreading species*:
  - *Anopheles culicifacies*
  - *Anopheles fluviateles*
  - *Anopheles stephensi*
  - *Anopheles sundaicus*
- *Mosquito-borne diseases*:
  - *Anopheles* — Malaria
  - *Culex* — Filaria, JE
  - *Aedes* — Dengue
  - *Mansonia* — Filaria
- Size of opening of mosquito net and screening of building—should be 0.0475 inch
- *Sticky fly paper in housefly control*:
  - 2 pound resin + 1 pint castor oil (heated to make paste)
  - Smear to a paper and hung in places
- Name of rat flea—*Xenopsylla cheopis*
- *Brain fever and monkey fever are transmitted*:
  - Brain fever—*Culex* mosquito
  - Monkey fever—Hard tick
- *Zoonoses*: Zoonoses are diseases of lower vertebrate animals/which man gets during the course of natural transmission.

14

Concept of Primary Health Care

INTRODUCTION

Primary health care is an outcome of an international conference on Primary Health Care, which was held in September 1978 in Alma Ata, the capital of Kazakh of erstwhile Soviet Socialist Republic.

DEFINITION

Primary health care is an essential health care made universally accessible to individuals and families in the community by means acceptable to them, through their full participation and at a cost that country and community can afford. It forms an integral part of the country's health system of which it is the nucleus and of the overall social and economic development of the community.

PRIMARY HEALTH CARE APPROACH

This concept is considered to be essential care based on practical, scientifically sound, socially acceptable methods and technology made universally available. At every stage self-reliance and self-determination of the community is considered.

Government has responsibilities to fulfil adequate and equitably distributed health and social measures.

This approach is expected to achieve an acceptable level of health throughout the world in foreseeable future as an integral part of social development in the spirit of social justice.

Primary health care addresses the main health problems in a community providing promotive, preventive, curative and rehabilitative services. Since these services reflect and evolve from the economic conditions and social values of the country and its communities, they will vary from country to country; however, will include at least:

- Promotion of proper nutrition
- Adequate water supply
- Basic sanitation
- RCH
- Immunisation against major diseases
- Prevention and control of local endemic diseases
- Education concerning prevailing health problems
- Appropriate treatment of common diseases and injuries.

PRIMARY HEALTH CARE AND DEVELOPMENT

Development implies progressive improvement in the living conditions and quality of life enjoyed by society and shared by its members. It is a continuing process that takes place in all societies; few would claim that development is complete.

Community Participation

A community consists of people living together in some form of social organization and cohesion. Its members share in varying degrees political, economic, social and cultural characteristics as well as interests and aspirations including health. Communities vary widely in size and socio-economic profile ranging from clusters of isolated homesteads to more organised villages, towns, cities and districts.

Self-reliance and social awareness are key factors in human development.

Thus, community participation has become a process by which individuals and families assume responsibility for their own health and welfare as well as for those of the community; and develop the capacity to contribute to their own and the country's development.

OPERATIONAL ASPECT OF PRIMARY HEALTH CARE

Primary health care is a component of health and other sectors, which contribute to the development of health.

Planning for primary health care has to be carried out by a nation.

Appropriate Health Technology

An important factor for the success of the primary health care is the use of appropriate health technology. Technology means "an association of methods, technologies and equipment which together with the people using them, can contribute significantly towards solving health problem". Appropriate means it is scientifically sound and acceptable to local culture.

HEALTH INSPECTOR IN PRIMARY HEALTH CARE SERVICES

At first contact care, a health inspector works in a team at PHC. He is a trained Paramedical worker who can take care of primary health care services in the community within available resources and at an acceptable level.

When a health inspector meets with a complicated case, advices on a complex problem, he is likely to be a staff who is trained at (more) high level.

Additional thought is given to referral facilities, which form the link next to primary health care in the health system chain.

Budgeting

Available and allocated budget should be sufficient for primary health care services. Preferential allocation should start from the community.

Control

Primary health care with its supporting services has to be controlled with the purpose of ensuring as far as possible that it is functioning in accordance with the national policy and national strategy.

PRINCIPLES OF PRIMARY HEALTH CARE

- Equitable distribution
- Community participation
- Intersectoral coordination
- Appropriate technology.

SECTION

2

Application of Public Health

15 Communicable Diseases, Noncommunicable Diseases and National Health Programmes

DISEASES TRANSMITTED THROUGH AIR

Smallpox

- It no longer exists in the world.
- India became free of smallpox in 1997.
- It was declared free in the world by a declaration on 8.5.1980 by the WHO.

Chickenpox

Vericella zoster virus causes chickenpox. Fever, malaise and rashes are characteristics of this disease (Fig. 15.1).

Incubation Period

It is 15 days.

Clinical Character

Fever and rash start together. Within one week, all stages are over and wean off. They are seen more on trunk. All stages like papule, vesicle and crust are seen at one time. We cannot see rashes on palm and sole (Fig. 15.2).

Very rarely chickenpox goes to complications.

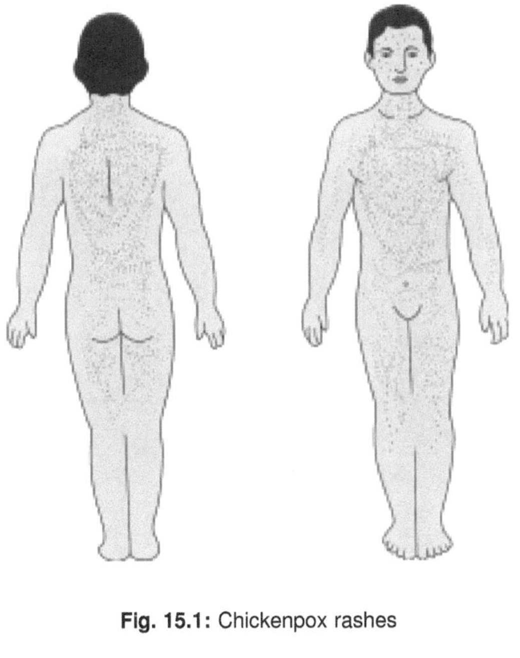

Fig. 15.1: Chickenpox rashes

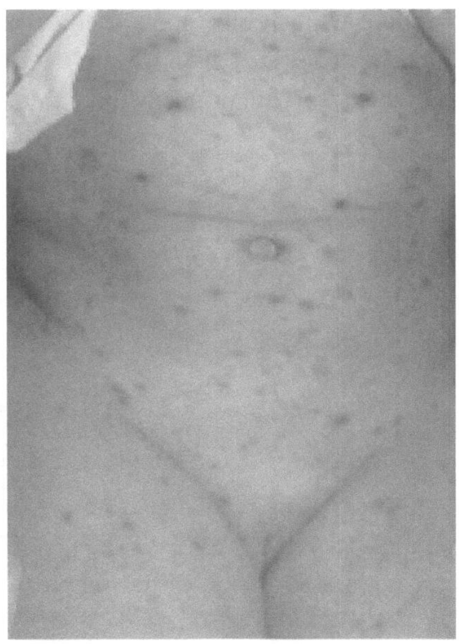

Fig. 15.2: Chickenpox rash in a child
(For colour version see Plate 1)

Epidemiological Character

- Common in children
- An attack gives immunity
- Commonly occur during March to May of the year.

Prevention and Control

- No specific treatment
- Notification
- Isolation for one week after crust.

Measles

Illness and deaths are associated with measles. It is severe among malnourished children. Measles vaccination is included under primary immunisation schedule for infants under the Universal Programme on Immunisation in India.

Clinical Character

The illness starts with fever, sneezing, cough, and eye redness. Later, dusky red skin rash develops on face, neck and body (Figs 15.3 and 15.4). Typical sign is small whitish blue spots seen on tonsil or buccal cavity. They are called Koplik's spots. They are seen when the patient opens the mouth.

As complications, lung infection (pneumonia) and diarrhoea are common.

Epidemiological Character

- Common disease of childhood
- More deaths are seen among malnourished children
- Spreads more in winter.

Incubation Period

It is 10 days. Child transmits the disease during 5 days earlier to rash appearance to 5 days after rash appearance.

Prevention and Control

Measles vaccine is given during 9 to 12 months of age under universal immunisation programme. It is one dose 0.5 ml subcutaneous route.

Isolation of cases for one week after the rash is done.

Mumps

Mumps is a viral infection attacking parotid glands (Fig. 15.5). Illness period is usually prolonged. Deaths due to mumps are rare in the community.

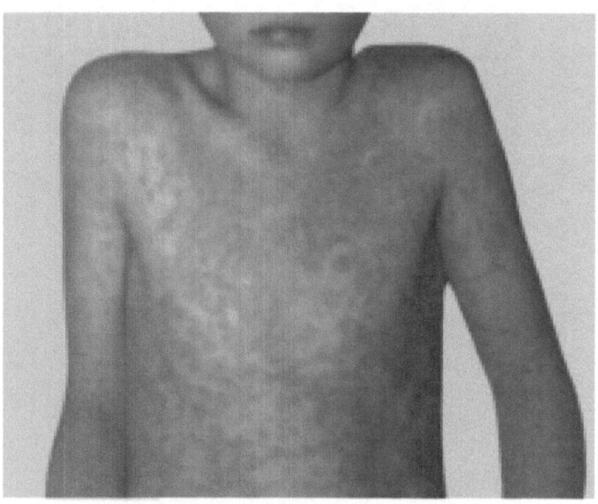

Fig. 15.3: Measles rashes on the chest
(For colour version see Plate 1)

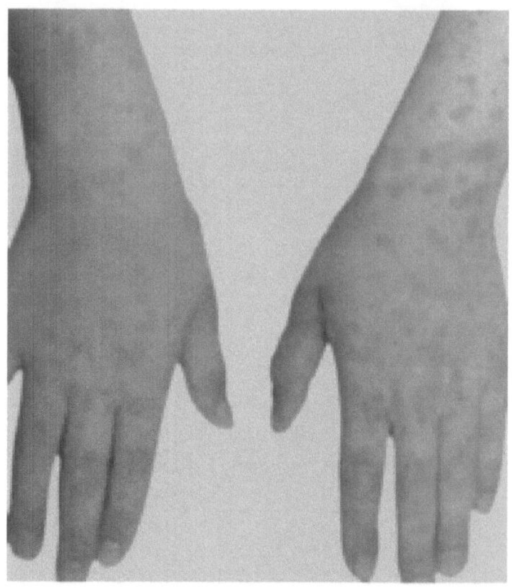

Fig. 15.4: Measles rashes on the hand
(For colour version see Plate 1)

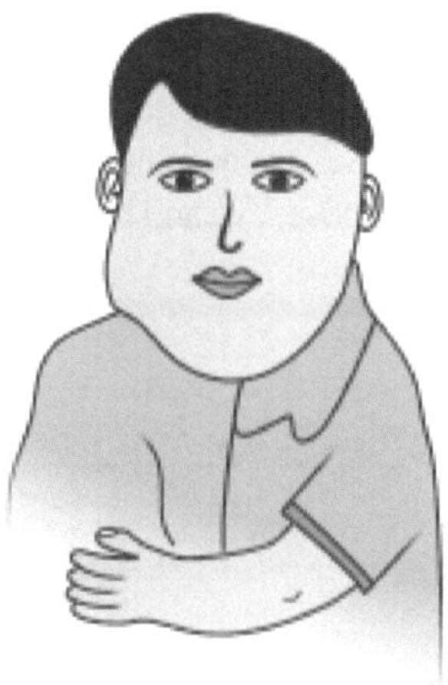

Fig. 15.5: Parotid gland swollen in mumps patient

Clinical Character

Pain and swelling start on the face, below and front of ears. Any ear-ache case should be looked for mumps. The patient experiences pain when he opens his mouth.

Severe case of mumps can lead to:
- Testes infection causing infertility
- Brain infection
- Heart muscle infection.

Epidemiological Character

- Quick spread is common causing more secondary attack rate up to 80 per cent.
- Case is infectious one week before and one week after parotid gland enlargement.
- Very common among adolescent age group.
- More cases occur in winter and spring.

Prevention and Control

Vaccination is the best measure in the prevention of measles. Measles vaccination before 12 months must be carried out or motivated to cover more per cent have fully immunised among infants in the community.
- Case is isolated for one week.
- Disinfections of infected articles are followed.

Diphtheria

Incidence of diphtheria has come down to zero level in recent days. Diphtheria used to kill many children before antibiotic era (Fig. 15.6).

Clinical Character

The patient suffering from diphtheria complaints of fever, sore throat and pain during swallowing. Examination by opening mouth show patch (Fig. 15.7). In severe cases, breathing becomes difficult and we may have to take the help of ENT

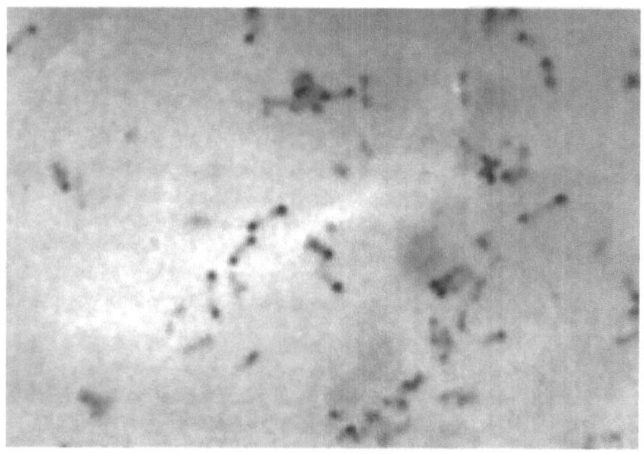

Fig. 15.6: Diphtheria bacteria in Albert Stain
(For colour version see Plate 1)

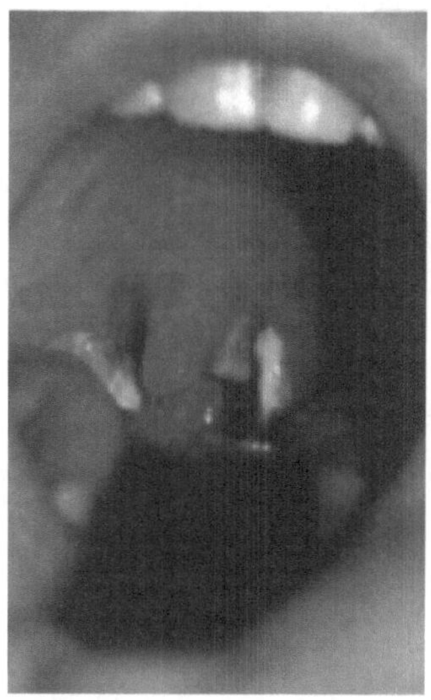

Fig. 15.7: Diphtheria patch seen in an opened mouth
(For colour version see Plate 1)

surgeons to get trachiostomy (cut the trachea and make provision to breath) done. Diphtheria also affects the heart function.

By doing skin test called Schick's test, we can find out the immunity status of a child.

Lymph nods are found enlarged and oedema of neck occurs. This character is called "bull neck".

Epidemiological Character

- Three types of bacteria cause diphtheria.
- Severe type used to be common in occurrence.
- Diphtheria case transmits infection to other children.
- Child will be infected up to one month after infection.
- Children are common victims.
- This disease used to occur more during the months of August and September of the year.

Incubation Period

It is 2 to 6 days.

Prevention and Control

Vaccination under UIP is best-suited preventive measure. DPT is given 0.5 ml deep intramuscular at one-month interval is suggested. This is given as per UIP schedule.

Other measures are:
- Early detection of cases
- Isolation of case for 15 days
- Treatment at isolation hospital with ADS and penicillin
- Diphtheria carriers are given Erythromycin tablets.

Whooping Cough

With UIP immunisation, incidence of whooping cough has come down remarkably. Continuous cough followed by whoop has given the name whooping cough.

Untreated whooping cough lives for 100 days; and hence, in olden days, whooping cough was called hundred-day cough.

Clinical Character

It is a bacterial infection causing infection of respiratory tract. Severe continuous cough giving rise to bleeding in nose, eye and hernia are common (Fig. 15.8).

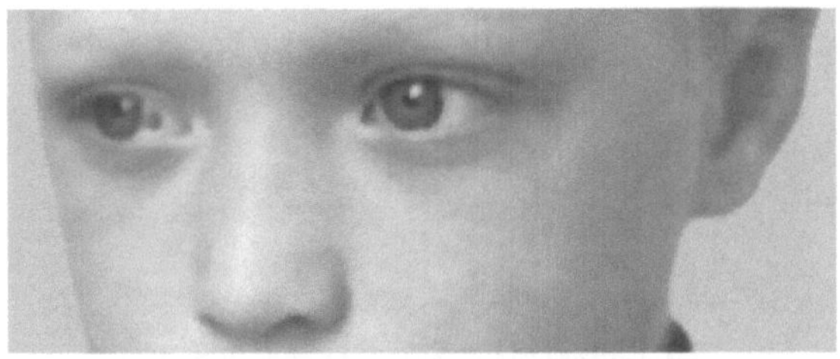

Fig. 15.8: Case of whooping cough showing bleeding in eye
(For colour version see Plate 2)

Epidemiological Character

Whooping cough is a disease of infants, but it is found to extend up to the age of 5 years of life. The case is infectious to others up to one month after infection. Many cases occur giving rise to high secondary attack rate up to 90 per cent.

The disease is more in winter and among overcrowded people.

Incubation period

It is 7 to 14 days.

Prevention and Control

Under UIP immunisation, the vaccine is given. This takes care of whooping cough among children.
- Case detection and isolation for 1 month is suggested.
- Contacts are given ampicillin treatment.
- Health education on the importance of UIP is one of the requirements in the prevention of whooping cough.

Acute Respiratory Infection

This is a very common infection and seen among children, causing discomfort, disability and school

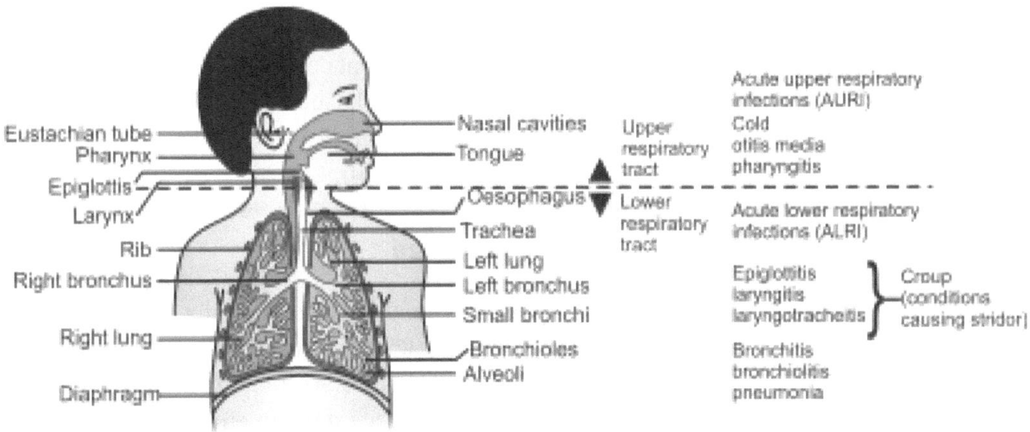

Fig.15.9: ARI classification according to the site of infection in the respiratory tract

drop-out. Depending upon the site of infection acute respiratory infection (ARI) is grouped under (Fig. 15.9).

- Upper respiratory tract infection (URTI)
- Lower respiratory tract infection (LRTI)

Many bacteria and many viruses are known to cause ARI among children.

Clinical Character

Illness starts with fever, running nose, sore throat, difficulty in breathing and ear infection (Table 15.1). Untreated ARI leads to pneumonia, which is often found to be common cause of death among children.

Table 15.1: Clinical characteristics of ARI

Severity	*Characteristic*
Mild cases	No chest indrawing No fast breathing Below 50 respiratory rate per minute among infants Below 40 respiratory rate per minute among 1-5 yr child
Moderate cases	No chest indrawing Fast breathing is present Above 50 respiratory rate per minute among infants Above 40 respiratory rate per minute among 1-5 yr child
Severe cases	Chest indrawing is present Not able to drink Fits might be present Abnormally sleepy Difficult to wake the child Associated with grade III or IV malnutrition.

Epidemiological Character

- Bacteria, virus or any organism can cause ARI
- Small children and grade III and grade IV die if not attended
- ARI is associated with overcrowding, poor nutrition, low birth weight and air pollution
- Common in winter months.

Case management (Tables 15.2 and 15.3)

Prevention and Control

- Improvement of living conditions of the family
- Advice on better nutrition
- Reduction of air pollution
- Good RCH care in the service area
- 100 per cent coverage of UIP primary immunisation in the area
- Home care instructions are given to mothers (Fig. 15.10).

Influenza

It is a viral infection causing epidemics. It starts with a few symptoms of common cold like illness, malaise, body ache, running nose, etc.; and within a few days, we start noticing thousands of cases of influenza causing epidemic. It is a public health problem. Hospitals start admitting thousands of

Table 15.2: Case management in the field

Severity	*Management*
Mild cases	• Assess for ear problem, throat problem • Advice home care • Treat fever with paracetemol • Advice health check up at PHC
Moderate cases	• Advice PHC visit for assessment • Advice antibiotics • Advice re-assessment once in 2 days during acute phase
Severe cases	• Transport the case to PHC • Make arrangement for treatment for fever, difficulty in breathing and for antibiotics

Table 15.3: Management of a case of pneumonia (cough and fast breathing)

Age	*Weight*	*Tablet*	*Syrup*
Below 2 months	3-5 kg	1 tab twice a day	½ spoon BD
2-12 months	6-9 kg	2 tab twice a day	1 spoon BD
1-5 years	10-19 kg	3 tab twice a day	1½ spoon BD

Note: 1 tablet contains
- Sulphamethoxozole 100 mg
- Trimethoprim 20 mg

1 spoon syrup contains
- Sulphamethoxozole 200 mg
- Trimethoprim 40 mg

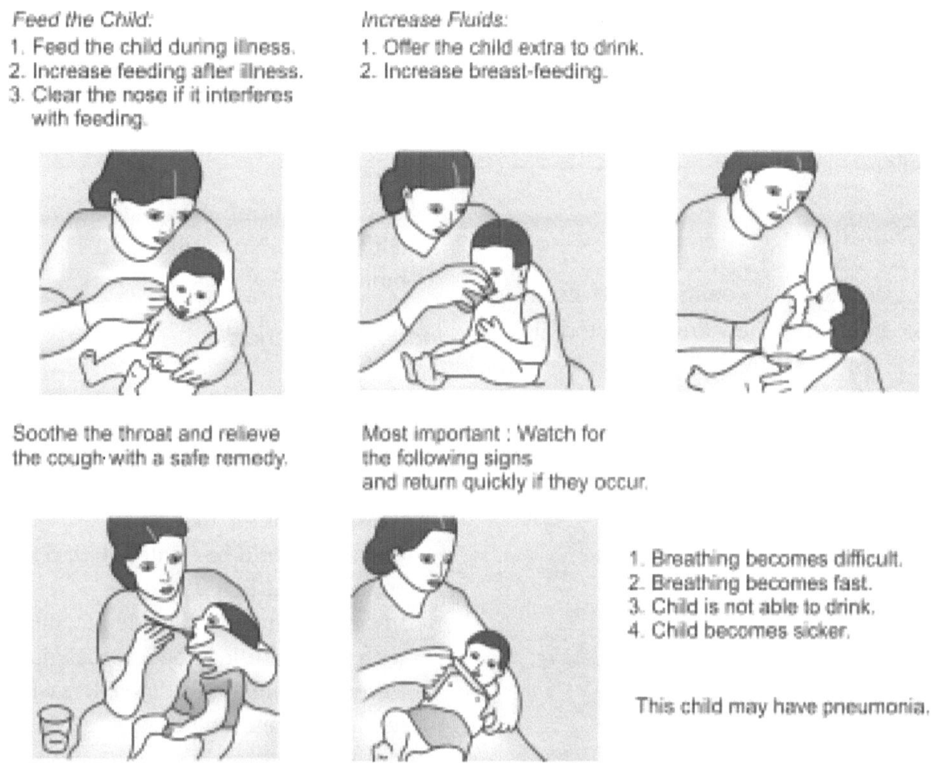

Fig. 15.10: Home care instructions to mothers

cases, schools show zero attendance, when there is an epidemic of influenza.

Clinical Character

Incubation period is 2 to 3 days. Cases show fever, chills, body ache, muscular pain, joint pain, cough and general weakness. Usually, everything settles in one week. In some of the cases, severe pneumonia causes deaths in influenza because of respiratory failure.

Epidemiological Character

There are three types of viruses that cause influenza. They are A, B and C influenza viruses.

In each epidemic, we come across a change in the character of virus. If it is sudden complete change, it is called antigenic shift. If it is gradual and incomplete change, it is called antigenic drift.

- Even animals and birds are known to suffer from influenza infection.
- More cases occur in winter and rainy season.
- Overcrowding helps in more secondary attack rate.

Prevention and Control

Little scope is available for influenza prevention. However, a few steps need consideration:

- Good ventilation
- Reduction in overcrowding
- Personal hygiene not to cough or sneeze on others
- Vaccine is of no use in developing countries like India

Meningitis

1. It is equivalent to brain fever caused by bacteria.
2. Serious outbreaks have occurred causing epidemics.

Clinical Character

Severe headache, fever, vomiting, stiff neck, not reacting to external stimuli are characteristics of meningitis (Figs 15.11 and 15.12). Usually, meningitis spreads in close circle of schools and slums of a community.

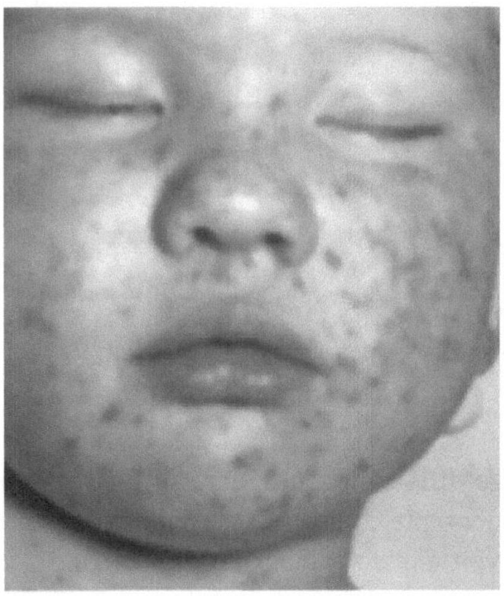

Fig. 15.11: Face of a child in meningitis showing skin bleeding *(For colour version see Plate 2)*

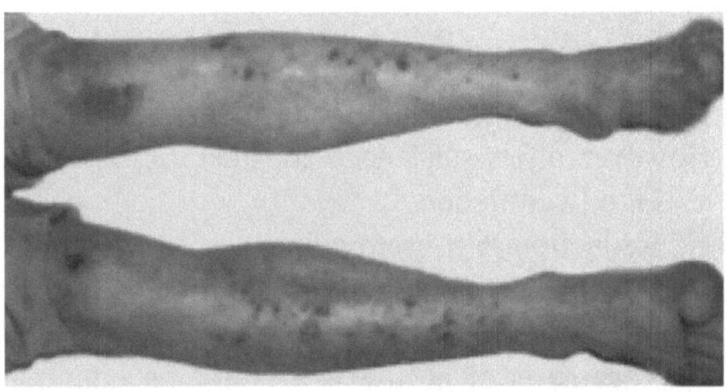

Fig. 15.12: Legs of meningitis case showing bleeding rash *(For colour version see Plate 2)*

Epidemiological Character

- Meningitis infection spreads quickly in the community
- Antibiotic treated case does not transmit meningitis
- Common during April and May (dry months) and during November and December (cold months).

Incubation Period

It is 3 to 4 days.

Prevention and Control

- Penicillin treatment cures meningitis and checks the spread of the disease.
- Carriers should be treated with other powerful antibiotics at PHC.
- In case of threatened epidemic, mass treatment with penicillin may be advocated.
- Vaccine is available for travellers who visit endemic areas. For example, Mecca, Medina pilgrims it is mandatory that they receive meningitis vaccine as a license to travel to that place.

Tuberculosis

Millions of people are developing tuberculosis in India. Among them, every year deaths by tuberculosis is seen to the extent of 5 lakh per year.

Tuberculosis is associated with HIV/AIDS infection and creating a new public health problem.

We have a good weapon of antitubercular drugs, which can cure the disease to the tune of one hundred per cent.

A Health Inspector is expected to note the following specific actions in the control of tuberculosis.

- He should work in local community to increase effective political commitment to create awareness for diagnosis and for treatment.
- He should help PHC responsibility of expanding RNTCP coverage.
- He should supervise and guide community health guide in antitubercular activities.

- He should involve community resources for observation and treatment.
- He should help PHC in recording, reporting and a check on regular drug supply.

Tuberculosis is a bacterial infection caused by *Mycobacterium tuberculosis*. It is being effectively treated with DOTS (Directly Observed Treatment Schedule) under RNTCP (Revised National Tuberculosis Control Programme) which has helped in bringing down remarkable changes in the implemented areas.

Clinical Character

Pulmonary tuberculosis causes persistent cough, continuous fever, chest pain and blood in cough-out sputum.

Nonpulmonary tuberculosis causes:

- Intestinal tuberculosis (Koch's abdomen)
- Brain tuberculosis (TBM)
- Bone tuberculosis (Osteomyelitis)
- Skin tuberculosis.

Epidemiological Character

Mycobacterium tuberculosis causes tuberculosis of lung and other organs. Sputum examination for AFB gives definite proof for the diagnosis. A person who suffers from pulmonary tuberculosis spreads the disease to others.

- Malnutrition predisposes tuberculosis infection.
- Tuberculosis is a social disease.
- It is associated with overcrowding, ignorance and poor quality of life.
- In the community, tuberculin test and Montoux test are done for the detection of exposure and confirmation of tuberculosis.

Prevention and Control

DTC gives training to PHC staff for the diagnosis and treatment of tuberculosis.

Case detection:

- Sputum examination (three samples—spot, early morning, and spot) of patients attending health facilities who have cough for 3 weeks or more.
- Promotion of awareness in the community and health staff regarding respiratory symptoms.
- Evaluation of household contacts of smear positive patients, in particular, children under 5 year of age.
- Evaluation of patients with abnormal chest X-rays.

Diagnosis: It is done by (Fig. 15.13):

- Smear from sputum examination (three samples) of patients seeking consultation for respiratory symptoms.
- Clinical and radiological investigations of smear negative patients who do not respond to a course of antibiotics (not including streptomycin or rifampicin).
- Clinical, X-ray and other methods of tests for extrapulmonary tuberculosis and tuberculosis among children.

1. *Pulmonary smear positive means*
   - Two sputum positive for AFB
   - One smear positive and X-ray abnormal
   - One smear positive and culture positive.
2. *Pulmonary smear negative means.*
   Three sputum negative for AFB.
3. *Extrapulmonary tuberculosis means.*
   Other organs involved (other than lung).

Treatment

New sputum positive cases, seriously ill AFB negative, and serious extrapulmonary cases are treated as category I cases for the purpose of treatment.

Retreatment of known pulmonary tuberculosis cases are treated as category II cases for the purpose of treatment.

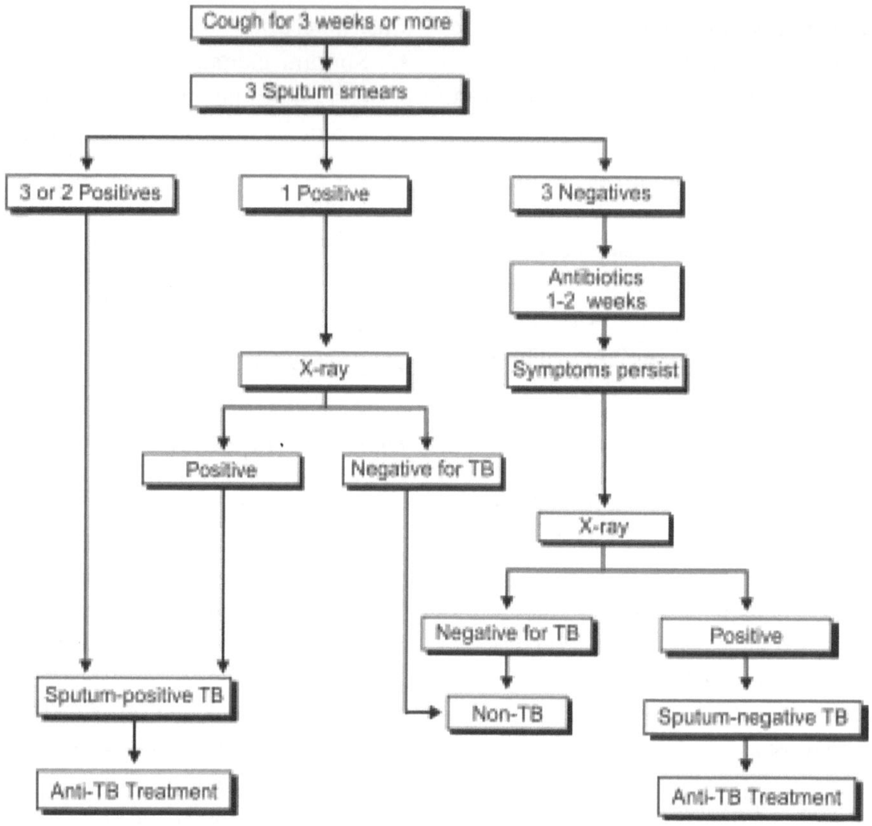

Fig. 15.13: Diagnosis and management of tuberculosis

New cases, not seriously ill, sputum negative and extrapulmonary cases are treated as category III cases for the purpose of treatment.

Common drugs (Table 15.4)

Table 15.4: Common drugs used in the treatment of tuberculosis

Common drugs used	*Abbreviations*
Isoniazid	INH
Rifampicin	R
Pyrazinamide	Z
Ethambutol	E
Streptomycin	S

When to do treatment evaluation?

- On quarterly basis
- On a cohort of patients (group)
- Two sputum exam per patient done
- Three times done:
  - 2nd or 3rd month
  - 4th or 5th month
  - At the end of treatment.

Words that are used in TB case evaluation under National TB Control Programme:

- *Cured* AFB smear negative after treatment
- *Completed* Completes the treatment but do not show evidence of cure

- *Defaulted* If there is 2 months break in the treatment
- *Failed* Who remain AFB positive even with full treatment or AFB negative becomes AFB positive with treatment
- *Died* Death during the treatment
- *Transferred* A patient is moved to other district.

Main forms and records that are used in RNTCP (Table 15.5):

- Identity card
- Treatment card
- TB register
- Lab register
- New treatment and retreatment cases quarterly report
- Sputum conversion quarterly report
- Result of treatment quarterly report
- Programme management quarterly report.

DOTS

DOTS is a strategy to enhance cure by giving TB drugs and confirming it on the spot. During intensive phase, a health worker watches the patient swallowing drug in his place. During continuation phase, one-week drug is issued in multiblister combipack of which I dose is swallowed in the health worker's presence. One week later; when the patient comes to collect the drug, the drug taken is checked.

BCG Vaccine

It is given under UIP Immunisation Programme. The doses of 0.05 ml intradermal to newborn and 0.1 ml intra dermal to older children are given. Tuberculin syringe (Omega micro stat syringe fitted with 1 cm steel 26 gauze intradermal needle is used.

Table 15.5: RNTCP regimen of tuberculosis treatment

Treatment	*TB patients*	*Intensive phase*	*Continuation phase*
1. *Category I*	New smear-positive New smear-negative (seriously ill) Extrapulmonary** (seriously ill)	$2\ (HRZE)_3$*	$4\ (HR)_3$
2. *Category II*	Sputum smear-positive: – Relapse*** – Failure*** – Treatment after default	$2\ (SHRZE)_3$ $1\ (HRZE)_3$	$5\ (HRE)_3$
3. *Category III*	New smear-negative (not seriously ill) Extra-pulmonary (not seriously ill)	$2\ (HRZ)_3$	$4\ (HR)_3$

* The number before the letters refers to the number of months of treatment. The subscript after the letters refers to the number of doses per week. H: Isoniazid (600 mg), R: Rifampicin (450 mg), Z: Pyrazinamide (1500 mg), E: Ethambutol (1200 mg), S: Streptomycin (750 mg). Patients who weigh more than 60 kg receive additional rifampicin 150 mg. Patients more than 50 years old receive streptomycin 500 mg. Patients in categories I and II who have a positive sputum smear at the end of the initial intensive phase receive an additional month of intensive phase treatment.

** Examples of seriously ill extra-pulmonary TB cases are meningitis, disseminated TB, tuberculous pericarditis, peritonitis, bilateral or extensive pleurisy, spinal TB with neurological complications and intestinal and genito-urinary TB.

*** Very rarely, patients relapse with extra-pulmonary or smear-negative pulmonary tuberculosis; such patients are considered as "Other" and treated with the Category II regimen.

DISEASES TRANSMITTED BY WATER

Poliomyelitis

Polio used to cause paralysis among infants; and hence, it is popularly known as infantile paralysis. It used to be common cause of lameness. With the ongoing IPPI (Intensive pulse polio programme), the disease is in the verge of eradication.

Clinical Character

Among 95 per cent of children, polio infection subsides without any manifestations. In about 4 per cent of cases, fever, body ache, pain in neck and back are observed. Recovery is rapid. In the remaining 1 per cent of cases, fever, followed by flaccid paralysis is seen. Nausea, vomiting, and headache may manifest. Within 4 days, paralysis is noticed. Very rarely, sudden death also occurs which is called bulbar polio paralysis.

Epidemiological Character

- There are three types of poliovirus that cause poliomyelitis
- Man is the only known reservoir
- Virus is found in the stool of patient
- Injection, injury and tonsil operation precipitate polio paralysis
- Contaminated water spreads the disease.

Prevention and Control

OPV is a specific vaccine available and found useful in the prevalence of polio. A dose of 3 drops is orally given in 3 doses during infancy under UIP.

- Line listing of reported cases is done to take steps
- Mopping up actions include door-to-door immunisation of all children up to 5 years of age
- PPI started in 1996 with every year NID (National Immunisation Days) is observed. Now IPPI is going on which follows:
  - One day booth immunisation, which is followed by
  - Two days house-to-house visit to cover the uncovered.
- A check on potency, safety and clarity is done by the introduction of VVM (Fig. 15.14).
- Now AFP (Acute Flaccid Paralysis) is going on as part of eradication strategy.

Hepatitis A

It is called infective hepatitis. Water contamination is causing epidemics of hepatitis A in the country. Characteristics of epidemic jaundice are:

- Slow raise of jaundice cases in the community
- Coverage of wide range of area by the disease
- Disease lasting for a few months
- Has common source of contaminated water.

Clinical Character

Fever, chills, headache, fatigue, general weakness, body pain, loss of appetites, nausea, vomiting and jaundice are characteristics of hepatitis A infection in the community. Disability lasts for a few months. Rarely, deaths are noticed in HAV infection.

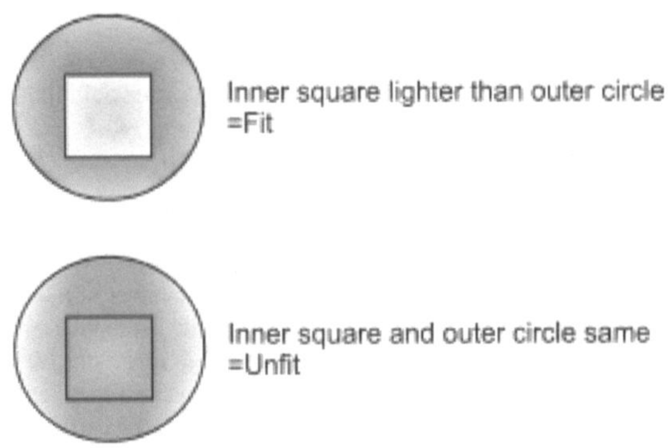

Fig. 15.14: VVM

Epidemiological Character

Stool containing hepatitis A virus gets contaminated with water. That contaminated water is responsible in the transmission of disease. Water filter and commonly used strength of bleaching powder do not kill hepatitis virus.

- Person will be infective for one week after jaundice.
- Rainfall is associated with hepatitis A epidemic.
- Poor sanitation and overcrowding give rise to water-borne epidemic.

Incubation Period

It is 15 days.

Prevention and Control

- Stool of infected person is to be disinfected with sodium hypochlorite (0.5%) solution
- Personal hygiene avoids water contamination
- Water purification helps in reducing transmission
- Vaccination is not found useful and not practicable.

Cholera

It is an acute diarrhoeal disease caused by bacteria *Vibrio cholerae*. Many epidemics have occurred in the world. Most of them are traced back from India and South East Asia region. New strains of bacteria have come up and are causing epidemics. Water and contacts play a vital role in the causation of cholera.

Clinical Character

Fever, body ache and loose motion are characteristics of cholera. In the beginning, acute diarrhoea that is profuse and painless (Rice water) produces severe dehydration. Because of dehydration, the patient collapses with loss of skin elasticity, low blood pressure, low pulse and lowered body temperature. Urine output comes down. Muscle cramps are observed. With treatment, the patient shows signs of quick recovery.

Epidemiological Character

Classical cholera occurred in a community will be severe in nature, deaths are more, very less secondary attack rate; whereas El Tor vibrio produces mild symptoms, no deaths are reported and more secondary attack rate is observed. One important character of El Tor vibrio will be that it has carrier state developed.

- Contaminated water is the vehicle of transmission of cholera.
- Population movement increases risk of exposure to infection.
- Poor environmental sanitation is the main reason of disease transmission.

Incubation Period

It is 5 days.

Prevention and Control

- Any loose motion should be suspected for cholera and should be checked for diagnosis.
- Cholera is a notifiable disease. Early detection can correct dehydration and can prevent deaths.
- Major need is ORS and is made available with advice as per PHC manual instructions.
- Severe cases should be admitted and treated in isolation hospitals. Tetracycline for children, tetracycline and doxycycline is used antibiotics in the treatment of cholera for adults as per the guidelines at isolation hospitals.
- Provision of protected water to the community. Side by side, food sanitation is advocated.
- Cholera vaccine, 1.0 ml subcutaneous for travellers travelling to notified areas are advocated. Otherwise, 0.5 ml subcutaneous 2 doses one month apart is suggested.
- Health education on ORS, proper treatment, food hygiene and potable safe water are given to the community.

ACUTE DIARRHOEAL DISEASES

Many bacteria and viruses cause acute diarrhoea in the community.

Definition of Diarrhoea

"It is loose liquid watery stool passed more than 3 times in a day."

Epidemic of gastroenteritis (GE) is a common experience where we see acute diarrhoeal diseases in the community.

Common virus causing diarrhoea is *rotavirus*. Common bacteria causing diarrhoea is *E. coli*.

Clinical Character

An attack of sudden onset of diarrhoea, lasting 3 to 7 days is caused by infection of the bowel (Fig. 15.15). GE (Gastroenteritis) is the described term for acute diarrhoea, which is watery stool diarrhoea. If blood is mixed with the stool, it is called dysentery.

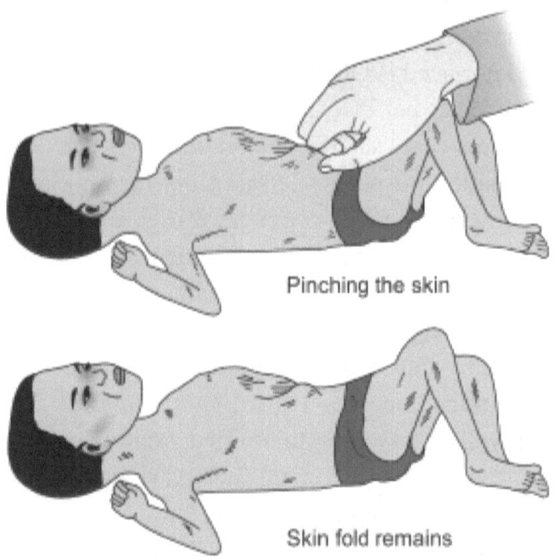

Fig. 15.15: Child with dehydration

Epidemiological Character

Common virus *rotavirus* and common bacteria *E.coli*, *Shigella* and *V. cholerea* cause GE epidemic in the community.

- Man is the main reservoir of infection.
- Children are common victims of this disease.
- Bacterial diarrhoea occurs in summer.
- Viral diarrhoea occurs in winter.
- Water is the main vehicle of transmission. It can also be transmitted through food.

Prevention and Control

ORS (Oral Rehydration Solution) and ORT (Oral Rehydration Therapy) are common words used in the case management of cholera, acute GE or in any diarrhoeal diseases (Figs 15.16 and 15.17). It can be safely and successfully be given to the patient, to the community through health workers.

- Breast feeding and appropriate feeds should be continued

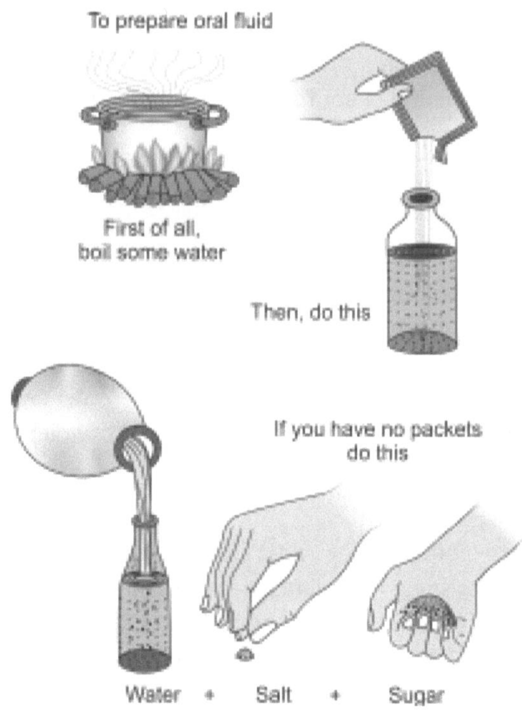

Fig. 15.16: ORS preparation

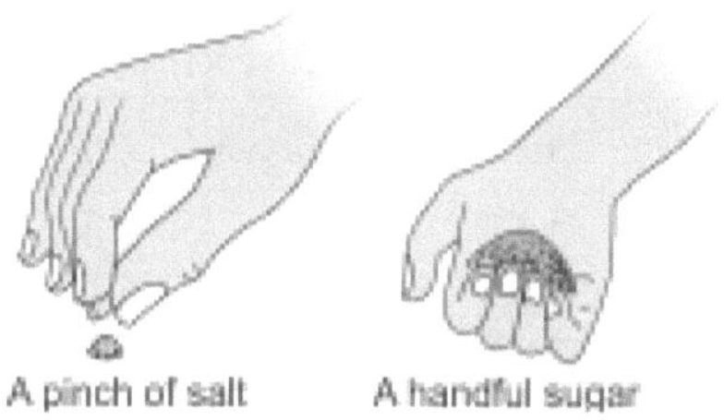

Fig. 15.17: Home measure for ORS

- Better RCH care
- Good water supply
- Improved excreta disposal
- Health education
- General sanitary measures in the locality.

Guinea Worm Infection

It is a parasitic infection. In India, guinea worm infection has reached zero incidences and is declared free of guinea worm infection.

Clinical Character

Skin changes, dermatitis, reactions, are ulcers are common manifestations of guinea worm infection. Adult worms below the skin in the legs produce disability in the person. No deaths are reported by guinea worm infection.

Life Cycle (Fig. 15.18)

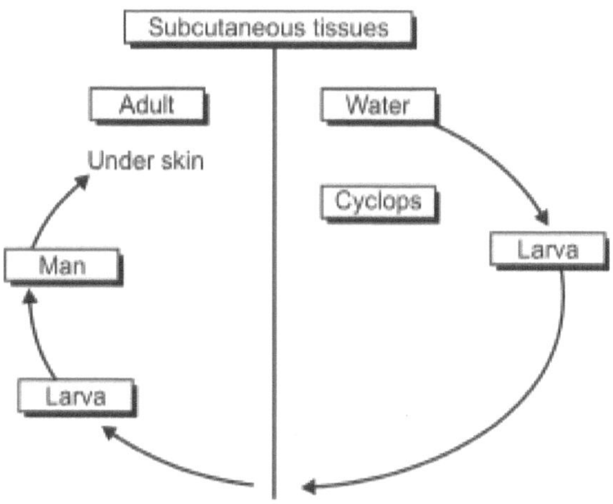

Fig. 15.18: Life cycle of guinea worm

Epidemiological Character

Adults inhabit below the skin of a person. When man reaches water source, guinea worm blister is ruptured and larvae enter water.

- Cyclops in water harbour the larvae
- Man acquires infection by drinking infected water
- Steps wells are mainly responsible in the transmission of guinea worm infection
- March and May months show peak occurrence of disease for guinea worm.

Prevention and Control

- Provision of piped water supply
- Control of cyclops
- Health education for: (i) boiling water and (ii) straining water in muslin cloth before drinking
- Search for new cases
- Treatment of cases.

ZOONOTIC DISEASES

Rabies

It is one of the highly fatal viral infections of man. Since patients show fear of water, it is called hydrophobia. Animals such as the dog, cat and wolf, transmit the disease rabies when they bite.

Clinical Character

Within 5 days of the bite by a dog, man develops headache, malaise and fever. Later, he cannot tolerate noise, light, cold and air. He shows increased muscle spasm, dilated pupil, increased perspiration and increased saliva. Mental make up changes to fear, anger and depression.

Epidemiological Character

- Rabies is virus, which will be present in the saliva of infected dogs.

- Hunters, laboratory workers, veterinarians are risk groups.

Incubation Period

It is 3 to 8 weeks.

Prevention and Control

ARV is a definite weapon to prevent rabies.

Case management Dog bite is divided into three categories for case management as in Table 15.6.

1. *BPL-inactivated vaccine*: Ideal site is abdominal wall, by deep subcutaneous route (Fig. 15.19). A fold of skin is lifted between the thumb and

Table 15.6: Categories of dog bite for case management

Class	*Dog bite*
I	Touch, and lick
II	Scratches, and abrasions
III	Many deep wounds

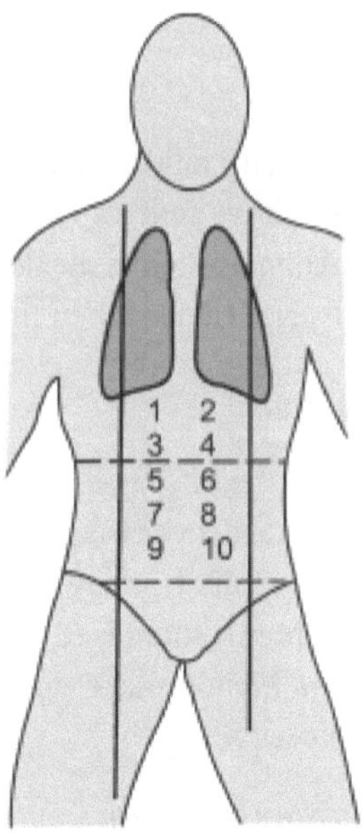

Fig. 15.19: Site of ARV injection (different 10 sites)

Table 15.7: The dosage schedule as per recommendation of Pasteur institute coonoor

Wound	*Adult*	*Children*	*Duration*
Class I	2 ml	1 ml	7 days
Class II	3 ml	3 ml	10 days
Class III	5 ml	3 ml	10 days

index finger and the vaccine is injected into the base of the fold by 37 mm long needle.

- *Dosage Schedule (Table 15.7)*
  - ARS (Anti Rabies Serum) is given for quick immunity which is called passive immunity.
  - 40 IU per kg body weight is calculated. 1/2 is infiltered around the wound. Other 1/2 is given intramuscular route.

2. *New ARV Vaccine:* New ARV (Rabipur) given 6 doses, 1 ml each on; 0, 3, 7, 14 and 28 days. Last booster dose is given on 90th day (Fig. 15.20).
3. *Other measures:* They include:
   - Control of street dogs as per the Municipalities Act
   - License and vaccination to pet dogs.

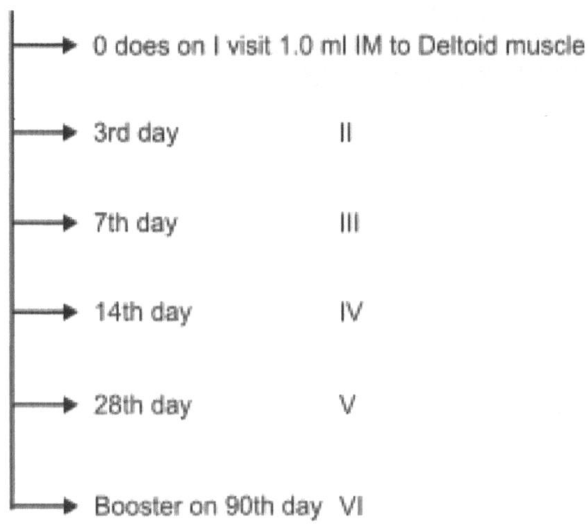

Fig. 15.20: New vaccine regimen in rabies case management

Anthrax

It is an acute infection of skin by *Anthrax* bacteria causing necrotic ulcer (Figs 15.21 and 15.22). Sometimes, it is followed by septicaemia and death. It is common among people who work in occupations like people who work with hides, hair, wool, agricultural workers, veterinary people and people who handle infected animals in slaughterhouse.

The agent is *Bacillus anthraces*, a gram-positive organism. It has a wide list of hosts like sheep, cattle and goats. Spore forms are seen.

Infective material is blood and other tissues of the diseased animals, the discharges from the human skin lesion and contaminated hair, wool and hides.

Incubation Period

It is 4 to 7 days.

Clinical Character

Spores get entry into the scratch on the skin and multiply at the site of entry. In skin anthrax, a papule develops which rapidly develops into vesicle and pustule and lastly, to necrotic ulcer with or without oedema. In inhalation anthrax, the onset is mild with the signs of upper respiratory tract infection. Inhalation anthrax is associated with high death rate.

Animal's immunisation is available. But immunisation of man is taken up and is now made available in the USA during the era of bioterrorism.

Preventive Measures

- Immunisation of workers at risk
- Isolation of infected animal and prompt treatment
- Disposal of infected carcasses by burning or deep burial with quick lime
- Personal protection by workers
- Sterilisation of finished products like shaving brush, etc.
- Notification.

Now terrorists use anthrax bacteria; and hence, the disease has become important under bioterrorism.

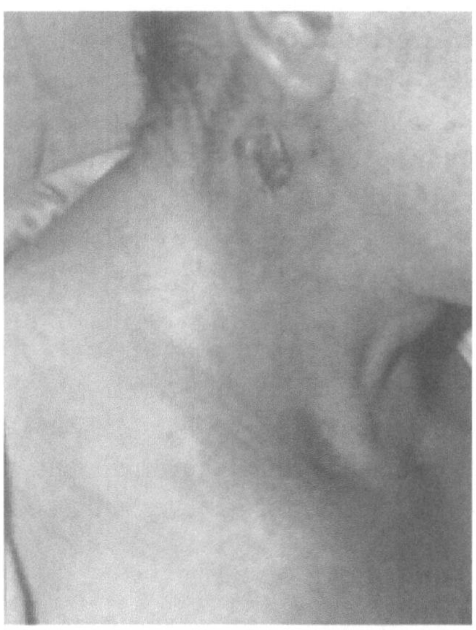

Fig. 15.21: Anthrax ulcer below the ear
(For colour version see Plate 2)

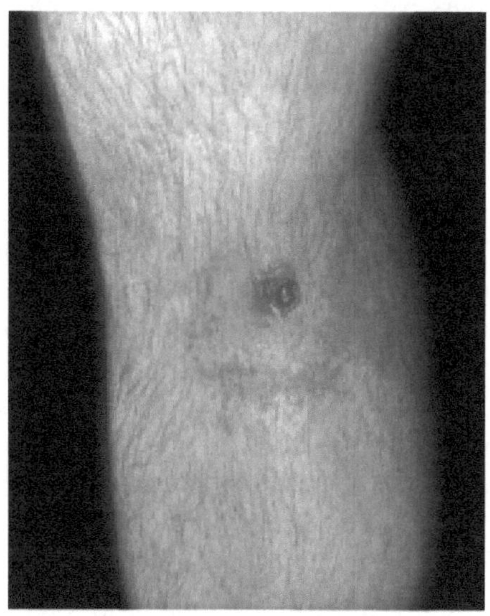

Fig. 15.22: Anthrax ulcer on leg
(For colour version see Plate 2)

DISEASES TRANSMITTED BY CONTACT

Scabies

Scabies person transmits scabies to others by contact. It is caused by itch mite called *Sarcoptes scabiei*.

In the infected patient, we see a rash or tiny cracks which are more in the finger webs, in front of wrist, elbow, armpit, waistline, thigh and external genitals. Itching is severe, especially at night.

Scabies is common among people who do not bathe regularly and is frequently seen in communities with poor personal hygiene. If you see a patient with scabies, you are likely to find that other members in the family also have scabies.

Treatment

Bathe with soap and water using a brush to open all the cracks.

While the skin is slightly wet, apply benzyl benzoate emulsion over the whole body except head and neck. The body is allowed to dry partly. A second layer of benzyl benzoate is applied on the body similar to first application. It is allowed for 24 hours. Next day morning, thorough bath is taken with soap and water. Clean clothes are put on. The treatment is repeated after 3 days.

Prevention and Control

- Diagnosis and treatment of all cases
- Treatment of all members of the family or contacts
- Contaminated clothes are washed in boiling water and soap
- Personal hygiene including regular bath and clean cloth wearing
- Health education to the community.

Pediculosis

Head louse infestation in the head, body louse infestation on the body and pubic louse infestation in the pubic area are very common contact transmitted infestation of man.

Overcrowding and poor personal hygiene are common causes of pediculosis.

Head louse and body louse transmit diseases like:

- Epidemic typhus
- Relapsing fever
- Trench fever
- Dermatitis.

Prevention and Control

Treatment of case is discussed under Chapter 13.

- Improvement of personal hygiene
- Good laundering of cloths
- Clothing should be washed in hot water and soap
- Health education to the community.

DISEASES TRANSMITTED BY INSECTS

Dengue Fever

Many states in India are experiencing epidemic of dengue and posing a public health problem. In Delhi, there was a big epidemic in the year 1996, which experienced heavy morbidity and even mortality. Rajasthan, Tamil Nadu, Karnataka and Gujarat are experiencing epidemic of dengue. The Government of India has given certain guidelines to control and prevent dengue.

Types of Dengue Manifestations

They are:

- Undifferentiated dengue fever
- Actual dengue fever
- Dengue haemorrhagic fever without shock
- Dengue haemorrhagic fever with shock.

Clinical Character

About 5 to 6 days after the exposure to the virus, a person develops malaise and headache. Later, fever, back ache, arthralgia, break bone fever (generalised pain), pain on eye movement, loss of appetite, nausea, vomiting and slow heart rate develop.

Fever lasts for 10 days.

Incubation Period

It is 5 to 6 days.

Epidemiological Character

- Increased transmission is seen with the rainy season
- Classical dengue is rare among indigenous people who have herd immunity
- Common mosquito-breeding places like discarded tin, broken bottle, fire bucket, flower pot, earthen pot, tree hole, tyre, overhead tank, water cooler, flower vase and defreeze container of refrigerators are responsible for heavy mosquito population and thereby spread of disease.

Prevention and Control

- Elimination of mosquito-breeding places
- Protection from mosquito bite by repellents and screening of houses
- Reporting to the authorities is obligatory
- Patient is isolated for 6 days from the onset of disease followed by insecticide spray to his house
- During epidemics, community survey, vector density study and antiaedes mosquito measures are to be undertaken
- Mosquito transfer through ships, aeroplanes and land transport are avoided by as per the international agreement of prevention of infectious diseases
- Health education activities.

Malaria

Malaria has come from the Italian word malaria meaning bad air. It is caused by malaria parasite, which is parasite, transmitted by the bite of infected anopheles female mosquito.

Species

Four species cause malaria in human beings. They are:

1. *Plasmodium vivax*
2. *Plasmodium malariae*
3. *Plasmodium ovale*
4. *Plasmodium falciparum.*

Morphology and life cycle are described in Chapter 13.

Malaria Problem in India

With NMEP, there was control over malaria up to 1976. Later, malaria reappeared with high malaria indices like API, ABER, SPR and SFR. Severe malaria due to *P. falciparum* is increasing.

Types of malaria vectors: Types of malaria vectors that are responsible in the transmission of malaria are as follows:

• In urban areas	*Anopheles stephensi* Breeds in used wells, overhead tanks
• In rural areas	*A. culicifacies* Breeds in stagnant water, slow running water
• In hilly areas	*A. fluviatilis* Breeds in slow running water
• In sea coastal areas	*A. sandaicus* Breeds in salt water
• In plantation areas	*A. mimimus* Breeds in slow running water
• In water logging areas	*A. philippensis* Breeds in high level subsoil water

Incubation Period

- *P. vivax* and *P. ovale* — 15 days
- *P. malariae* — 30 days
- *P. falciparum* — 12 days

Clinical Character

Vivax and ovale malaria Fever on alternative days, starts with rigour. The patient feels cold but body temperature rises to 40° C. Hot phase follows for 30 minutes. Later profuse perspiration occurs. And fall of temperature occurs.

Malariae malaria: Produces mild symptoms. Fever appears on every third day.

Falciparam malaria: Malaise, headache, vomiting, diarrhoea, cough, bleeding tendency. Liver and spleen are enlarged and painful. In later state, confusion and drowsiness can occur. It involves organs like:

- Brain
- Lung
- Kidney
- Heart
- Liver.

Malaria smear making, staining and examination are described in Chapter 15 and Appendix 20.

Malaria Measurement in the Community

- *Spleen rate*: Percentage of children 2 to 10 years who show splenomegaly
- *Parasite rate*: Percentage of children 2 to 10 years who show MP smear positive
- *Infant parasite rate*: Percentage of infants who show MP smear positive
- *Proportional case rate*: It is the number of malaria cases out of 100 attending hospital patients.

Malaria indicators

- API (annual parasite index)

$$= \frac{\text{Confirmed cases during 1 year}}{\text{Population under surveillance}} \times 1000$$

- ABER (annual blood examination rate)

$$= \frac{\text{No. of slides examined}}{\text{Population}} \times 100$$

- AFI (annul falciparum incidence)
- SPR (slide positive rate)
- SFR (slide falciparum rate).

Epidemiological Character

- Anopheles female infected mosquito transmits malaria through bite
- Man and mosquito both are reservoirs
- Period of communicability is 5 days after appearance of asexual parasite in the blood
- Economic status, immunity and population movement determine malaria transmission
- High incidence occurs during July to November every year
- Man-made malaria is an environmental factor, which can be prevented.

History of Malaria Control in the Country

- NMCP 1953
- NMEP 1958
- Focal outbreaks 1961
- Resurgence of malaria 1976
  Because of:
  a. Administrative failure
  b. Technical failure
  c. Operational failure
- Modified plan of operation launched 1977
- Malaria action programme initiated 1995:
  - To create public awareness
  - To encourage community participation
  - To conduct malaria month
- Roll back malaria, a World Bank assistance 1998:
  - For delivery, insecticide, training and drugs
- Focus on epidemiological types of malaria:
  - Urban malaria
  - Rural malaria
  - Tribal malaria

- Border malaria
- Project area malaria.

Prevention and Control

Under malaria surveillance, case detection is done by MP smear examination.

Active surveillance: Fortnightly visit by a health worker, who detects fever, collects blood smear for MP smear staining and examination.

Passive surveillance: All health care institutions detect fever cases, collect blood smear for staining and examination.

Treatment

PT in low-risk and high-risk areas (Tables 15.8 and 15.9).

RT for malaria and severe malaria (Tables 15.10 and 15.11).

Table 15.8: PT in low-risk areas

Age	*Chloroquine*	*Remarks*
Below 1 year	75 mg (1 tab)	Blood smear taken to all
1-4 years	150 mg (1 tab)	PT is given after food
4-8 years	300 mg (2 tab)	
8-14 years	450 mg (3 tab)	
Above 14 years	600 mg (4 tab)	

PT for chloroquine resistance cases

- Amodiaquine 600 mg or sulphaline 1000 mg
- Pyrimethamine 50 mg.

RT for chloroquine resistance cases

- Sulphaline 1000 mg
- Pyrimethamine 50 mg
- Primaquine 45 mg—as single dose.

Table 15.9: PT in high-risk area

Age	*Chloroquine (mg)*			*Primaquine (mg)*	*Remarks*
	I day	II day	III day	I day	Blood smear taken to all
Below 1 years	75	75	37.5	–	
1–4 years	150	150	75	7.5	PT given after food
4–8 years	300	300	150	15	
8-14 years	450	450	225	30	No primaquine for pregnant and infants
Above 14 years	600	600	300	45	

Table 15.10: RT for malaria

Age	*Chloroquine (mg)*	*Primaquine (mg)*	*Remarks*
Below 1 year	75	–	
1-4 years	150	2.5	
4-8 years	300	5.0	No primaquine for pregnant and infants
8-14 years	450	10.0	
Above 14 years	600	15	

Table 15.11: RT for severe malaria

Age	Chloroquine (mg)			Primaquine (mg)	Remarks
	I day	II day	III day	I day	
Below 1 yr	75	75	37.5	-	
1-4 yr	150	150	75	7.5	No primaquin for pregnant and infants
4-8 yr	300	300	150	15	
8-14 yr	450	450	225	30	
Above 14 yr	600	600	300	45	

Malaria Chemoprophylaxis

A person should take any one of the following till he moves in endemic areas:

1. Chloroquine 500 mg weekly
2. Chloroquine 300 mg weekly + proguanil 200 mg daily
3. Chloroquine 300 mg weekly + Pyrimethamine 50 mg daily

Public health measure to be attended by the health inspector:

1. *Area with API above 2*
   - Spraying 2 rounds DDT or 3 rounds HCH
   - Entomological assessment
   - Surveillance
   - Case management
2. *Area with API below 2*
   - Focal spraying
   - Surveillance
   - Case management
   - Follow-up
   - Epidemiological investigation

Integrated vector control: Major measures through integrated vector control are:

- Residual spray
- Antilarval measures
- Personal protection
- Control of breeding places by intermittent irrigation and source reduction.

Plague

It is known as Black Death. It is a zoonotic disease transmitted by infected rat flea. Clinical entities are:

- Bubonic plague
- Pneumonic plague
- Septicaemic plague
- Plague causing meningitis, pharyngitis, tonsillitis
- Asymptomatic plague.

Clinical Character

Bubonic plague: Rigour, high fever, dry skin, severe headache, lymphnode enlargement in groin, rapid pulse, low blood pressure, mental confusion and spleen enlargement.

Septicaemic plague: Meningitis, pneumonia and blood stained sputum.

Pneumonic plague: Sudden onset, cough, difficulty in breathing, copious sputum, cyanosis, X-ray patch present and death.

Incubation Period

It is 1 to 3 days for pneumonic type and 2 to 7 days for other types.

Interconnection with Man, Rat and Rat Flea (Fig. 15.23)

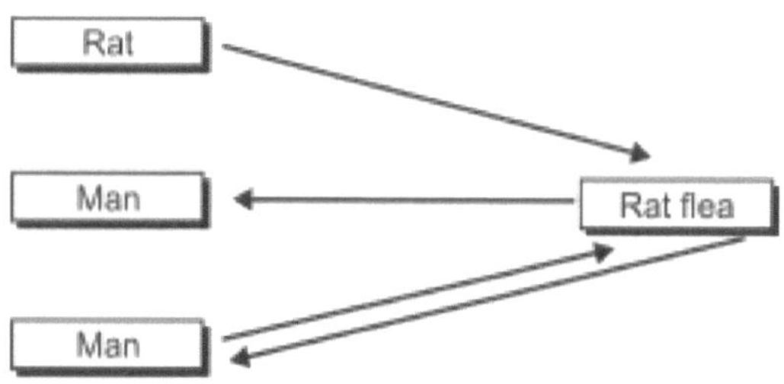

Fig. 15.23: Man, vector and rodent interconnection

Field Indicators in Plague

- Total flea index $= \dfrac{\text{No. of rat flea counted in rats}}{\text{No. of rats examined}}$
- Cheopis index $= \dfrac{\text{No. of X cheopis counted on rats}}{\text{No. of rats examined}}$
- Cheopis % $= \dfrac{\text{No. of X cheopis}}{\text{Total no. of rat flea counted}} \times 100$
- Burrow index of Cheopis

$$= \frac{\text{No. of X cheopis counted}}{\text{Total burrows examined}}$$

Public Heath Measures in the Control of Plague

When report of unexpected deaths of rats in the area is received, the following actions are mandatory:

- Collection and forwarding rats to nearest laboratory
- Autopsy of rats is done
- Plague bacteria in them are demonstrated
- Appropriate public health measures are taken
  - Early diagnosis and specific treatment are substituted
  - It is notified to the health authorities
  - Disinfection of sputum, articles of patients are carried out
  - Dead bodies are carefully handled
  - Specific rat flea control and rat control measures are undertaken
  - Contacts are given Tetracycline 2 g. per day or cotrimaxazole 1 tablet per day given for 7 days
  - Health education in the area
  - Surveillance in the area
  - Plague vaccine 0.5 ml subcutaneous as first dose and 1.0 ml. At 14th day as second dose given
  - Single injection of 1.0 ml dose given during epidemic

OTHER DISEASES OF PUBLIC HEALTH IMPORTANCE

SARS

Severe acute respiratory syndrome (SARS) is a droplet infection by new corona virus, highly contagious and high SAR and high CFR.

In India, suspected cases are reported from Manipal, Kerala, Pune and Goa. NICD New Delhi has observed 10 out of 12 are negative and that all flu are not SARS. No single case fits to the WHO criteria; and hence, India is SARS free country.

During the duty in public health, the following are points to suspect a case of SARS:

- High fever above 38 degree C
- Cough or breathing difficulty
- Close contact with a suspect or probable case of SARS
- History of travel to an affected area.

SARS Initiative Programme

- Health education
- Masks and PPE
- Environmental protection by disinfections
- Reporting of suspected cases
- Safe disposal of biohazard waste.

Leprosy

It is a chronic bacterial infection caused by *Mycobacterium leprae.*

Types

There are two major types of leprosy:

1. Infectious type which is called lepromatous type
2. Noninfectious type which is called tuberculoid type.

Clinical Character

Hypopigmented anaesthetic (senseless) patches and thickened nerves are seen. Nodules are seen on skin, face and ears. Later stages, loss of fingers, nasal depression, foot drop, claw toes and planer ulcers are seen. In the field collection of slit and scrape tissues for diagnosis is described in Appendix.

Epidemiological Character

- Source is infectious case of leprosy
- Infective material is nasal discharge and ulcerated skin
- Overcrowding is an associated cause.

Prevention and Control

- Leprosy campaign in the community
- Staff training at PHC and subcentres
- Detect hidden cases by active house-to-house search for 6 days or at fixed centres
- Confirm and treat all detected cases.

Leprosy elimination campaign: This include the elements like:

- Capacity building measures for local health workers to improve MDT (Tables 15.12 and 15.13)
- Increasing community participation
- Diagnosis and curing leprosy patients.

SAPEL

It is Special Action Projects for Elimination of Leprosy (SAPEL) for services to access areas or situation or to those belonging to neglected population groups.

Table 15.12: Grouping for MDT regimen in the field

Lesion	*Single skin lesion (Patch) PB*	*Paucibacillary PB*	*Multibacillary MB*
Skin lesion	1	2-5	6 and above
Nerve involvement	No	Only one	More than one
Skin smear	Negative	Negative	Positive

Table 15.13: MDT regimen

	Drug	*Dose*	*Frequency*	*Criteria for cure*
Single	Rifampicin	600 mg		
Skin	Ofloxacin	400 mg		
Lesion	Minocyclin	100 mg	Single dose	Single dose treatment
PB	Rifampicin	600 mg	Once monthly	Completion of 6 monthly
	Dapsone	100 mg	Daily	pulse within 9 months
MB	Rifampicin	600 mg	Once monthly	Completion of 12 monthly
	Dapsone	100 mg	Daily	pulses within 18 months
	Clofazimine	300 mg	Once monthly	
		50 mg	Daily	

Surveillance of Leprosy by the Health Inspector

- Single patch and 1 to 5 patch are followed once a year up to 2 years
- 6 and above 6 patches are followed once a year up to 5 years

Leprosy control unit (LCU): It takes care of coverage in the area where prevalence is 1%. It is a control unit with 1 MOH and 12 paramedical workers. It covers a population of 150000.

Survey education and treatment unit: It takes care of coverage in the area where prevalence is between 0.5 to 1.0 %. It is a subcentre for activity with one nonmedical supervisor and 5 paramedical workers covering a population of 10000.

Sexually Transmitted Diseases (STDs)

They are contagious bacterial, viral, protozoa, and fungal and ectoparasitic infectious diseases of man whose principal mode of transmission is by intimate sexual contact.

Following are the list of STD under the control programme:

- First generation STD
  - Syphilis
  - Gonorrhoea
  - Chancroid
  - LGV
  - GI
- Second generation STD
  - TV infection
  - Scabies of genitalia
  - Thrush
  - Herpes simplex
  - Warts
- Third generation STD
  - HIV/AIDS.

Clinical Character

- Syphilis produces ulcer, lymph node enlargement, and skin rashes are seen in skin. Mucous membranes and bones are involved. Congenital syphilis is known.
- Gonorrhoea produces urithritis, cervicitis, fallopian tube infection, and eye infection.
- Chancroid produces painful ulcer and lymph node enlargement.
- LGV produces painless ulcers on genitals and lymph node enlargement.
- TV produces urithritis.

Epidemiological Character

- Urban migration and low socio-economic status has an influence on STD.
- Prostitution, broken home, easy money, travel, independence, social stigma and alcoholism have found association.

Prevention and Control

- Case detection, contact tracing, cluster testing
- Case treatment
- Health education.

STD Surveillance

It is the continuous scrutiny of factors involved in the distribution and trends of STD through systematic collection, consolidation and evaluation of mortality and other relevant data. This is linked to a system of feedback and action.

Syndrome approach: Where diagnosis and treatment is based on a group of symptoms and signs. It is targeted to all diseases that cause a symptom.

- Genital ulcers (no speculum examination)
- Vaginal discharge (with speculum examination)
- Urethral discharge
- Lower abdominal pain in the female (PID).

These are available in PHC manual and are referred in the field.

Typhoid

Typhoid and paratyphoid are common causes of fever in India. It is transmitted by faecal-oral route.

Directly by ingestion of contaminated water, food, or flies and indirectly by contaminated hands.

Clinical Character

Fever, malaise, headache, myalgia, low heart rate, constipation, diarrhoea and vomiting in children are common. During the second week of infection, skin rashes, spleen enlargement and abdominal distension are seen. Complications lead to mortality unless treated with antibiotics.

Epidemiological Character

- Source of infection is always a cause of typhoid
- Carrier state is present who transmits disease without their sufferings
- During September of the year it is high
- Poor environmental sanitation, open field defaecation and poor hygiene are associated factors in the causation of typhoid.

Prevention and Control

- Case management by early diagnosis
- Selective isolation till three stool exams are negative for bacteria
- Contaminants are disinfected with 5% cresol
- Carriers are given one course of drugs as suggested under case management
- Health education on personal hygiene
- Sanitation under:
  - Water purification
  - Food hygiene and
  - Environmental hygiene
- Immunisation by typhoid vaccine. TAB vaccine 0.5 ml subcutaneous at an interval of 6 weeks. Booster dose is needed once in 3 months.
- Oral Typhoral enteric-coated capsule are given on 1st day, 3rd day and 5th day one hour before meal in tepid water gives protection from 15th day to 3 years.

Amoebiasis

It is a very common intestinal parasitic infection seen in day-to-day practice.

Amoebic dysentery has the following characteristics:

- 6 to 8 motions per day
- Copious quantity at each loose motion
- It has offensive odour
- Colour is dark red
- Stool contains blood and mucus
- pH is acidic in nature
- It does not have adherence property
- On microscopy examination RBC shows clumps
- There will not be any pus cells
- There will not be any microphages.

Clinical Character

With an incubation period of 15 days to few years, grumbling abdominal pain, constipation and diarrhoea and above-mentioned stool characteristics are present. There may be acute bowel symptoms.

Epidemiological Character

- Contaminated food and drink transmits the disease
- Composting of human excreta is associated with amoebiasis
- All households get the disease
- It is high during the rainy season
- Poor socio-economic status and poor sanitation are associated with the disease
- Early diagnosis and prompt treatment of cases
- RCA latrine and good sewerage system in the society
- Health education.

NONCOMMUNICABLE DISEASES

Definition

When the cause of disease is not known, and only risk factors are known, when onset of illness is slow and usually stay latent, and which are not communicable to other, the disease is called noncommunicable disease.

Terminologies

- *Risk factor*: Disease agent is not known; hence, cause is described by risk factors, for example, lack of exercise for heart diseases, smoking for lung cancer.
- *Primordial prevention*: Prevention of development of risk factors in population in whom they have not yet developed, for example, eating habit and exercise to prevent obesity.
- *Impairment*: Loss of structure or function in human body, for example, loss of foot by accident, defective vision in diabetes.
- *Relative risk*: It is the ratio between the incidence of NCD among exposed persons and incidence of NCD among nonexposed.

$$RR = \frac{\text{Incidence of NCD among exposed}}{\text{Incidence of NCD among nonexposed}} \times 100$$

- *Cohort*: Group of people who share a common characteristics or experience within a given period is called a cohort, for example, (1) All births on 1.1.2004 is a cohort (one day newborn both sexes), (2) All vaccinated on 1.1.2004 (women aged 20-40 years vaccinated with AIDS vaccine), (3) All girls married on 1.1.2004.
- *Screening*: When a test is done on normal individuals or a group, not for diagnosis or treatment, based on one criterion, it is called screening. For example, VDRL in pregnancy, Pap smear test in women.
- *Ischaemic heart disease (IHD):* Inadequate blood flow to the heart leading to poor heart function.
- *Stroke:* Brain function is affected by blood clot, leading to nerve paralysis.
- *Rheumatic heart disease (RHD):* It is a crippling disease of heart due to rheumatic fever causing damage to connective tissue of the heart.
- *Tumour*: Any cancerous growth in the body leading to pressure symptoms is called a tumour.
- *Pap smear*: It is cervical smear test to detect cervical cancer.
- *Breast self-examination (BSE)*: It is breast self examination to detect cancer of the breast.
- *Diabetes*: A noncommunicable disease where glucose metabolism is deranged in the body.
- *Obesity:* It is an abnormal growth of fat tissue giving rise to overweight.
- *Blind:* Vision is below 3/60, i.e. inability to count finger in daylight at a distance of 3 metres is called blindness.
- *Accident:* Unexpected injury causing damage or death, for example, road accident.

Public Health Importance of Diabetes Mellitus

Four per cent of people are found diabetic in the world. If it is not diagnosed or adequately treated, it causes or leads to:

- Heart problems
- Kidney problems
- Eye problems
- Premature death.

Risk Factors

Following environmental risk factors need special mention in case of diabetes:

- Sedentary lifestyle
- Obesity by overeating is associated
- PEM in child can damage insulin secretion cell of the pancreas to cause diabetes
- High intake of cassava and certain beans that are called cyanide-producing foods can damage insulin-secreting cells in pancreas to cause diabetes.
- High social lifestyle is seen associated with diabetes.

Approach

Primary Health Care approach through PHC:
- Urine examination
- Blood sugar examination
- Health education on diabetes like:
  - Avoid sedentary life style
  - Check over nutrition
  - Check alcohol consumption
  - Check smoking
  - Annual health check-up for the elderly.

Public Health Importance of Hypertension

Basic aspect of high blood pressure and measurement of blood pressure in the field by a health inspector are highlighted in Chapter 1.

About 5 per cent in urban and 3 per cent in rural are showing elevated blood pressure in India.

If it is not diagnosed early or if it is inadequately treated, it leads to:
- Heart attack
- Kidney failure
- Heart failure
- Early death.

Risk Factors

Following risk factors are found associated with high blood pressure:
- Overweight
- High salt intake
- High fat intake
- Alcoholism
- Sedentary lifestyle
- Mental stress.

Approach

Primary Health Care approach through PHC:
- Dietary change for low fat diet, low salt intake and avoidance of alcohol
- Moderate exercise everyday to avoid sedentary life
- Behavioural change by disallowing smoking and alcohol
- Annual health check-up for risk group.

Public Health Importance of Blindness

One per cent of population is found blind in developing countries like India.

Common Causes

Common causes of blindness are:
- Cataract
- Eye infection by trachoma (viral infection)
- Vitamin deficiency
- Glaucoma (High eye ball pressure)
- Eye injury.

  If early detection is not done and if untreated, they lead to following health problems
- Irreversible damage to eye organs
- Loss of vision

Risk Factors

Following risk factors need special attention:
- Old age when eye-lenses become opaque
- Malnutrition leading to vitamin A deficiency which causes eye dryness, Bitot's spot
- People working in fumes, gas, radiation and welding are prone to eye injury
- Ignorance and treatment by quacks can make person blind.

Approach

Primary Health Care approach through PHC:
- Primary eye care like eye protection, better nutrition, early diagnosis, prompt treatment for eye illness
- Vitamin A prophylaxis programme
- School eye care programme
- Trachoma infection control programme
- Eye camps for screening and cataract operation

Public Health Importance of Cancer

Cancer incidence is gradually increasing in India. About 100 to 110 people out of 100000 seem to be suffering from cancer in India.

Common Cancers in India

They are as under:
- Lung cancer
- Stomach cancer
- Liver cancer

a. *Men*: Among men following are common cancers:
   - Lung cancer
   - Stomach cancer

b. *Women*: Among women following are common cancers:
   - Breast cancer
   - Cervical cancer

If the cancer is not diagnosed or treated in early phase, (early phase is called Ca. *in situ*), cancer progresses and involves other organs. This biological process is called *secondaries*. This reduces the lifespan of the person. The person dies of organ failure or pressure symptoms.

Risk Factors

Known risk factors in the causation of cancer are:
- Tobacco chewing and smoking
- Alcohol consumption
- Food additives and food contamination may be carcinogenic
- Working conditions with chemicals (benzene, asbestos, etc.)
- Hepatitis B and hepatitis C viruses infecting liver.

Approach

Primary Health Care approach through PHC is as follows. Cancer screening programme for early diagnosis and prompt treatment is the only hope for cancer control. Other approaches suggested are:
- Control of tobacco consumption
- Control of alcohol consumption
- Avoiding exposure to radiation
- Enforcing PFA Act
- Treatment of precancerous lesions
- Cancer education giving danger signs of cancer like:
  - Unexplained weight loss
  - Swelling not reducing but growing
  - Severe blood loss
  - Unwanted uterine bleeding
  - Persistent cough
  - Persistent hoarseness of voice
  - Bleeding per rectum
  - Hard lump in the breast.

Public Health Importance of Coronary Heart Disease (CHD)

It is called heart attack, which is caused by lowered blood supply to heart muscle, by some obstruction.

Severe chest pain, severe perspiration, heartbeat irregularities, heart failure or sudden death after severe chest pain indicates CHD, which is also called IHD (Ischaemic Heart Disease)

In India, about 4 to 5 per cent of population seems to suffer from CHD.

If early diagnosis and prompt treatment are not available, it leads to sudden death. Heart attack has 55 per cent death rate within first hour of attack. Sudden death rate due to heart attack is about 25 per cent.

Risk Factors

Following risk factors seem to be significantly related with CHD:
- Cigarette smoking
- High blood pressure
- High blood cholesterol
- Sedentary way of life
- Type A personality who show loosing temperament and impatient.

Approach

Primary health care approach through PHC:

- Risk factors are controlled in the entire population. This is called *population strategy*.
- Prohibition of smoking
- Regular physical activities
- Suggested good dietary habits.

Health Education for Noncommunicable Diseases

- HE in diabetes mellitus
  - Genetic counselling
  - No change in lifestyle
  - Reduce risk factors like smoking, hypertension, elivated serum cholesterol
  - Diagnosis and treatment are got done early
  - Self-care by diet and drug and administration of insulin
  - Home blood glucose monitoring
  - Diabetic therapeutic diet
- HE in hypertension
  - Genetic counselling
  - No change in lifestyle
  - Reduce risk factors like salt, fat high calorie
  - Obesity control
  - Active physical exercise
  - Self-care
  - Early diagnosis and prompt treatment
- HE in cancer
  - Reduce smoking
  - Reduce alcohol
  - Reduce radiation
  - Treatment of precancers
  - Motivate early diagnosis and prompt treatment
  - Emphasise warning signs like
    - Lump in the breast
    - Change in birth mole
    - Cough and hoarse voice
    - Blood in sputum
    - Bleeding per vagina
    - Bleeding per rectum
    - Loss of weight
  - Cooperation for cancer screening
  - Oral hygiene
  - Self-examination of breast
- HE in CHD
  - Importance of not changing lifestyle
  - Reducing smoking
  - Reducing alcohol
  - Active life (exercise and active ageing)
  - Cooperation for screening programme.

NATIONAL HEALTH PROGRAMMES

All National Health Programmes are being carried out through the peripheral unit of health PHC and subcentres in the country. Health problems of India are classified into five categories as under:

- Population problem
- Health care problem
- Environmental sanitation problem
- Nutritional problem
- Communicable disease problem

Above health problems are tackled through present health care system in the country by specified National Health Programmes. They are tabulated in Table 15.14.

National Malaria Effective Control Programme

- The Health inspector visits every house in his area once in 15 days according to a field schedule. During the visit he enquires:
  - Whether there is at present any case of fever in the house.
  - Whether there has been any case of fever in the house since his last visit.
  - Whether there have been any guests in the house and if so, whether any of them had fever.
  - Whether any inmate or guest in the house who had fever has since gone to any other place and if so, where

Table 15.14: Specified National Health Programmes

Population problem
National FP programme
Health care problem
Primary health care
Environmental sanitation problem
National water supply and sanitation programme
National accelerated rural water supply programme
Nutrition problem
- Applied nutrition programme
- Mid-day meal school programme
- Vitamin A prophylaxis programme
- National nutritional anaemia prophylaxis
- National iodine deficiency disorder control
- Integrated development service scheme
- Prevention of Food Adulteration Act
- National programme for the control of blindness

Communicable disease problem
- Malaria action programme
- National filaria control programme
- National TB control programme
- National cholera control programme
- Modified leprosy elimination campaign
- National AIDS control programme
- Universal programme on immunisation

Maternal and child health problem
- Reproductive child health programme

Welfare problem
- Minimum needs programme
- 20-point programme

- He will enter his visit on the stencil in the house visited
- If there is a case of fever, he will take a blood smear
- He will give presumptive treatment to the fever case by giving 4 tablets of chloroquine to adults and for other age group according to the schedule given from PHC.

- In case of confirmation of malaria by smear examination, he will give radical treatment to the fever case as specified viz.,

– For *P. vivax* and *P. malariae*	• Chloroquine 600 mg	Single dose
	• Primaquine 15 mg	for 5 days
– For *P. falciparum*	• Chloroquine 600 mg	Single dose
	• Daraprim 509 mg	Single dose

- For various age groups, it is mentioned under the disease malaria discussion.
  - He should give precaution that the drug should never be taken on an empty stomach; otherwise, it can cause cramps, nausea and vomiting
  - Before giving daily dose of primaquine, he should check for the presence of bluish colouration of gums and lips; and later, fingernails or smoky pink coloured urine. If present, take the help of MOH
  - Primaquine should never be used in infants and pregnant

Under the programme, the following items are considered by the health inspector:

- Fever surveillance
  - Home visits
  - Blood smears
  - Presumptive treatment
  - Records
  - Laboratory reports
  - Radical treatment
- Spraying operations including mopping-up operations
- Contacting the drug distribution centres and fever treatment depots in their areas
- Health education
- Community participation.

Spraying Operations

The measures under spraying operations consist of the following:

- Draw up an advance programme
- Repair and collection of spraying equipment
- Store of insecticide at appropriate place
- Training of spraying personnel
- Preparation of suspension of insecticide
- Actual spraying
- Records of spray done

- Monthly report on form MF-6 indicating balance stock of insecticides, antimalarials and detail of spraying operations

Supervision

Supervision at the time of spraying is as follows:

- Advance notification
- Schedule of spraying operation
- Turn out of spray crew
- Condition of pumps
- Nozzle tip discharge rate
- Suspension preparation
- Spray technique
- Number of houses locked
- Records maintained.

Consecutive supervision, i.e. supervision after completion of the spray operation, either on the same day, next day or next week done with specified observations as per PHC manual.

Mopping-up Operations

After the spraying operation, a spray squad follows the main team in order to ensure that the houses left unsprayed are attended to. When the refusal rate is high or a large number of houses are found locked as nay happen during the rice transplantation season, harvest season, or weekly bazaar days, the main team may leave behind many unsprayed houses. This cannot be avoided, as the main team has to move on in order to maintain its schedule of operations. In such cases, the main team should send back a message for the mopping-up team to visit the area within a few days, not after a month or more, and certainly not after completion of the round. Occasionally, the main team may stop for the night in a particular area or leave behind a squad to ensure *mopping-up* on the next day.

Antimalaria Operations

Tackle the problems during the antimalaria operations:

- Mud plastering following spray : By health education
- No advance programme notified : It should be made as advance notification
- Negative attitude for malaria : Health awareness campaign
- No killing of mosquito a belief : Health education
- Caste prejudice for the crew : Give badge as official, or recruit some from the same community
- Grains are stored : Provide polyethylene sheets to protect grains
- Women of house with pardah : They can move to one room
- Complaints bedbug increases : Convince that it also kills bedbug

National Filaria Control Programme

Filaria control units, survey units and filarial clinics are functioning under the scheme.

Annual single dose therapy with DEC along with NFCP strategy is followed in endemic areas.

It is combined with malaria control because of uniformity in control measure and proper effective use of resources.

- DEC do not kill adults and hence repeated to kill microfilaria larvae. The dose is 6 mg per kg body weight for 12 doses to be completed in 2 weeks (6 days in a week).
- Protection by mosquito net and use of repellents are advised.
- Early detection of positive cases by night blood smears taken from apparently healthy persons in endemic areas.
- All positive cases are given DEC treatment.
- Vector control includes insecticide spray by BHC, malathion, pyrethrum, diazinon or dieldrin.
- Vector control includes larvicide like Mosquito larvicidal oil (MLO), baytex, abate, etc.

- Removal of aquatic plants by shell weedkiller.
- Improvement of environmental sanitation (underground drainage, closed drains, elimination of water collections).
- Health education is given on.
  - Need to cooperate in night blood smear survey
  - Need to take early and complete treatment
  - Need to cooperate in insecticide spray, larvicidal treatment and improvement of environmental sanitation
  - Need to protect against the bite of mosquitoes.

National Tuberculosis Control Programme

In 1962, NTI was established for long-term and short-term programmes.

Long term—checks at new case occurrence and reducing prevalence rate below 1 per cent.

Short term—diagnosis, treatment, BCG vaccination and integrated health care service.

There are 446 District TB centres functioning in the country.

1. *Case finding is by*
   - Sputum exam
   - MMR
   - Tuberculin test
2. *Treatment is by*
   - Domiciliary care by motivation and treatment
3. *DTC staff*

• DTO	1
• MO	1
• Lab technician	2 (LT)
• Health visitor	2
• X-ray technician	1 (XT)
• Nonmedial team leader	1 (NMTL)
• Statistician	1 (SA)
• Pharmacist	1

4. *DTC functions*
   - Case finding by:
     - Sputum examination
     - Tuberculin test
     - MMR
   - Record maintenance
   - RNTCP treatment (DOTS)
   - BCG vaccination
   - Preventive treatment
   - Rehabilitation
   - Surveillance

Method of Sputum Collection

Sputum is from lung, bronchi, larynx and pharynx and is by coughing, and is mixed with saliva.

1. After registration, the serial number is entered to the person on the sputum cup as well as on the lid, especially if there is more than one patient in the household.
2. Sputum should be collected in an open space, to guard against the danger of infection. The patient should stand facing the wall away from the breeze.
3. Give the patient confidence by explaining to him the reason for the examination. The patient should preferably be asked to rinse the mouth, so that the specimen is not mixed with food particles, betel or tobacco.
4. Health inspector should stand behind the patient.
5. The patient should be advised to place both his hands on the hips, take a deep breath and cough forcefully. At the same time, he should lean forward slightly so as to bring out the sputum easily and spit out the sputum into the sputum cup, which is kept close to his mouth. To get solid sputum, he should repeat two times.
6. There must not be any soiling at collection.
7. Sputum cup must be burned for proper disposal.

DOTS programme detail is given with the disease.

National Cholera Control Programme

Under the programme, stool specimen is collected by any one of the following methods:

- *Rectal swab method*
  - A cotton swab is prepared
  - Passed into the rectum for 2 to 4 cm
  - It is removed and immersed in the bottle of transport media provided by PHC
  - Break off the end of stick and screw on the cap of the bottle.
- *Catheter method*
  - Sterile rubber catheter is taken
  - Lubricated with liquid paraffin and passed into the rectum for 4 to 5 cm
  - Hold the outer end of catheter over the bottle for 2 to 3 ml liquid stool
  - After use, wash and sterilise catheter by boiling.
- *Blotting paper method*
  - Place blotting paper in a plastic packet
  - Pour watery stool on the blotting paper
  - Seal the plastic pocket to transmit for exam.
- *Surveillance*
  Investigation of all cases and reporting to PHC
- Early detection of case and isolation of the case
- Disinfections of stool, vomit, clothing, bedding, utensil, floor, furniture, dead bodies
- Improvement of environmental sanitation by safe water supply (chlorination of sources, boiling drinking water), sanitary disposal of human excreta (RCA latrine), safe food (protection from flies, clean food, food handlers examination), fly breeding control (disposal of garbage), personal hygiene (handwash), immunisation (vaccine and health education to the community under the programme).

National Leprosy Control Programme

Under the programme, the Health Inspector undertakes the following:

- Survey and case finding
- Case holding
- Case treatment
- Follow-up
- Referral
- Health education of individual and group.

Village Survey

- All houses are examined.
- Absentees are examined later.
- Villages are taken up by turn.
- Done on two consecutive days in a week. from 6.30 to 10.30 am and 3.30 to 6.30 pm.
- Minimum of 95% of village is done before going to next village.
- Detected cases are listed to the centre.
- Contact survey must be done.
- Resurvey is to be done once in 5 years.
- All contacts are given annual check-up.

School Survey

- Done in all schools
- All children, all staff and all teachers are examined
- Teacher's help is taken in writing the names
- There must be good daylight for examination
- Confidentiality is maintained for the detected cases
- Other steps are similar to village survey

Records to be maintained are—survey book, map, school survey book, contact register and individual case card.

Data are analysed for prevalence, incidence and child prevalence rates.

Reports to be submitted are monthly progress report, quarterly progress report, and annual progress report.

Health Education Talking Points

- Similar to other disease.
- It is a bacterial disease.

- It is not disgraceful.
- Not a curse and not a disease of beggars.
- It is not by any food.
- It is not hereditary.
- It is not by sexual contact.
- It is not associated with age, sex and social status.
- Separation of infant at birth from leprosy patient is needed because children are susceptible to get the disease.
- All cases are not infectious.
- Segregation is not necessary, they can be at home.
- Cure is possible if diagnosed early.
- Deformities occur at late stage of disease.
- Reconstructive surgery is there for deformities.
- They are acceptable for feasible employment.

National AIDS Control Programme

National STD control programme is linked with the National AIDS control programme.

- Blood safety programme is taken care of in the programme by mandatory testing procedures.
- HIV test is done on voluntary basis with planned counselling.
- Diagnosis and treatment of all STD cases are done on syndrome approach.
- Condom promotion is included in the control programme.
- AIDS surveillance is carried out.
- HIV surveillance is carried out.
- IEC activities for the health awareness are undertaken.
- Early diagnosis and treatment of RTI and STD have become the theme of family health awareness campaign.

AIDS day theme since 2000 AD:

2000 AIDS: Men make a difference
2001 I care do you?
2002 Stigma and discrimination
2003 Stigma and discrimination
2004 Women, girls, HIV and AIDS
2005 Stop AIDS: Keep the promise
2006 Stop AIDS: Keep the promise—Accountability
2007 Stop AIDS: Keep the promise—Leadership.

National Programme for the Control of Blindness

- Strengthening services to provide the following is done:
  - Transplantation of donated eyes
  - Refractive error correction among school children
  - Follow-up of all cataract-operated cases without fail
  - Providing treatment for glaucoma.
- Fixed facility surgical approach is being provided under the programme.
- Conventional surgery is replaced with IOL implantation surgery. This gives better quality of postoperative vision in operated patients.
- World Bank facilities are expanded for:
  - Construction of dedicated eye operation theatre
  - Construction of eye wards in district level hospitals
  - Training of eye surgeons in eye surgery
  - Supply of ophthalmic instruments to all hospitals.
- Participation of NGO is stressed and their area is demarcated.
- Government agency area is demarcated.
- Identification of bilateral blind patients is done under the programme.
- Village-wise and area-wise blind registers are maintained to give preferences to bilateral blind patients for surgery.
- District blindness societies with multidisciplinary structure with Government, non-Government and private agencies work together for the control of blindness.

Iodine Deficiency Disorders Control Programme

The essential components of the programme are:
- Use of iodised salt in place of common salt
- Monitoring
- Surveillance
- Manpower training
- Mass communication.

Universal Immunisation Programme

UIP provides immunisation to infants as primary immunisation, to mothers to protect the newborn from neonatal tetanus and to children up to the age of 16 years.
- Minor illness including mild fever, cough, cold and mild diarrhoea as well as malnutrition, are not a contraindication to immunisation.
- No child should be returned due to nonavailability of any vaccine.
- A child can be given more than one vaccine at the same time such as BCG, DPT, OPV and measles.
- The site of injection should be different.
- The vaccine should be injected by using a separate sterile syringe and needle for each injection.
- No child should be returned unimmunised just to keep wastage rates of vaccines low.
- An effective surveillance system is established to find out the reduction of vaccine preventable diseases.

Routine immunisation is highlighted in the Chapter 10.

Components

Under the programme, the following components are taken up by the PHC:
1. Preventive services:
   - Routine immunisation programme
   - Mop-up rounds
   - IPPI campaigns
   - Disease surveillance
   - Investigation and management of outbreaks of vaccine preventable diseases (VPD).
   - Adverse reactions following immunisation
2. Curative services:
   - Correct case management of VPDs
   - Treatment to all vitamin A deficiency
3. Provision of logistic and other support:
   - Cold chain maintenance
   - Proper indenting of vaccine
   - Supply to requirement points
   - Maintenance of cold chain equipment
   - IEC activities
4. Monitoring and supervision.

Depending upon the need of the area the following types of sessions are arranged:
- Fixed centre session
- Outreach sessions
- Mobile sessions

Conduct of immunisation session is done as per the PHC manual provided.

UIP has taken up the following campaigns in the country:
- Urban measles campaign
- Neonatal tetanus elimination campaign.

RCH Programme

It is integration of all ongoing health programmes that are concerned with young women and young children. UIP, National FP programme, ORT, CSSM, ARI programme, etc. are combined to make more meaningful and more effective.
- Child components are:
  - Immunisation
  - Vitamin A prophylaxis
  - ORS
  - ARI control
- Mother components are:
  - ANC
  - TT
  - Safe delivery
  - Anaemia control

- Family welfare
- RTI/STD control
- Reproductive hygiene

National Water Supply and Sanitation Programme

Problem village is identified, when there is no source of safe water or water is available within a distance of 1.6 km or where water is available at a depth of more than 15 metres or where water source has excess salinity, iron, fluorides and other toxic elements or where water is exposed to the risks of cholera.

- 40 litres of safe water per head per day is planned in the programme
- One hand pump for every 250 person is planned in the programme
- One spot source of water for every 250 person is planned in the programme
- IEC activities
- All existing dry latrines to be converted to low-cost sanitary latrines
- Evolve viable sewerage system in cities.

National Family Welfare Programme

Objectives

The objectives of NFPP is adopted to suit the objectives of NPP 2000. They are:

- Basic RCH services are provided
- Free and compulsory education up to 14 years of age
- IMR reduction to 30
- MMR reduction to 1
- UIP to all
- Age at marriage 20 for girls
- 80 per cent institutional deliveries
- 100 per cent by trained staff
- Cafeteria approach for family planning methods
- Provide RTI and STI management
- Indian system of medicine is included to reach all
- Small family norm for achieving replacement level of total fertility rate
- Made people centred programme with social and welfare schemes.

Minimum Need Programme

It is for the social and economic development of the community in the country.

Components

Its components are:

- Rural health
- Rural water supply
- Rural electrification
- Elementary education
- Adult education
- Nutrition
- Environmental improvement of urban slums
- House for landless labourers.

20-Point Programme

Restructured 20-point programme emphasises the following:

- Eradication of poverty
- Increase of productivity
- Reduction in inequalities
- Removing social disparity
- Removing economical disparity.

Aims

The programme aims at:

- Poverty alleviation
- Provision of safe and wholesome water
- Health care for all
- Small family norm
- Free education to all
- Healthful housing to all
- Slum improvement in urban areas
- Environmental sanitation and environment protection.

16

Investigation of an Epidemic

EPIDEMIC

Diseases when start occurring more than our expectations in a community, when many cases start occurring excess of normal expectation during a specific duration of time, we call it as epidemic.

Common Diseases

Common diseases in epidemics in public health practice are:

- GE epidemic
- Cholera epidemic
- Typhoid epidemic
- Dengue epidemic
- Jaundice epidemic (hepatitis)

Epidemics are occurring widely in nature. Investigations of such epidemics have given us opportunity to learn about the disease spread and disease control.

Many people die and many will become invalid by epidemics. Hence, it is important to tackle the epidemics on urgent basis. District Health authorities like DH and FWO, District Collector (Deputy Commissioner or District Magistrate) have powers to take measures to contain and control the epidemic of a disease.

To prevent high mortality (deaths) and high morbidity (disability), there is a strong need for investigation of an epidemic.

Investigation

Investigation of an epidemic helps us in the following way:

- It defscribes the time of occurrence, place of occurrence and people involved in an epidemic.
- We get an idea about factors responsible for an epidemic.
- Investigation identifies the source of infection.
- Investigation helps us to know the mode of transmission of disease.
- Immediate control measures are to be taken based on investigation report.
- Investigation also helps us to take preventive steps to prevent the further occurrence of epidemics.

Normally, by the time we understand that it is an epidemic; it would have come to a peak. Hence, fieldwork in investigation of epidemic requires flexibility, little modification in the practical procedure of investigation of epidemic. We may have to do certain things simultaneously.

Practical Steps in Investigation of An Epidemic

Step 1: As soon as the report of epidemic is received the area must be visited along with Medical Officer and report made by public, newspaper or community is verified. Lay people call this on the spot diagnosis, which verifies the report.

Step 2: Verification is done for more number of cases than expected, for the area because commonly occurring illnesses cannot be called an epidemic.

Step 3: After steps (1) and (2), we should specify the area and population exposed. It is called defining the population at risk. Preparing spot map and population census of the area are done.

Step 4: With the help of a proforma, all old and new cases are visited and recorded. The data recorded is called "epidemiological case sheet". In this stage, as many cases as possible should be visited. Case detection should also be done with contacts at home, school, neighbourhood, workplace, etc.

Step 5: Analysis of data for the following is done:

a. Time distribution of cases
b. Place distribution by spot map
c. Person distribution for age, sex, occupation and risk factors.

Step 6: A decision is taken for source of infection, cause, spread and environment. This is called puttingforth "hypothesis".

Step 7: The decision in step (6) is tested to prove the cause.

Step 8: By knowing source, cause, spread and environment, we can take measures to prevent further epidemic.

Step 9: Screening, surveillance and survey are continued to do full detail investigation.

Step 10: Report is prepared and submitted.

An Illustration with Investigation of an Epidemic of GE in a Town

Step 1: When report of GE is received immediately, it is visited along with MOH. GE (Gastroenteritis) is also called food poisoning. The condition (GE) is verified by:

- Vomiting and diarrhoea among many at the same time.
- All affected people will have common symptoms and signs.
- There will be history of common food consumption.

Step 2: Since many other conditions like PEM, measles, indigestion, etc. also cause diarrhoea; and that they do not show common symptoms and signs, verification is done by visit to find out hundreds of people with same complaints.

Step 3: Population of affected city or village is counted by quick survey. This gives an idea of population at risk for GE. A spot map is prepared for the area, which should give correct picture of clustering of GE cases, and water supply of the area.

Step 4: Epidemiological case sheet is prepared and information on contact at home, school, neighbour, and workplace are collected.

Step 5: Time distribution (on which date more cases?), place distribution (in which area more cases?), person distribution (which age and which sex has more?), occupation and risk factors are collected for analysis.

Step 6: Postulation of hypothesis is done for source, cause, spread and environment is done.

Step 7: Decision on step (6) is taken, for example, contamination of drinking water caused GE.

Step 8: Measures are taken to provide protected water supply, environmental sanitation and health education, apart from treating all cases.

Step 9: Survey, screening and surveillance are continued till zero case is reported.

Step 10: A report on investigation of epidemic is prepared and submitted to DH and FWO for action and advice.

With regard to GE, the following conditions should be kept in mind by the health inspector:

- Food poisoning (bacterial)
- Cholera (severe and deaths will occur)
- Arsenic poisoning

Specific procedure in GE epidemic:

- You should prepare the list of cases and keep them readily available.
- Get the food, vomit, and stool, examined at laboratory.
- A request is made for blood test.

4. Inspection of all eating places done.
5. A check on food handlers is done.
6. Sanitary survey of water source is done.

Common Terms

Common terms used in the investigation of an epidemic:

- CFR (Case Fatality Ratio)

$$= \frac{\text{Number of deaths due to GE}}{\text{Total number of GE cases}}$$

- Attack Rate = $\frac{\text{Number of GE cases}}{\text{Total population at risk}} \times 100$

- *SAR (Secondary Attack Rate)*: It is the number of GE cases occurring after first (primary) case.

MUNICIPALITIES ACT 1964

Duties at the time of threatened outbreak of epidemic or actual outbreak of infectious disease is given under chapter IX section 248 and 249 of Municipalities Act. This book is made available by the Department of Law and Parliamentary Affairs in Municipalities, office of the DH and FWO and Primary Health Centres for office references.

Special Note on Investigation of An Epidemic

In recent days, when a disease is fully controlled and is on eradication list, then even one case (single case) detection becomes an epidemic. Current public health relevance is with poliomyelitis because IPPI is going on for eradication of polio since 1995. Hence, epidemiological investigation in one case of polio occurrence is treated on par with outbreak of epidemic.

Investigation

This single case of polio prompts an urgent investigation as under:

a. Stool sample of all polio cases or all suspected polio cases are collected and sent for laboratory test.
b. Following checklist is used in investigation of epidemic of polio (even one case):
   - Name of the area or locality where investigation of epidemic is being done
   - Date of first case reported in the area
   - Period of investigation from .... to .....
   - Number of paralytic cases detected:
     - By clinical diagnosis only
     - By laboratory confirmation
     - By types of virus isolated
   - Number of deaths from paralytic polio
   - Number of paralytic cases of polio by age:
     - Below one year
     - 1 to 4 years
     - 5 to 9 years
     - 10 to 14 years
     - 15 to 19 years
     - 20 years and above
   - Number of contacts of paralytic polio case examined by household contact examination and by others (to be specified)
   - Brief description of the investigation
   - History of vaccination practice in the locality including the dates of last vaccination to the community-by-community vaccination programme and the type of vaccine used.
   - Name of the investigator and the name of the laboratory.

17

Maternal Health, Child Health and Family Welfare

MOTHERS AND CHILDREN

Mothers and children form more than 60 per cent of population of India.

- Women of 15 to 45 age group = 23%
- Children below 15 years = 38%.

Mothers and children are susceptible for ill health because they are vulnerable to diseases. Widespread infection and malnutrition make the things still worse.

Taking care of this huge group, it is necessary for the progress of the country, we need specific group health care services which is available as MCH care.

To consider mother and child as one unit, the following are the reasons:

- Growing foetus in the womb is part of mother
- Mother's health influences child health.
- Feeding practices and weaning practices determine child health.
- Health begins at home and mother is first teacher to the child.

MOTHER AND CHILD HEALTH

Words used in Maternal and Child Care

- *MCH*: The concept of mother and child health as one unit came to implementation after 1950. It is the brainchild of Bhore Committee Report.
- *MCH and FP*: Family planning incorporated in mother and childcare. It is the brainchild of Mukherjee Committee Report.
- *CSSM*: It is child survival and safe motherhood. It is the brainchild of National Health Policy during 1983.
- *RCH*: All matters concerned with reproduction and child health is called RCH. It is the brainchild of Planning Commission of India.

History of MCH Movement

The Christian Missionary started giving training to community *dais* that used to conduct deliveries. This dates back to 1866.

In the year 1919, the All India League for MCH was established. This also started training of health visitors in the community.

During 1955-56, MCH services was linked with Primary Health centre and became major function of PHC.

After the Indian Factory Act, we noticed development of Day Care centres that are also called crèches for the childcare.

In the year 1966, FP became a component of MCH. And that is how we have now the word MCH and FP.

In the year 1975, the Government of India planned an Integrated Child Development Service scheme, which is popularly known as ICDS, is another milestone in the history of MCH care in India.

During 1992-93, all programmes of mothers and children were taken up under CSSM (child survival and safe motherhood).

After 1994, conference on population and development in Cairo, we noticed RCH, which is a reorganised MCH care, in the year 1997.

National strategy for HFA (Health For All) 2000 gives major components of MCH and FP in health care services.

Present Organisation

Following is the present organisation set up in functioning for the care of mothers and children in the country (Fig. 17.1).

MCH and FP services are major functions at central health care through state health and family welfare services. Since 1997, RCH wing in each state is coordinating welfare of mothers and children.

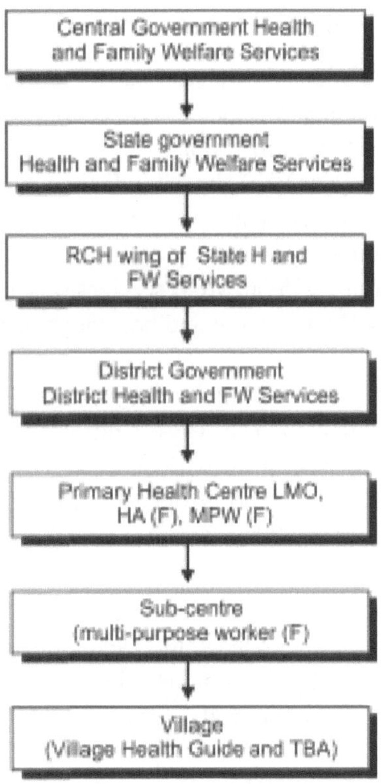

Fig. 17.1: Organisational set up for MCH and FW in India

District RCH officer is in charge of all MCH and FP activities in the district, which is supervised by ADHO of the district (Asstt. District Health and FW Officer).

One of the main functions of PHC is MCH and FP with various activities, targets and reports.

Job responsibilities are given to LMO and HA (F) to supervise, guide and give MCH and FP care to the PHC areas through subcentre activities.

Job responsibilities are given to MPW (F) to chalk out MCH and FP activities in her subcentre area.

Every village is attended by village health guide and traditional birth attendant (VHG and TBA). They are trained and give substantial help to cover MCH and FP in the village area.

Other Agencies for MCH and FP

Various voluntary health organisations have given their hands in the ongoing MCH and FP services in the country. They are:

- Family Planning Association of India (FPAI)
- Indian Red Cross (IRC)
- Indian Medical Association (IMA)
- Rotary club
- Lions club
- Christian Missionaries in India
- General Practitioners Association (GPA).

At International level, the following agencies work for MCH and FP care services:

- UNICEF
- IPPF (International Planned Parenthood Federation)
- UNFPA (United Nations Fund for Population Activities)
- USAID (United States Agency for International Development)
- Population Council
- Ford Foundation
- World Bank.

Before knowing the MCH services, it is required that we should know common MCH problems that are seen in the country.

MCH PROBLEMS

Main MCH problems are unregulated fertility, infections of mothers and children and malnutrition of mothers and children. They are enumerated as under.

Unregulated Fertility

Though birth rate in India is 26 per 1000 midyear population, still reproduction rates are high leading to poor progress in socio-economic development of family, society and the country.

The fertility indicators that show still higher level of fertility in India are given in Table 17.1.

High growth rate of population in India is causing health problems, which needs intervention.

- Birth rate — 26
- Death rate — 9
- Growth rate — 1.93% as per 2001 census

So, actual bearing of children per woman is more, which is responsible for the following health problems both in mothers and children:

- Low birth weight babies are more
- Many women are anaemic
- Abortions are more
- Bleeding before delivery causing health problems
- Deaths among mothers
- Deaths among children.

Infections in Mothers and Children

Many types of infections influence both mother and growing foetus. Common among them are:

- Urinary tract infection
- Herpes viral infection
- Toxoplasma infection
- Cytomegalovirus infection

Children in developing countries are known to suffer from ARI, diarrhoea and skin infections. It is not just a single infection, but many episodes of infections cause child morbid. Tuberculosis and malaria still make the thing worse. These infections cause the child to suffer from malnutrition and anaemia.

Common childhood infections are:

- ARI
- Diarrhoea
- Skin infections
- Tuberculosis
- Malaria
- Measles
- Whooping cough
- Chickenpox
- Mumps.

Table 17.1: Fertility indicators

GFR (General fertility rate)	1.8
TFR (Total fertility rate)	3.5
GRR (Gross reproduction rate)	1.7
NRR (Net reproduction rate)	1.5

Malnutrition in Mothers and Children

All categories viz, pregnant women, lactating mothers and children up to 15 years of age are known to suffer from malnutrition which are caused by many factors (multifactorial causation).

The sequences of malnutrition in them are given in Table 17.2.

Table 17.2: Sequences of malnutrition

Mothers	*Children*
Anaemia	LBW
Toxaemia	PEM (marasmus, kwashiorkor)
PPH	Vitamin A deficiency
Goitre	Rickets Anaemia Goitre

PRENATAL SERVICES

Prenatal period is commonly called **Antenatal period**. The care given is popularly known as ANC (antenatal care). After fertilisation, from the development of foetus till delivery, the period is crucial; and hence, much care is given for antenatal period in MCH care services.

Antenatal Care

Antenatal care includes the care given to pregnant women from the time of conception till delivery. The government of India has stipulated the following objectives for a good antenatal care:

- Protecting the health of pregnant women
- High risks are detected
- High risks are given attention
- Removing fear about pregnancy in women
- Help mother to take up proper child care
- To have spacing
- To have small family

Criteria for Good Antenatal Care

Following are the minimum services and health care to say that pregnant woman received good ANC.

- Three antenatal visits at
  - Pregnancy noticed
  - 8th month beginning
  - 9th month for obstetrical check-up
- Urine examination is done.
- Weight recording is done.
- Blood test is done for:
  - Haemoglobin percentage
  - Blood grouping
  - Rh grouping
- Iron folic acid tablets minimum 100 tablets taken during pregnancy
- TT immunisation is done.

Risk Cases of Pregnancy

When there is abnormality expected or when abnormality exists, we group pregnant women under risk category and give MCH services under risk approach. These situations are:

- Primi gravida above 30 years of age
- Primi gravida who are short in their height
- Abnormal foetal presentation
- Bleeding tendency in pregnancy
- Oedema, high BP, and convulsions
- Anaemia
- Twin pregnancy
- Too much liquor omni (hydromnios)
- Past bad history of delivery
- Woman who has passed beyond the expected date of delivery
- Heart diseases
- Kidney diseases
- Diabetic woman
- Tuberculosis
- Liver diseases.

Responsibilities of Health Inspector in MCH care as Supervisor under Duties and Responsibilities of HA (M)

- Identify and refer woman with abnormal pregnancy, medical problems, and gynaecological problems to PHC through HA (F).
- Immunisation of pregnant woman with TT. Also, help HA (F) in this context.
- Help HA (F) in referring difficult labour and problem with newborn.

Health Inspector's participation in general activities pertaining to MCH care:

- Assessment of growth and development of infants in the area.
- Take suitable action in poor milestone and poor growth of infants
- Health education of community about MCH care through talk (interaction), group discussion, exhibition, film show, etc.

Health Inspector's participation along with HA (F) for MCH care in the area:

- Registration of pregnancy and health care throughout pregnancy

- History taking should include:
  - General health
  - Past illness
  - Family health
  - Living condition of family
  - Past delivery history
  - Present pregnancy—normal or abnormal.
- Urine examination for sugar and Hb% estimation at home visit, at clinic and at PHC
- Height recording
- Weight recording
- BP recording
- Examination for pallor (anaemia)
- Advice to pregnant women on: (i) regular health check-up, (ii) balanced diet and (iii) TT
- Case reference to PHC when abnormalities are present.
- Minor ailments and complications are to be noted and to be attended (Table 17.3).
- Required help to HA (F) and MPW (F) and *dais* in home deliveries and difficult labour
- Problems of newborn
- Follow-up of cases

Prenatal Clinics (Antenatal Clinics) at PHC, Subcentre, MCH Centre, and Private Clinics

Every week on specified days, MCH clinic is run in any of the above centres and helps LMO in conducting prenatal clinics.

Table 17.3: Minor ailments and complications

Minor ailments	*Complications*
Morning sickness	Abortion
Heart burn, nausea	Bleeding
Backache	Urinary infection
Constipation	Premature rupture of membrane
Varicose veins	Abnormal presentation
Piles itching of vulva	Ectopic pregnancy
Fungal infection	Too much liquor omni

At these clinics, the following cases will assemble:

- All pregnant women in the area
- Women with IUD
- Risk pregnant women
- Risk children

Though conducting and arranging is the sole responsibilities of HA (F), it is obligatory on the part of Health Inspector [HA (M)] to know the procedures and responsibilities while conducting MCH clinics.

Usually, MCH clinics will be MCH and FP clinics.

Organisation of the Clinic

One day in a week, according to local convenience is kept for MCH and FP clinic. This should be done in one monthly programme-planning schedule.

Health staff should be punctual in time and should not make pregnant woman tired.

MCH and FP clinic preparation should be ready before beneficiaries arrive.

These preparations are:

- Cleanliness of clinic centre
- Arrangement of clinic room
- Sterilised instruments should be ready
- IUD should be ready
- Drug, dressing, vaccine, glove, linen, etc. should be procured well in advance and be made available
- Case cards, registers and referral forms must be ready
- Drinking water facilities should be made.
- Seating arrangements (at least a mat to sit) should be ready for beneficiaries.
- Health education material are made available

Holding the Clinic

LMO is assisted by allowing one by one in the clinic, allowing the sick on priority, collecting urine specimen and taking care of children brought by mothers are attended.

Filling cards, taking weight and height assisting in TT giving, medicine dispensing and distribution of contraceptives are done.

HA (F) and MPW (F) will help LMO at clinic examination and at IUD insertion.

In case of pregnant women, check the following at the end of the clinic:

- History
- BP
- Weight, height, urine result, Hb% done
- General examination done
- Abdominal examination done
- Advice and referral slip given.

In case of IUD women, check the following at the end of clinic:

- Eligible couple register entry
- IUD insertion entry
- Advice and medicine taken.

ADDITIONAL JOBS IN MCH CLINICS

Following additional jobs are to be carried out since they are felt need of the society:

- Examination and treatment of minor ailments
- UIP primary immunisation of children

Training of *Dais*

Though it is the jurisdiction of HA (F) and MPW (F), Health Inspector is expected to know for organisation and help as team member in training.

Objectives of Dais Training

Main objective is to give delivery help and promotion of small family norm to the community at affordable cost and in their own environment.

Specific objectives during its course of main objective that are met can be mentioned as under:

- Sepsis and antisepsis are understood by *dais*
- Aseptic procedures in delivery is possible
- Develop skill to help deliveries
- Understands when to call help from subcentre and PHC
- Play role in promotion of FP programme
- Accepts as a health team member.

Criteria for Selecting *Dais* for Training

- She must have conducted deliveries in the community
- She is from the local community.

Venue for Dais Training

It can be in:

- PHC
- Subcentre
- MCH clinics

Duration of Training

Total duration is 30 days.

In a week, she visits PHC/subcentre/MCH clinics for 2 days and accompanies MPW (F) for the remaining 5 days.

During training, she conducts 2 deliveries under the supervision of HW (F) and HA (F).

Content of Dais Training

- Anatomy of female pelvis; reproductive organs; menstruation; fertilisation; growth of foetus.
- Definition of asepsis and sepsis; antiseptics; sterilisation technique; how to sterilise scissors and cord ties
- Prenatal care; registration of prenatal cases; prenatal examination; urine testing; importance of immunisation against tetanus.
- Abnormal conditions during pregnancy; complications of pregnancy; timely recognition of abnormal pregnancy; indications for referring cases for medical advice.
- Mechanism of normal labour
- Preparation for normal delivery; preparation of use of *Dai's* kit

- Management of normal labour; giving an enema; accidents arising from ill-advised intervention during labour.
- Postpartum haemorrhage—causes, prevention and first aid.
- After care following delivery—care of the perineum; care of the breasts.
- Care of the newborn—cleanliness; cord care; importance of breastfeeding; weaning foods; immunisation
- Causes and prevention of illness and deaths among mothers and infants. Reporting births and deaths
- Methods of contraception
- Role of *Dais* in Family Welfare Planning programme—Maternal and Child Health and FP.

Method of Training

- Simple local language is used
- Discussions are allowed
- Too much information is not given in one session
- Model, obstetrical manikin, foetal doll should be used
- Local models are developed for the training; for example, a cloth bag with a purse string to demonstrate how cervix dilates to allow the foetal head to come out, etc.
- Always use copper T, oral contraceptives, nirodh, foam tablets putting in water, applicator with vaginal jelly as demonstration rather than lecture
- During session on preparations for normal delivery, the following should be made available:
  - *Dai* kit
  - Stove
  - Clean vessel for water
  - Set of baby cloths
  - A small room for delivery
- *Dai* should practice the following under supervision:
  - Prenatal examination
  - Perinatal care
  - Cord dressing
- How to motivate mothers for child care should be demonstrated
- Training programme should be casual and not as a classroom
- At training, *Dais* words are respected when she tells on:
  - Delivering the baby
  - Breastfeeding
  - Using nirodh, etc.
- Any mistake committed must be corrected at a later stage when she is alone.

Facility for Dais Training

Teaching equipment:

- OBG manikin
- Foetal doll
- Model of newborn baby
- Model of female reproductive organ
- Birth atlas
- *Dai's kit*
- Nail file.

Dai's kit:

Dai's kit contains the following:

- Aluminium kit box – 1
- Stainless steel straight scissors (blunt pointed) – 1
- Stainless steel teaspoon – 1
- Enamel irrigator with rubber tubing and ebonite nozzle – 1
- Enamel bowl (large) – 1
- Aluminium bowl – 2
- Mackintosh sheeting (90 cm square) – 1
- Hand towel – 2
- Soap dish with soap – 1
- Nail brush – 1

- Absorbent cotton wool (sterilised) – 1 pkt
- Gauze (sterilised) – 1 pkt of 12 pieces
- Umbilical cord tape (sterilised) – 6pieces
- Dusting powder in a plastic container – 1
- Antiseptic lotion, e.g. dettol – 1 bottle

Stipend and Payment to Dais

- During training Rs.10 per day is paid as stipend
- After training Rs.3 per delivery conducted by her in her area

Health Inspector will help HA (F) and MPW (F) on the following:
- Oral and practical examinations at the end of the Dais training.
- Guidance and support to TBA training
- Monthly report collection in the prescribed form.

Diet Supplements

Pregnancy requires supplementation of:
- Calories
- Protein
- Iron.

It is necessary for a healthy woman who is pregnant, for gain in weight of 12 kg during her pregnancy, for good birth weight of newborn, for child survival, for good iron, for newborn store for required growth and development.

Therefore, apart from balanced diet recommended for adult woman, (See Chapter 7) pregnant women require the following diet supplements, every day:
- Cereals – 35 g
- Pulses – 15 g
- Milk – 100 g
- Sugar – 10 g

Above items give additional calories of 293 to pregnant woman.

Home Visiting

Health staff paying visit to the family of pregnant woman, lactating mother, newborn baby, infants, children for environmental evaluation and for medical advice is called home visiting.

In case of MCH and FP, HA (F) and MPW (F) and TBA (trained) are expected to make home visiting as a part of their duties and responsibilities under MCH care services. However, as team member, Health Inspector has to know the role of home visiting, at the time of emergency call, or on duty on behalf of a person on leave.

Free and fair information are available at home visiting because woman feels free at home and responds casually without anxiety.

The health worker needs home visiting for:
- Information collection on health status
- Information collection on social condition
- Information collection on environmental condition
- When woman cannot visit PHC or subcentre due to poor transport facilities and poor economic conditions (not affordable)
- Home visiting is mandatory even to those pregnant woman who attend regularly ANC clinics

Home delivery planned by the health worker makes the home visiting double importance in MCH care services.

Delivery Services

When everything is normal, delivery will be a smooth natural process. In normal delivery also at most care for 5 cleans are maintained. They are:
- Clean surface for delivery
- Clean hands of the attendants
- New blade for cutting cord
- Clean tie for cord
- No application on cord stump

Disposable Delivery Kit (DDK)

It is a simple kit containing essential items required for conducting a clean delivery. This includes the following:

- A piece of soap
- A new razor blade
- Two pieces of thread
- Two pieces of gauze
- Two cotton swabs

Main idea of good delivery service is to eliminate the following:

- Sepsis during delivery
- Complications during delivery
- Neonatal tetanus
- Safe delivery

Maternity Hospitals and Nursing Homes

They should be equipped with minimum requirement for better delivery services. These requirements are enumerated below:

- Sterilising instruments
- Linen supply
- Antiseptic solution
- Soap
- Cleaning material
- Towel
- Drapes
- Sterile gloves
- Essential drugs

Hospitals and nursing homes including maternity homes are geared up to deal with any complications like APH, prolonged labour, convulsions of mother, abnormal presentations, cord prolapsed, etc.

These Institutions also have facility for resuscitation of newborn, care of the cord, care of eyes of newborn and special care of newborn at delivery.

DOMICILIARY MIDWIFERY

In India, 78 per cent of population live in rural situations. Most of them are poor enough to afford delivery cost, unable to reach because of no transport facilities and many a time they may be out of reach. Indigenous *dais* has helped them for over centuries. Now that they are trained, we can expect good MCH care in these areas. MPW (F) is responsible for health care services in her area.

All most all-normal deliveries are taking place at homes and *domiciliary midwifery service* is a major component of delivery care services (intranatal care).

Conducting normal deliveries at their homes with proper planning and periodic visits by health worker is called *domiciliary midwifery service.*

Advantages

There are many advantages of domiciliary midwifery services. They are:

- Home is a familiar surrounding.
- It is not associated with fear.
- There is no chance of cross infection.
- Mother can take care of her scheduled domestic affairs.
- Mother can take care of other children.
- Pregnant mothers do not have mental tension at home (at the time of delivery).

Disadvantages

Disadvantages of domiciliary midwifery services are as follows:

- There is less medical supervision.
- There is less nursing supervision.
- Mother gets exhausted with other household duties.
- Mother does not take care of her diet and instead takes care of husband and children.
- Sometimes minimum facilities like privacy, good water, etc. may not be available.

Salaried Midwifery Services

A health worker (female) from subcentre attached to PHC forms a salaried midwife. She is a government servant to cater health and family welfare services to her catering area. She is responsible for domiciliary service without any expectations from mothers. She is adequately trained and given continued education at PHC.

A salaried midwife is better informed to recognise danger signal during labour. In case of emergency, she arranges transport and shifts the case to the hands of LMO at PHC.

She is expected to guide and supervise all private midwives in the catering area.

Under domiciliary midwifery service, the following are attributed as danger signals:

- High fever at delivery
- Heavy bleeding at delivery
- Collapse or unconscious mother
- Unseparated placenta even after 30 minutes of delivery
- Foetal distress as seen by the absence of foetal heart sound and maternal distress as seen by mother's collapse or unconsciousness
- Liquor omni is meconium stained and irregular foetal heart rate
- No pain even after rupture of membrane

For effective domiciliary midwifery, there must be good coordination and good referral system between salaried midwifery service and maternity hospital services.

Private Midwifery Practice

Local *dais* are called indigenous *dais* who conduct deliveries for over many generations. They are well-accepted by local people. They are called "traditional birth attendants (TBA)". One cannot expect safe delivery in their hands unless they are trained.

The government of India has realised that training local dais or training the TBAs is almost at most emergency that to for regaining the better MCH care in the country.

These private midwives are trained by MPW (F), HA (F) and LMO for 30 days. Trained TBAs are safe under the supervision of salaried midwives of the area. This link is important for an effective referral system in case of emergency and to save the life of mother or child.

POSTNATAL CARE

After the delivery, care of mother and care of newborn form post-PNC, which is required on the following grounds:

- To help mother to restore to her normal health
- To prevent any postnatal complications
- To provide health education
- To provide FP service
- To help in feeding practices.

Usual complications after deliveries are sepsis. It is called puerperal sepsis because genital infection occurs within 3 weeks after delivery. Next common infection is infection of veins of legs called thrombophlebitis. Any bleeding from vagina from 6 hours to 40 days is secondary haemorrhage. Urinary tract infection and breast congestion also are common. They should be looked into during PNC services.

Common postnatal check-up by HA (F) and MPW (F) include the following:

- Umbilical cord
- Temperature
- Pulse
- Respiration
- BP
- Breast condition
- Uterus involution
- Any discharge
- Checks urine and bowel
- Anaemia
- Mental make up.

Postnatal Advices

They include the following:

Dietary Advice

For lactating period, repair, involution and newborn feeding, mother requires additional diet, apart from suggested balanced diet. Allowance during lactation includes (per day).

- Cereals – 60 g
- Pulses – 30 g
- Milk – 100 g
- Fat/Oil – 10 g
- Sugar – 10 g

The above items yield 521 calories.

Postnatal Exercise

For housewife, this aspect is taken care because of her household duties and her movement stabilises her body similar to postnatal exercise. MPW (F) will give (her learnt skill) postnatal exercises idea to bring back the stretched muscles of pelvis and stretched muscles of abdomen back to normal.

Exclusive Breastfeeding Advice

Breast milk being the best food for newborn, it is advisable to give only breast milk till 4th to 6th month of age and not allowing any other feed, constitutes exclusive breastfeeding. The practice of excusive breastfeeding helps to prevent infection in the child. Soon after delivery, the milk comes out of breast which is called colostrum. Feeding colostrum should be encouraged. Unless there is a specific indication like inverted nipple, etc. bottle-feeding should be discouraged, since it is nutritionally poor, and it causes bacterial infections.

Infant and Preschool Services

Infant Care

Up to one year of age from birth, the period is called infancy. At birth, doctors and nurses take care of the following:

- Soon after delivery, air way is cleaned for proper breathing
- By score method, the newborn is assessed whether it is normal or not. The method is called APGAR'S score. In this, 5 items are considered:
  - Heart rate
  - Respiratory effort
  - Muscle tone
  - Reflex response
  - Skin colour

  Normally, APGAR'S score must be between 7 and 10 in a healthy child.
- Care of the umbilical cord is undertaken
- Care of eyes are undertaken
- Soon after birth, the body of the newborn is covered with turkey towel to maintain its body temperature. Too much of exposure to outside coldness leads to a condition called hypothermia, which may turn out dangerous.
- Common infections of newborn, like neonatal tetanus, congenital syphilis, hepatitis B and HIV infection are checked and taken care of.
- Birth weight is recorded which should be above 2.5 kg. Otherwise, it will be LBW baby.
- Following conditions are considered dangerous to infant. They are called at-risk children.
  - Birth weight below 2.5 kg
  - Twins
  - A child born to multipara
  - No breast milk given
  - Repeated severe diarrhoea
  - Broken home born baby.

Low Birth Weight (LBW)

Without considering the age of foetus or period of gestation, the birth weight if below 2.5 kg, the child is referred to as LBW baby. In India, it is about 26 to 28 per cent. Common causes of LBW are:

- Twins
- Severe infections
- High BP
- Poor nourishment.

The problem of LBW can be overcome by good ANC, good MCH care at delivery and after delivery.

Growth Chart

The infant growth is checked by recording weight every month or at least once in three months and recording in the growth chart available in subcentre of PHC. This is called growth monitoring. The common growth chart used is at *anganwadi* provided under ICDS services (Fig. 17.2).

Growth monitoring will help to group infants under following categories:

- Normal
- Grade I } mild malnutrition
- Grade II
- Grade III } severe malnutrition
- Grade IV

Supplementary nutrition to normal children and mild malnutrition children are advocated.

Therapeutic nutrition (double the quantity of supplementary nutrition) is advocated to severe malnutrition children.

Preschool Child Care Services

Preschool child constitutes 1 to 4 age children. Among them, it is very common to see malnutrition like kwashiorkor and marasmus, infections like diarrhoea, ARI, measles. Vitamin A deficiencies are also commonly seen among preschool children. Thus, common health problems of preschool child are enumerated as under:

- LBW
- Kwashiorkor and marasmus (Table 17.4)
- Diarrhoea, ARI, measles
- Accidents
- Poisoning
- Behavioural problem.

Protein Energy Malnutrition (PEM)

It is seen among preschool children to the extent of 2 per cent. It is associated with infection and they are interrelated with each other (Fig. 17.3).

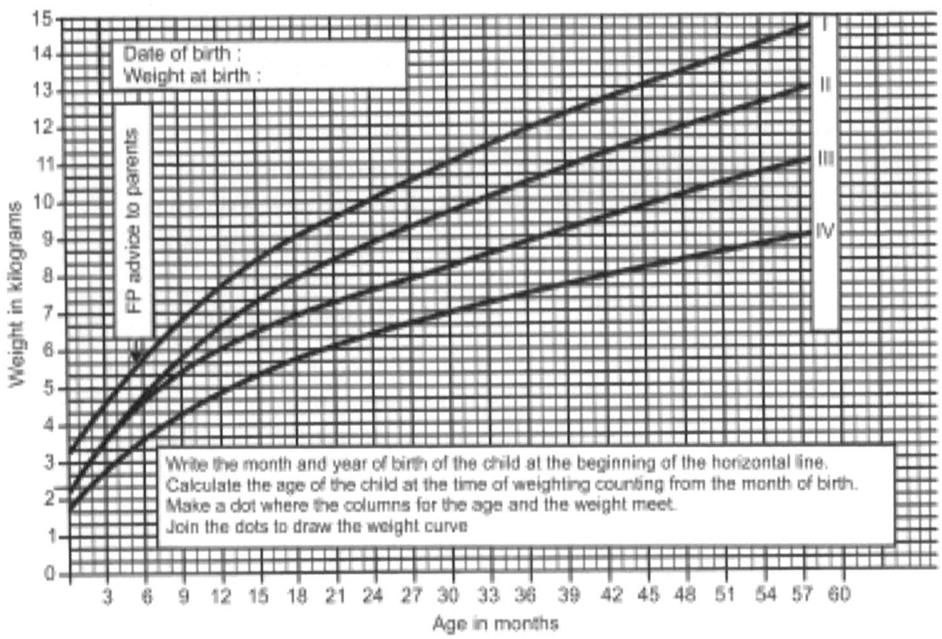

Weights of average well-fed healthy children should be above the uppermost line I.
Children whose weight falls between lines I and III are under-noureished and require supplementary feeding at home.
Children whose weight falls below line III are severely malnourished. Consult the doctor and follow his advice.
Children whose weight falls below line IV will have to be hospitalized for treatment.

Fig. 17.2: Growth chart used under ICDS services

Table 17.4: Differences between kwashiorkor and marasmus

	Kwashiorkor	*Marasmus*
Muscle wasting	No	Yes
Fat wasting	No	Yes
Oedema	Yes	No
Weight	Low	Very low
Nature	Irritable	Quiet
Appetite	Poor	Good
Skin changes	Yes	No
Hair changes	Yes	No
Liver changes	Yes	No

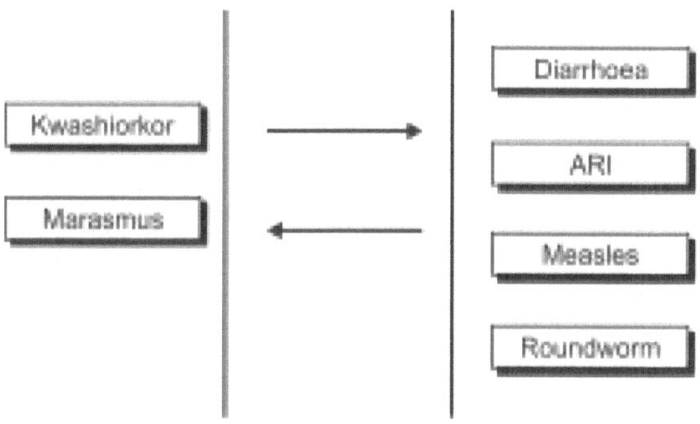

Fig. 17.3: Inter-relationship between malnutrition and infection in preschool child

PEM is called by poor MCH care, failure of lactation, no exclusive breastfeeding, poor child rearing practices, poor weaning practices and over crowding in the families (Fig. 17.4).

Since infection, culture, socio-economic status, food production and availability of health services influence PEM, they are also called *ecology of malnutrition.*

Vitamin A Deficiency

This is a common cause of preventable blindness in the country. Hence, there is the National Programme of vitamin A prophylaxis programme to prevent preventable blindness.

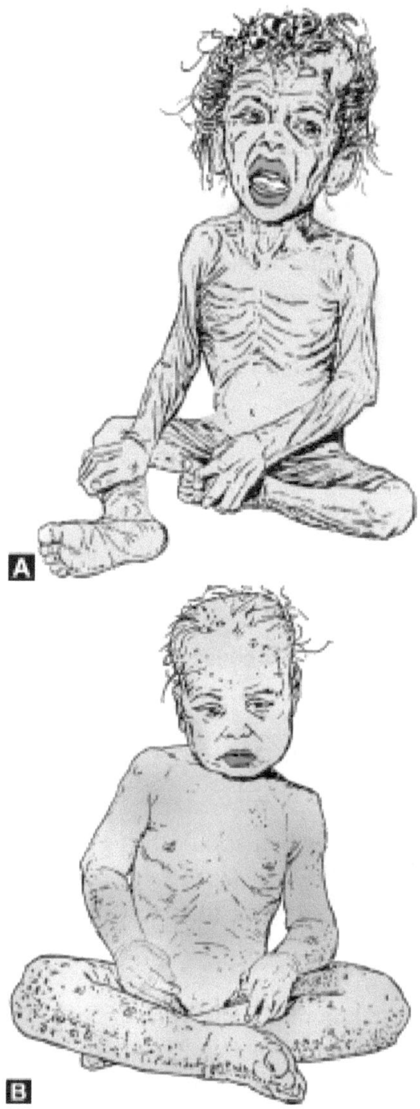

Figs 17.4A and B: Kwashiorkor and marasmus children

Infections

Diarrhoea due to bacteria and virus are common causing dehydration and even deaths among children. Other preschool child diseases are ARI, measles, whooping cough which need careful attention.

Accidents and Poisoning

It is common to see falls, burns and chemical poisoning and drowning among preschool children. They need great attention by the parents.

Behavioural Problems

Depression, overacting, criminal act of behaviour, hurting elders and injuring others are usual behavioural problems of preschool children. Family attention and child welfare activities can overcome these problems.

Under Five Clinics

This is a recent concept of combination of fewer than five childcare services. It is also called a comprehensive health service for the under five children.

Under five clinics concept makes provision for curative and preventive health services (Fig. 17.5).

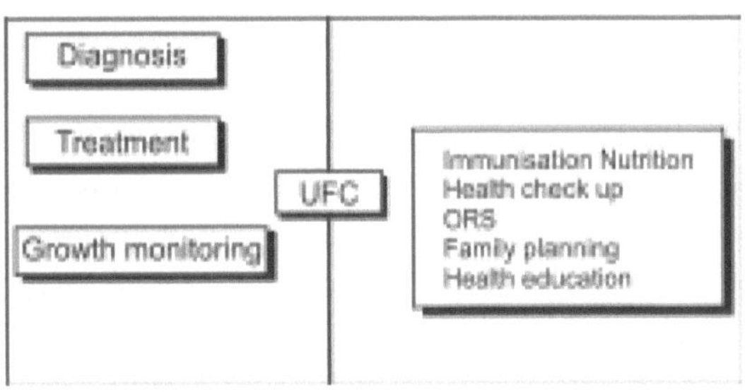

Fig. 17.5: Functions of under five clinics

INDICATORS OF MCH CARE (RCH INDICATORS)

MCH services given should bring out required changes in the health status of mothers and children. They are assessed by the following indicators (See Chapter 5):

- MMR
- Perinatal mortality rate
- Infant mortality rate
- One to four mortality rate
- Under five mortality rate
- Child survival rate.

REPRODUCTIVE HEALTH

Definition

"A state of complete physical, mental and social well-being and not merely the absence of disease or infirmity in all matters relating to the reproductive system and its functions and process. Reproductive health, therefore, implies that the people are able to have satisfying and safe sex life and that they have the capability to reproduce and the freedom to decide, if, when and how often to do so. Implicit in this last condition are the right of men and women to be informed of and to have access to safe, effective, affordable and acceptable methods of family planning of their choice, as well as other methods of their choice for regulation of fertility which are not against the law, and the right access to appropriate health care services that will enable women to go safely through pregnancy and childbirth and to provide couples with the best chance of having a healthy infant."

Basic Elements of Reproductive Health

- Family planning
- MCH
- Safe abortion services
- Effective control of STD and RTI
- Prevention and management of infertility
- Prevention, detection and treatment of reproductive malignancies.

Factors Affecting Reproductive Health

- Socio-economic conditions
- Status of women
- Education opportunities
- Family environment
- Nutrition
- Gender relationship
- Family pattern

REPRODUCTIVE AND CHILD HEALTH (RCH)

RCH is defined as, "People have the ability to reproduce and regulate their fertility, women are able to go through pregnancy and childbirth safely, the outcome of pregnancies is successful in terms of maternal and infant survival and well-being and couples are able to have sexual relations free of fear of pregnancy and of contracting disease" (*Ministry of H and FW*).

Components of RCH

- Child survival
- Safe motherhood
- Family planning
- Prevention and management of RTI/STD/AIDS

Ongoing RCH Activities for Better MCH Care

- 24-hour delivery services at PHCs, essential obstetrical care and emergency obstetrical care are mooted in the RCH activities.
- ARI control, vitamin A prophylaxis, immunisation (UIP), ORT and essential newborn care are mooted in the RCH activities.
- Control of RTI and STD is incorporated in RCH activities.
- RCH has taken up the supply of drug and equipment kits to CHC, PHC and subcentres.

DEMOGRAPHY

It is the study of human population with respect to size, type, composition, pattern and distribution.

Population Education

It is a health education, which provides for a study of population situation in the community, country and world with the purpose of developing rational and responsible attitude among present generation towards FP behaviour.

Major Sources of Demographic Data

- Registration of births
- Registration of deaths
- Registration of marriages
- Registration of migration
- Census
- Hospital records
- PHC records
- Notification diseases.

Effects of Overpopulation

- Obstructs national development
- Produces unemployment
- Poor housing
- Nonavailability of health care services
- Poor environmental sanitation
- Fast development of slums

Demographic picture of the World:

- World population – 6054 million
- Annual growth rate – 1.4%

Demographic picture of India:

- India population – 1027 million
- Rural population – 72.2 %
- Urban population – 27.8 %
- Male population – 51.7 %
- Female population – 48.3 %
- Dependency ratio – 68 %
  (8% and 60% for 65+ and below 15 age respectively)
- Density of population – 324 person/sqkm
- Average family size – 3.4
- Literacy – 65.38 %
- Life expectation
  - Male – 62.9 years
  - Female – 63.9 years

Age structure of India is best represented as pyramid. The age pyramid of India has broad base and a tapering top (Fig. 17.6).

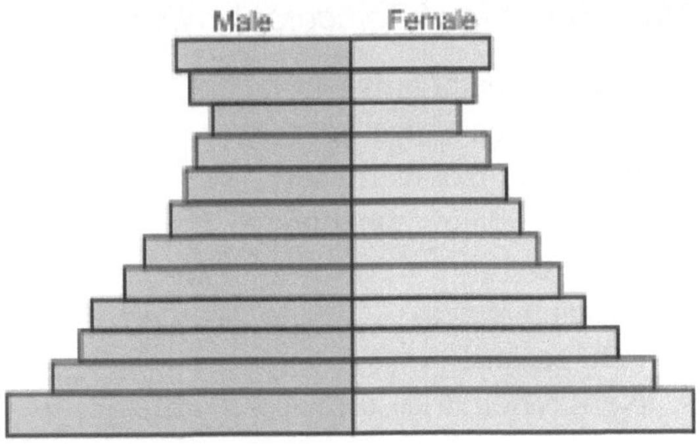

Fig. 17.6: Age pyramid of India

Increase of population is calculated by natural increase method by the following formula:

Current population = Census + (Births – Deaths) + (Immigration – Emigration)

FAMILY WELFARE

Family welfare is a key intervention for improving the health of women, children, family, society and even the nation. Women are protected from unwanted pregnancies and unsafe abortions. By better care it saves life of children. Family can lead better life. Nation shows socio-economic development.

Definition of Family Planning

Now it is called Family Welfare Planning.

It refers to practices that help individuals or couple to attain objectives like:

- Avoiding unwanted pregnancies or births
- To bring about wanted pregnancies or births
- To regulate birth spacing
- To determine the size of the family.

Small Family Norm

To stabilise the country with two children per family and to help achieving NRR to ONE, which is to be made acceptable to our lifestyle is called small family norm.

Spacing

Postponing pregnancy to maintain 3 to 4 years difference between children is called spacing.

Eligible Couple and Target Couple

Eligible couple in India is 150 per 1000 population.

When we consider age group of 15 to 45 years of married men and married women, they are called target couple.

When we say eligible couple, it means that married couple who are eligible for adopting FP methods. When we deduct the following from target couple, we get eligible couple:

- Primary sterility
- Secondary sterility
- Early menopause

Couple Protection Rate

It is an indicator of FP. It is the percentage of eligible couple protected against childbirth by approved methods of FP.

Incentive in FP

Following incentives are available for FP acceptances:

- Tubectomy – Rs. 200.00
- Laparoscopy – Rs. 145.00
- Vasectomy – Rs. 180.00
- Motivation of tubectomy – Rs. 10.00
- Motivation of vasectomy – Rs. 40.00

Present FP Organisation

District is the main unit and PHC is peripheral unit for FP activities (Fig. 17.7).

MTP (Medical Termination of Pregnancy) Act 1971

MTP is a safe, legal abortion made universally available for FP in the country.

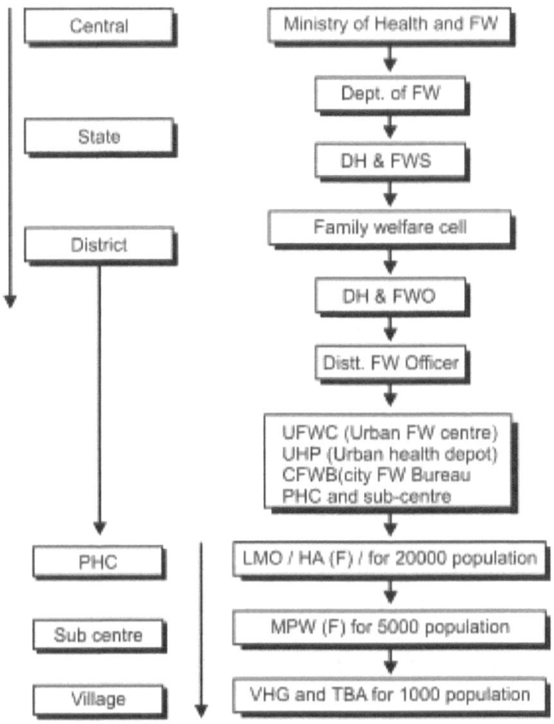

Fig. 17.7: FP organisation in India

Indications

- Medical when pregnancy causes injury or death to mother
- Eugenic when abnormal growth is established
- Humanitarian when rape has caused pregnancy
- Socio-economic when socio-economic cause can lead to death or injury to mother
- Failure of contraceptive when failed FP methods cause pregnancy.

Person to Perform MTP

- By RMP, if below 12 weeks of pregnancy
- By 2 RMP opinion, if above 12 weeks of pregnancy
- Place to perform
- DH and FWO can certify the place of conducting MTP

FP Depot Holders Scheme

Depot holders scheme is provided to ensure that supplies of nirodh, contraceptive jellies, foam tablets and OC tablets are available to people in villages.

It also enlists the assistance of the depot holders in motivating couples in their areas to use contraceptive methods or to undergo sterilisation.

Orientation training of depot holders is responsibilities of health inspectors of the area.

Place, time and date are fixed for a 3-hour programme of training. As per training manual, content is selected and done by group discussion method.

Emphasis is laid on the role of depot holders as under:

- Procuring supplies
- Storage of supplies
- Dispensing supplies
- Maintaining simple records and submitting regular reports
- Motivating couples to accept a contraceptive method
- Encouraging acceptors to be regular users
- Referring couples to the PHC or subcentre for sterilisation, IUD, or oral contraceptives, or for any complications following sterilisation or the use of contraceptives.

Role of Health Inspector in Education and Motivation for FP and Sterilisation Camps

Step I: The approach to the community is planned.

Step II: Community Health volunteers and trained TBAs are visited in the area

Step III: Meet the leaders in the community and plan with them a programme for education and motivation of the community for family planning. For example, the planning could cover any or all of the following points depending on the decision of the group.

Step IV: Methods followed are:
- Eligible couple survey
- Targets set by group itself
- Group meetings for men, for women or mixed groups
- Individual talks with couples
- Exhibitions and film shows are arranged
- Selection and training of depot holders is done
- Referral of cases for IUD, CC, vasectomy or tubectomy
- Deciding on responsibilities during vasectomy camps or tubectomy camps.

Contents for the Health Education

They can be:
- Need for small families
- Talking points on contraceptive methods
- Services available
- Sterilisation camps
- MTP
- Infertility

Following activities need to be done:
- Referrals are formulated
- Replenishment of depot holders' stock in the area
- Updating of eligible couple register

Report of the camp shall be prepared as per the procedure.

Checklist for the Health Inspector for the Selection of Oral Pill Acceptor

In case of any positive findings to the checklist, the MO must examine the case before putting on to OC.
- Woman must be below 35 years
- Not pregnant
- Not lactating
- Not malnourished
- Not obese
- No jaundice
- Not a smoker
- Not a diabetic
- No frequent headache
- No visual disturbances
- No convulsions
- No lump in the breast
- No oedema of extremities
- No pain in abdomen
- No breathlessness on exertion
- No irregular vaginal bleeding
- No history of PET\
- Pulse rate is normal
- No skin rashes

FAMILY PLANNING METHODS

Natural FP Method

Avoiding vaginal sex completely during fertile time. This is called periodic abstinence (Fig 17.8).

Vaginal Methods

They are spermicidal, diaphragm, cervical cap and vaginal sponge (Fig. 17.9).

Spermicidal include foaming tablets or suppositories, foam tablets, jelly and cream.

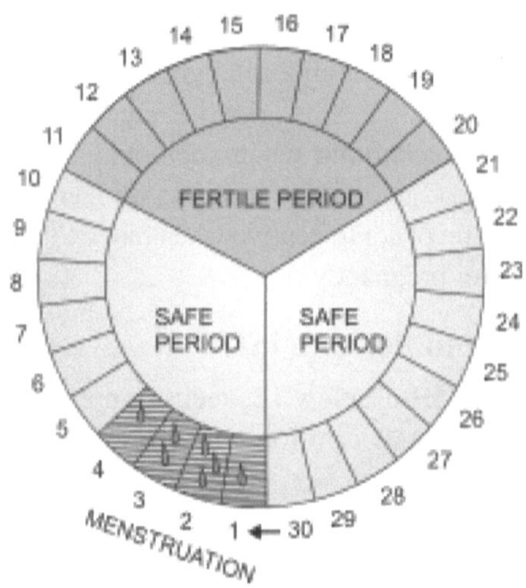

Fig. 17.8: Fertile period in menstruation

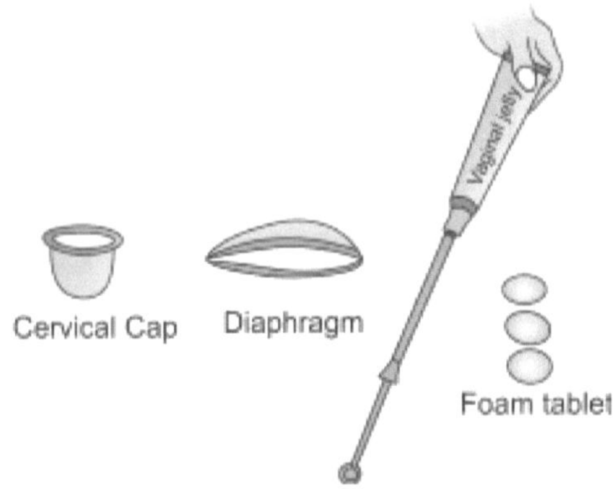

Fig. 17.9: Vaginal methods of FP

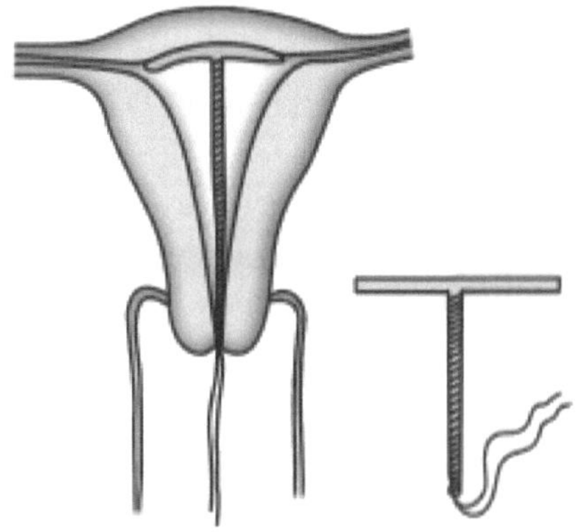

Fig. 17.10: IUD in position

They inhibit oxygen intake of sperms. Diaphragm is rubber cup that covers the cervix. Cervical cap is similar to diaphragm but smaller.

Vaginal sponge is available under trademark "Today".

Intrauterine Device (IUD)

Copper T is the present IUD that is used in the FP practice (Fig. 17.10). The user can check that the OUD is still in place by touching the strings. A nurse can remove the IUD by pulling gently on the strings with forceps.

Advantages of IUD

- Low expulsion rate
- Low side effect
- Easy to insert
- Better tolerated
- High protection rate
- Useful as postcoital contraceptive

It is not to be put in:

- Acute pelvic infection
- Chronic pelvic infection
- Menorrhagia

Most ideal time for IUD insertion is during menstruation or within 10 days of the beginning of a menstrual period. Post-puerperal insertion has several advantages.

Condom

It is made up of latex rubber. The government for free supply supplies them (Fig. 17.11).

Nirodh needs specific advice and correct use. Otherwise, it shows higher failure rate.

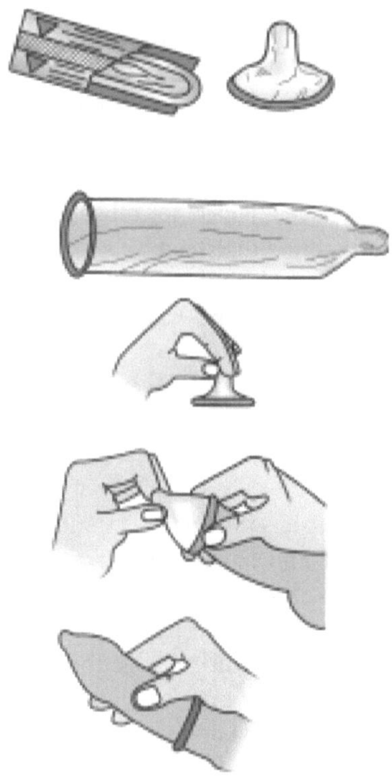

Fig. 17.11: Nirodh and its use

Its advantages are simple, reliable, no examination by a doctor is necessary, there are no complications, protects against STD, available at no cost by health centre.

Its limitations are it may tear off; needs self-discipline for use and it may interrupt intercourse, as it has to be put on after erection.

Female Sterilisation (Tubectomy)

It is a permanent contraception for women who do not want more children. It is safe and simple surgical procedure (Fig. 17.12). It is done in local anaesthesia and light sedation. There are two methods used:

- Minilaparotomy
- Laparoscopy.

Tubectomy

- This is an operation in woman in which the two tubes leading to the uterus are cut and tied so that the sperms cannot reach the eggs (Fig. 17.12).
- The tubectomy can be done either soon after delivery or it can be done at any other time convenient to the woman.
- When you select a case for tubectomy, look to the following requirements:
  - Her age must be between 20 and 44 years or she should still be having her menstrual periods.
  - The husband should not be below 25 years or over 50 years.
  - The couple should have two or more living children.
  - The couple should not want any more children and should understand the full implications of sterilisation.
- Advantages are:
  - After operation, no other action is necessary for FP
  - The operation is done free of charge in any government hospital or PHC.

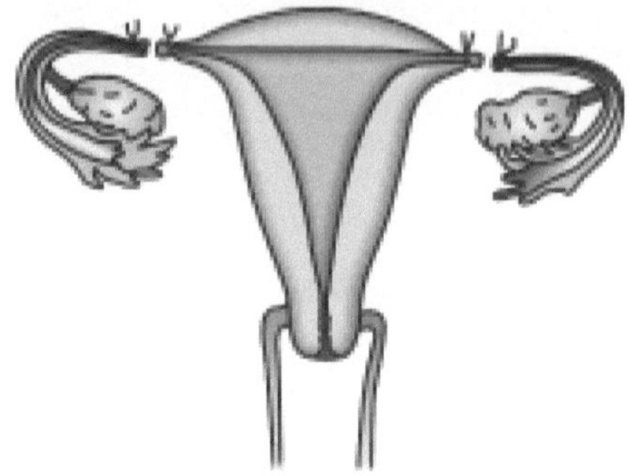

Fig. 17.12: Tubectomy procedure for sterilisation for woman

- The limitations of tubectomy are woman has to stay in hospital for 1 week—reversal operation, if woman wants baby wants baby, is difficult.

Minilap Operation

Minilap operation is safe, efficient and easy and is used in tubectomy camps. It is suitable for postpartum tubal sterilisation.

Male Sterilisation (Vasectomy)

It is a permanent contraception for men who decide they will not want more children. It is safe, simple, quick surgical procedure (Fig. 17.13). It can be done in a clinic, a camp. Guidance and counselling at

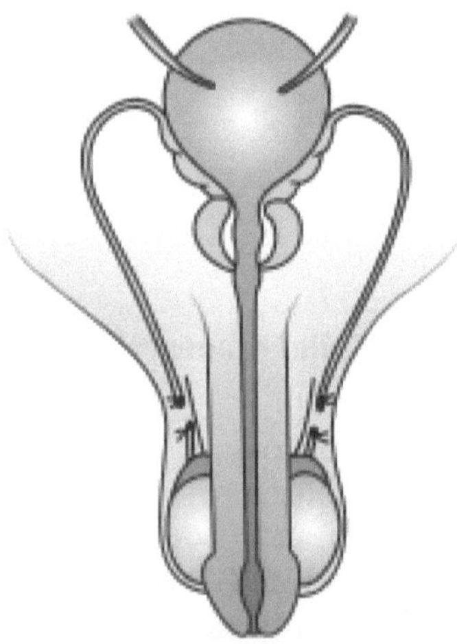

Fig. 17.13: Male sterilisation

nursing care require telling that it is not castration and it does not affect testes or it does not affect sexual ability of the man.

Indications for Vasectomy

- The man should not be below 25 years or above 50 years.
- The wife should not be below 20 years or above 44 years or she should be having her menstrual periods.
- The couple should not want any more issues and should understand the implications of sterilisation.

Advantages

- After the initial 12 ejaculations following the operation, no further action is needed to prevent conception.
- There is no need for hospitalisation.
- No interfere with sexual desire or with intercourse.
- No cost involved since it is done free.

Limitations

- Reversal is difficult.
- Pregnancy will occur in first 12 ejaculations.

No Scalpel Vasectomy (NSV)

It is a special procedure and has the following considerations:

- Use of a small puncture instead of 2" incision in the scrotum
- Special anaesthesia technique needs only one needle puncture instead of 2 or more
- Advantages are less pain, less bruising, short recovery time and less operating time.

Oral Contraceptives

They are effective contraceptives when properly used, which have 100 per cent effectiveness (Fig. 17.14).

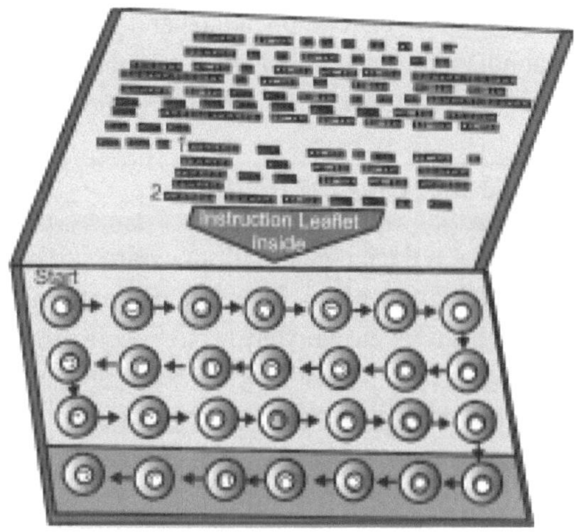

Fig. 17.14: Oral contraceptives

Combined Pills

Mala N (free supply through Health and FW Department) contains:

- Norgestrol 0.3 mg
- Ethinil oestradiol 0.03 mg

Mala D (21 active and 7 brown placebo) is made available under social marketing at low cost.

- Norgestrol 0.3 mg
- Ethinil oestradiol 0.03 mg

Oral contraceptives are taken by a woman to prevent the release of eggs from her ovaries. The first course of pills should be started on the 5th day of the menstrual cycle by taking the tablet from the pocket marked start. Everyday she should take one tablet, following the arrow on the card. As soon as one pack is finished, she should start with new pack.

Advantages are effective, no interference with sex life, can be discontinued for pregnancy.

Limitations are nausea, mild headache and dizziness.

By preventing ovulation, it prevents conception. It produces midcycle spotting, breast tenderness, facial pigmentation and nausea in first month.

Medially significant complications are:

- Jaundice, thromboembolism, severe headache, cervical erosion, and fibroid enlargement.

Progesterone Only Pill (POP)

They do not reduce breast milk; they are suitable for breastfeeding woman. There are no contraindications. This is taken everyday at one specific time.

ROLE OF HEALTH INSPECTOR IN MCH AND FP

Guidance, supervision to health worker (M) and health worker (F) in implementation of National FP programme.

- Education of community about various aspects of FW programme and benefits to them
- Involvement of community and members of other sectors in the form of block and village level committees for planning, implementation and evaluation of national FP programme
- Coordination of other agencies and sections in PHC activities
- Management of camps and campaigns
- Childcare services
- ICDS activities
- UIP activities
- Supplementary nutrition and therapeutic nutrition under childcare activities

General Activities of Health Inspector in Primary Health Centre FP Activities

- Utilise the information from the eligible couple and child register for the FP programme.
- Spread the message of FP to the couples in his area, motivate them for family planning individually and in groups and educate the community on the availability of services for medical termination of pregnancy.
- Distribute conventional contraceptives to the couples.
- Provide facilities and help to prospective acceptors of family planning services, if necessary by accompanying them to hospital.
- Provide follow-up services to FP acceptors, identify side effects, give treatment on the spot for side effects and minor complaints, and refer those cases that need attention by the MOH.
- Establish depot holders, help the PHC staff in training them, and provide a continuous supply of conventional contraceptives to the depot holders.
- Identify those women requiring help for MTP and refer them to the nearest approved institution.

18

Health Education and Communication

INTRODUCTION

All health and FW services are integrated with health education and communication. All medical, paramedical and local health workers are responsible for giving health education to the community; thereby the country can improve their health.

When once people are made to understand, they help themselves by their own actions and efforts. Community shows and develops responsibility for its own betterment as individual, as family member, as community member and as citizen of the country.

Like general education, health education is also a learning process, which is concerned with changes in knowledge, feelings and behaviour.

We provide facts, figures and available data, which can be called *information.*

In addition to providing facts and figures or information, if we emphasise on conduct by motivation, it is called *education.*

Very often for selfish motto or for commercial purpose, ideas are spread. They are called *propaganda.*

For the success of health education, the person who gives health education (communicator) should interact effectively. This interaction is called *communication.*

Communication is done through speaking, writing, facial expression, eye expression, body gesture or movement.

HEALTH EDUCATION OPPORTUNITIES FOR HEALTH INSPECTOR IN HIS WORKPLACE

- At OPD when the patient and his relatives visit PHC, subcentre or hospital
- Selected group of people who visit antenatal clinic
- Selected group of people who visit postnatal clinic
- Selected group of people who visit well-baby clinic
- Selected group of people who visit FP clinic
- Selected group of people who visit TB clinic
- Selected group of people who visit leprosy clinic
- Wards when the patient is admitted
- Individual counselling for:
  - Family planning
  - Chronic illness like TB, leprosy
  - Mothers with children having diarrhoea
- Field visit:
  - When fever case is approached
  - When scabies case is approached
  - When pregnant woman is approached
  - When an anaemia case is approached
- Informal group:
  - Need of water (near a well)
  - Need of food hygiene (near tea stall)

Definitions

Health Education

"Health education is a process that informs, motivates and helps people to adopt and maintain healthy practices and lifestyles, advocates environmental changes as needed to facilitate this goal and conducts professional training and research to the same end."

"Health education is part of health care to promote healthy behaviour."

Communication

"Communication is an interaction which takes place between two persons or among many persons through talking, writing, expression through body language. "

Philosophy

In health education, the main philosophy lies in changing behaviour of a person or of a family, or of a community to influence the behaviour of individual or a group. One has to go to the health problem of that person or group and on the acceptable methods in the country.

Health education increases knowledge and thus reinforces the required change of behaviour. Education also can have greater influence on health education in the community.

Scope

The scope of health education is many. It aims at carrying message to public by which one can change human behaviour. The scope lies in the following:

- Building healthy lifestyle
- Modifying individual behaviour
- Modifying social environment
- Make people to participate
- Make people to involve
- Make a person self-reliant
- Community also can be made self-reliant

HEALTH EDUCATION APPROACH

There are four known approaches in health education. They are:

- Information is conveyed by things, rules and regulations, for example,
  - Scooter helmet
  - Car seat belt
  - No smoking
  - No child marriage

  In this regulating approaches care is taken to see that human right is not taken off.
- Information is conveyed while giving health services, for example,
  - At bore well provision site
  - At the provision of RCA latrine

  While giving the health education at the doorstep, under service approach, one should take care of the need of the community.
- Information is conveyed by planned health education session and exposure of public in it. Here main health problems are considered, for example,
  - Role of small family norm
  - How to prevent HIV/AIDS
  - How to safeguard from water-borne diseases?
  - Importance of early detection of cancer

  This encourages human choice though it is a slow approach. It is possible to change behaviour pattern through mass media and social organisation.
- By conveying the information, the community through their active involvement on the problems of PHC, becomes self-reliant and gets required information from health worker (Table 18.1).

Content of Health Education

- *Information on health services*: There is no limit to the content of health education. It can include

Table 18.1: Health education and propaganda

Health education	*Health propaganda*
Knowledge is acquired and learnt	Knowledge is forced
People think	People do not think
Human behaviour	Animal behaviour
Reasoning present	Emotion present
Affects behaviour	Do not affect behaviour

any matter, which relates or produce interest in the minds of people, for example,
  - Immunisation session
  - FP camp
  - Cancer screening
- *Information on disease prevention and control:*
  - DDT spray on the walls of houses to kill mosquitoes
  - Iodised salt use to control endemic goitre
  - Use of potable water to prevent diarrhoea, cholera, polio, hepatitis
- *Information on family health:*
  - Child rearing practices
  - Child bearing practices
  - Self-care by elderly
- Information on personal hygiene, for example, bath, hand wash, toilet, nail clean, teeth care, oral hygiene
- Information on environmental hygiene, for example, food store, sanitary latrine, borewell use, waste disposal
- Information on good food, for example
  - Balanced diet
  - Diet in fever, heart disease
  - Prevention of malnutrition
- Information on accident prevention, for example
  - Road safety education
  - Occupational safety education
  - Prevention of home accident
- Information on mental health, for example
  - Assurance to family members at death of sole earner of the family
  - Economic loss of person when occurs
  - When a person is suffering from incurable cancer
- Information on human cycle, for example,
  - Human body structure and function
  - Information on habits like sleep, rest, exercise
  - Exclusive breastfeeding.

Principles of Health Education

At the outset, one should know that health education involves human psychology, touches human social component and is built on human behaviour. Hence, the following basic principles should be followed in every act of health education:

- It should be based on scientific knowledge.
- The topic must be useful to people. When it is useful, it creates interest.
- If a man starts thinking of health problem, thinks of his solution, he starts participating in health education.
- There must be some motivation for knowing the unknown, for example
  - Hunger makes man to eat
  - Fear of punishment prevents a person from stealing
  - Tubectomy undergone women can motivate their group
- Health education should be to the level of knowledge and education status of the person, for example, a tribal women is told about a pinch of salt rather than ½ a spoon of salt.
- Repeated health education makes a person to keep remembering the required healthy habits.
- Examples should be always from known objects
- It is advisable to make a person who knows a thing to tell others. This is called learning by doing.
- The person who gives health education should set examples to the community, for example
  - A person who has one child, telling about small family norm is welcome.

- A person who does not smoke telling on ill effects of smoking is welcome.
- It is always advisable to take help of local leaders, religious leaders, etc. in health education.

EDUCATION IN RELATION TO ENVIRONMENTAL SANITATION PROGRAMME

Chlorination of Water for Drinking Water

- Common sources are pond, tank, reservoir, river, lake and wells
- Human excreta, bathing, animal wash, storing in unclean utensil and pollute water
- Materials required for chlorinating a well like bleaching power, bucket and rope
- Method of preparing the bleaching powder solution for well-disinfections.

Soakage Pit

It is a hygienic method of disposal of wastewater, cheap and easy to construct (Fig. 18.1).

Kitchen Garden

Easy and useful method of disposal of household water to garden where fruits and vegetable can be grown.

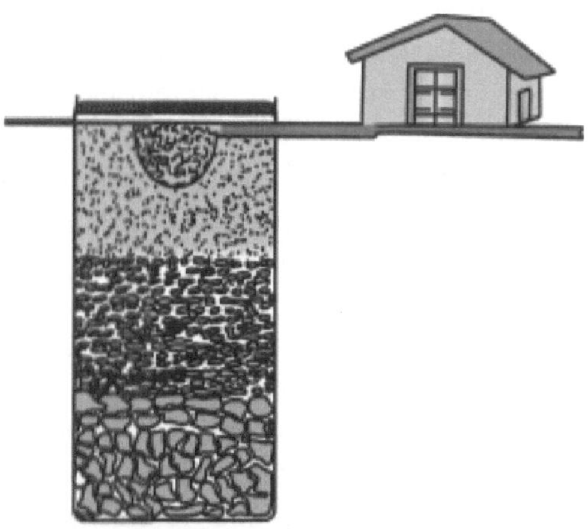

Fig. 18.1: Soakage pit

Compost Pit

Cow dung, horse dung and other animal excreta along with ash and refuse can be hygienically disposed in a pit, which gives compost manure.

RCA Latrine

Sanitary latrine is primarily the responsibility of owner of a house. It is simple, cheap and easy to maintain. BDO assistance is available for RCA latrine construction (Fig. 18.2).

Smokeless Chulhas

It reduces eye irritation, eye infection and is economical. House walls are not damaged.

HEALTH EDUCATION MATERIAL ON ENVIRONMENTAL SANITATION

Safe Drinking Water

Sanitary Open Well (Fig. 18.3)

- If water from unprotected sources is consumed, it can lead to diarrhoeal disease, typhoid and cholera.

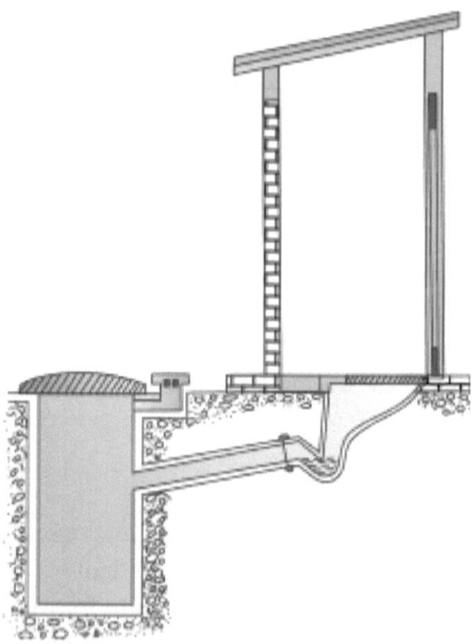

Fig. 18.2: RCA latrine

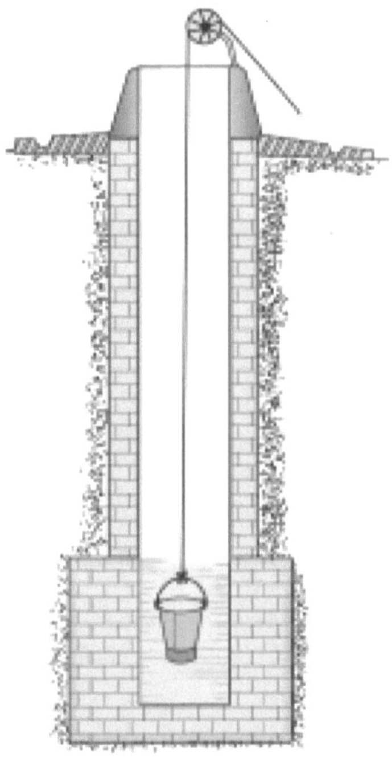

Fig. 18.3: Sanitary open well

- Water collected from ponds, tanks, etc. which have not been chlorinated should be boiled before drinking. This is particularly so during the rainy season.
- Well should be protected from contamination by (Fig 18.3):
  - Constructing a parapet 1 metre high around the well
  - Constructing a platform 2 metre around the well sloping downwards to the outside
  - Constructing a gutter around the outer edge of the platform to lead the waste water to a soakage pit
  - Using a clean bucket on a pulley for drawing water
  - Not washing clothes and utensils nor bathing near the well
  - Not allowing the well to fall into disrepair
- Although chlorinated water tastes different, it is safe to drink.

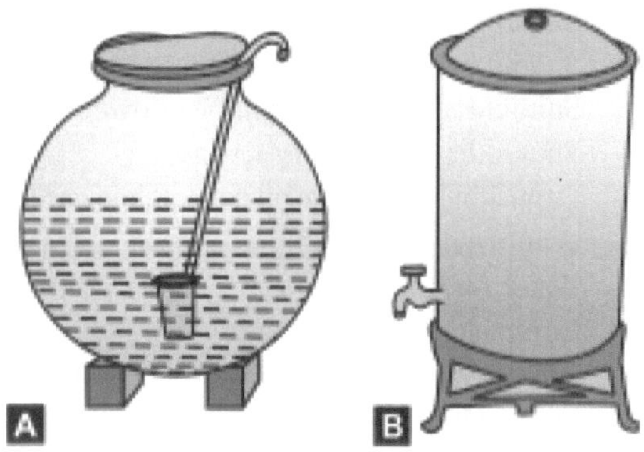

Figs 18.4 A and B: Storing and drawing water

- Water should be stored in clean containers and drawn in a hygienic way (Fig. 18.4).
- It is the responsibility of the whole community to see that their sources of drinking water are kept clean.

Sanitary Method of Disposal of Liquid Waste

- Water collection around the houses is a health hazard as it leads to mosquito-breeding.
- Collection of waste water gives rise to unpleasant odours
- Waste water can be safely disposed by constructing:
  - Soakage pits
  - Kitchen gardens

Solid Waste Disposal in Sanitary Way

- Solid waste attracts flies, dogs and produces unpleasant smell
- If dumped in drains, water gets stagnated and causes mosquito-breeding
- Composting, burning and burying are best methods
- It gives good fertiliser.

Home Sanitation

- Clean at home, keep all healthy
- Healthful housing means:
  - Well-built with concrete roof

- Smooth wall and floor for easy cleaning
- Should have good ventilation
- Sunlight and natural light be allowed
- Should have a sanitary latrine
- Provision for soakage pit and kitchen garden is allowed
- Water for drinking must be stored properly
- Compost pit should be provided
- Cowshed must be away from the house
- Smokeless chulha is advised
- Food grain storage must be proper

• Regular whitewash is advocated

Kitchen Garden

• Provides fruits and vegetables
• Waste water is easily disposed
• Cheap to have at home

Use of Sanitary Latrine

• Avoids fly breeding
• Sanitary method of night soil disposal
• No rubbish should be allowed in it
• Good maintenance is advocated
• It is a way of healthy life habits

Smokeless Chulhas (Fig. 18.5)

• Prevents eye irritation and eye infection
• Neat kitchen can be maintained
• Easy and cheap to construct
• It is fuel efficient

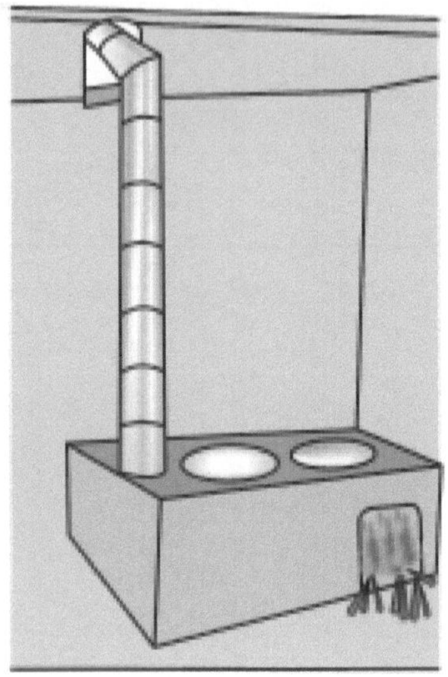

Fig. 18.5: Smokeless chulha

Food Hygiene

• Should be protected from rats, flies, etc.
• Need good protection (Fig. 18.6)
• Raw fruit or vegetable should be washed before eating
• Storing cooked food should be avoided since it ferments
• Rat proof bin is provided for food grain

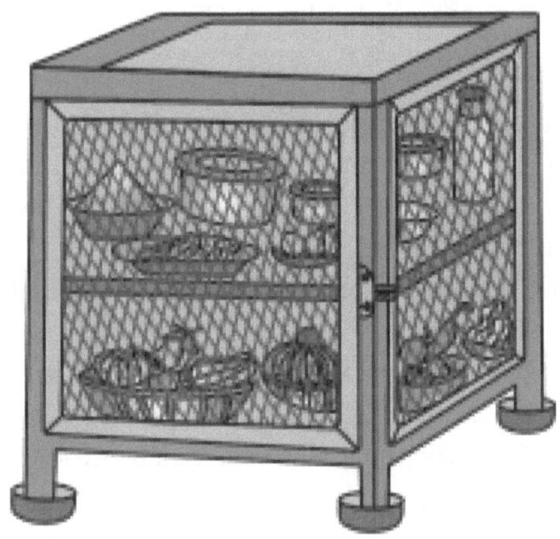

Fig. 18.6: Food store

Control of Insects, Dogs and Rodents

• Breeding of insects should be controlled.
• Stray dogs should be collected and killed as per the Municipality Act.
• Rodents are killed with poison.

Education on Personal Hygiene

- Clean personal habits
- Teeth care by brushing, rinsing and health check-up
- Attending to clean hair
- Head louse in children is to be attended
- Skin care
- Cloth cleanliness
- Hand and nail cleanliness
- Eye protection from dust, dirty cloth, dirty stick and foreign body
- Care at spitting, coughing and sneezing
- Ear care from stick, foreign body or hairpin

APPROACH

Sanitary Inspectors' Approach to Village Health Problems for Organising Education Programme

The approach to health education in a village is a carefully planned approach under health education programme. Before carrying out health education programme in the village, one should prepare checklists of all the steps to be taken by health inspector and other staff of primary health centre. Based on repeated health education activity, the health inspector can get many flexible forms of action-oriented activities.

Steps

The steps are enumerated below:

Step I: Health problems of the village are identified.

Step II: Health needs of the village are identified.

Step III: The problems and needs are discussed with PHC staff.

Step IV: Village leaders are identified (senior citizen, village head, religious heads, government agency representatives, etc.).

Step V: Village leaders are visited and a preliminary discussion is held with them.

Step VI: List out priority items, available facilities and problems that can be solved.

Step VII: Help of village leaders is taken in each step.

Step VIII: Village leaders help in: (1) topic for health education, (2) date and venue for health education, (3) available resources, (4) allotting responsibilities to public, (5) help in identification of problems, (6) help in solving problems, (7) preparation of talking points, (8) decide audio-visual aids, (9) orient village leaders on the given topic, (10) implement health education, (11) do follow-up, and (12) get feedback from village.

Tips

Following are tips for the health inspector for the health education in the village:

- Give only required information during health education
- Topic must be on current problem and on current need
- See to the convenience of the community for place and time of session
- Use local language
- Talk first and demonstrate later
- Allow questions at health education session
- Do not criticise anyone
- Do not loose temperament
- Let health education be short and sweet
- At the end do not forget to give the summary.

AUDIO-VISUAL AID IN HEALTH EDUCATION

AV aid helps the medical and paramedical in effective health education. Without AV aid any health education is incomplete. There are many AV aids that are used in health education activities.

Common and feasible AV aids are enumerated below:

- Radio
- Tape recorder
- Mike
- Chalk board
- Leaflet
- Poster
- Chart
- Model
- Specimen
- Television
- Cinema projection.

Above AV aids help in the following way. They are called principles in the use of AV aids.

- Create interest
- Depict clear ideas
- Saves time of the person who gives health education
- Presentation will become lively
- Presentation is made attractive
- They are remembered well by the audience
- They stimulate the audience to ask questions

Health education materials, like charts, posters, and photos, are available with BEE and with Deputy Health Education Officer from whom they can be procured.

By using paint, paper, card, scissor, string and glue, one can prepare local indigenous AV aids.

Place of AV Aids in Health Education

They are used in:

- Individual approach
- Group approach
- Mass approach.

Here folk media like *harikatha*, folk song, dance, drama, *gazelles*, *kawali*, *keerthan*, mono-acting, and puppet show are used as instruments of better health education.

Tools and Techniques in Health Education

For individual health education:

- Contacted in person
- Counselling done
- Home visit paid
- Correspondence by letter done

For selected group health education:

- Lecture is given with the help of a blackboard
- Demonstration done with chart, model and cases
- Group discussion done by using flipchart, flannellograph, exhibits and charts
- Role play by socio-drama is found appealing

For mass health education:

- Cinema projection
- Radio programme
- Local newspaper
- Poster distributions
- Health exhibition.

Utilising Community Resources for Health Education

- Media acceptable in the locality is assessed. One may find *Powada*, *Katha*, *Tamasha* or puppet more popular.
- With imagination and ingenuity, using paper, paint, card, scissors, string, and gum, cut outs are made, photos of magazines can be taken and newspaper cuttings can be used (local language) (Fig 18.7).
- One can make own glove puppet to use them to illustrate a health story or for a health song. Local folk story or folkway song can be selected.

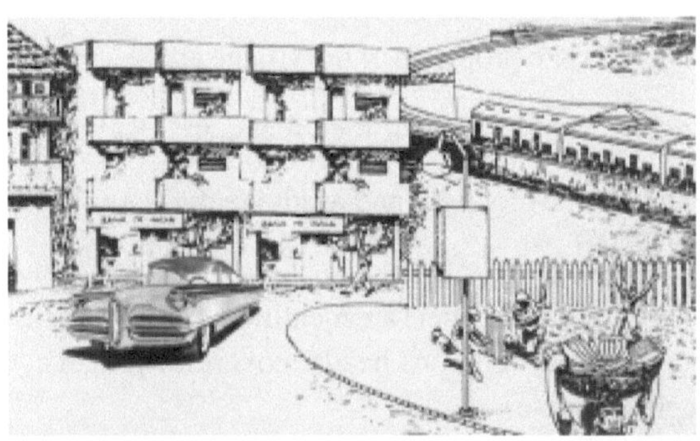

Fig. 18.7: Gathering the information of a clean city

- *Chitra katha*, a folk art is used by series of pictures on cards to tell a story.
- Aids done by local community traditions and culture are very well-accepted.

A mud wall can be smeared with a smooth layer of cow dung. One can draw picture by white wash on it. When another picture is to be written, the wall is smeared with fresh cow dung to erase it.

Education through Primary Health Centre

Waiting time of patient and relatives attending OPD is used. Various topics are selected for:

- Antenatal clinic
- Postnatal clinic
- Well baby clinic
- Family planning clinic
- Tuberculosis clinic
- Leprosy clinic.

Field Visits

- During field visit for attending a fever case, a scabies case, a pregnant woman, and individual talk are useful.
- During well disinfections, informal group can be given information. The group receives health education on safe use of well water better.
- At hotel, an informal group can be told about sanitary food storage to prevent food-borne diseases.
- At school visit, informal and formal talk to teachers and schoolchildren about safe water, handwash, not eating exposed food, proper disposal of waste in school are found useful.
- OTC camps on Health and Family Welfare for leaders are arranged at PHC.
- During eye camp, tubectomy camp, vasectomy camp, IUD camp education is found very useful.

Campaign

Campaign for H and FW Service activities like:

- FP fortnight
- WHO day celebration
- AIDS day celebration
- Antimalaria campaign
- Leprosy month celebrations are welcome.

Health education and communication can be summarised as in Figure 18.8.

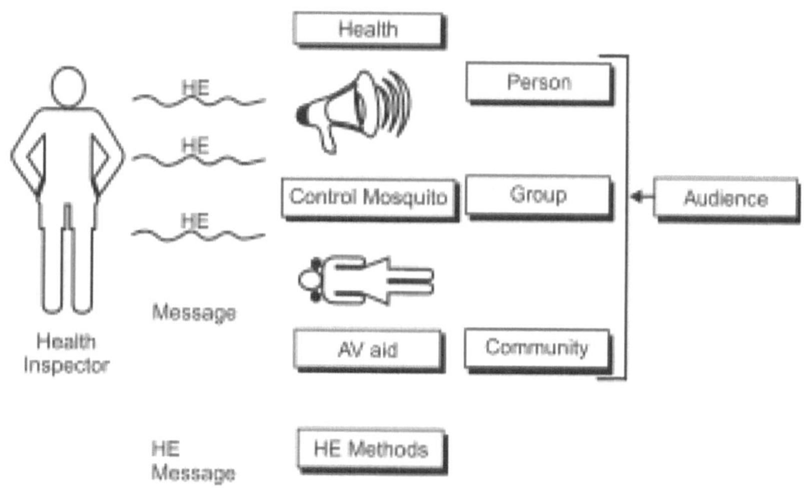

Fig. 18.8: Health education (HE) and communication (summary diagram)

COMMONLY USED TERMINOLOGIES IN HEALTH EDUCATION

• One-way communication	– HI speaking to villagers
• Two-way communication	– Group discussion
• Obstacle or barrier of communication	– Cannot hear – Language not understood – Too much noise
• Counselling	– It is a process to make a person to understand his problem who is emotionally disturbed
• Oldest method of health education	– Folk method
• Latest method of health education	– Internet
• Mass approach	– It is the education of general public through newspapers posters, AVD, TV, museums and exhibitions
• Folk media	– It refers to *Harikatha*, *Yakshagana*, Monoact, drama, folk song, folk story, and puppet show, *Gazzal*, *Khawali*

ORGANISATIONS INVOLVED IN HEALTH EDUCATION IN THE COUNTRY

- CHEB (Central Health Education Board, New Delhi)
- State Health Education Board
- District Health Education Board
- DAVP (Directorate of Advertising and Visual Publicity)
- AIR (All India Radio)
- Doordarshan
- Indian Red Cross
- Branches of International Union for Health Education.

19

First Aid

There is nothing more exciting or wonderful in the world than doing or giving first aid to safeguard man's life from damages that have occurred by accident, fall, injury and acute manifestation of diseases.

OBJECTIVES OF FIRST AID

The main objectives of first aid are:
- To save life
- To prevent further injury
- To prevent further complications
- To produce improvement
- To prepare and get medical treatment
- To assist the doctor by giving first hand information.

In all cases of first aid, the health workers should cultivate certain qualities like self-confidence, tactfulness, judgement, organising ability and sympathy.

DROWNING

Drowning is a common cause of obstruction of air passage causing failure of breathing. Brain and heart are affected. Death can occur within minutes. Early rescue and application of artificial respiration without delay gives best chance for recovery. Exposure to cold and drop in body temperature are also to be attended.

Immediate Action

As soon the person is taken to air from water, immediate action is taken for the following:
- Clearing air passage
- Immediate artificial respiration
- Heart massage if required
- Body protection from cold
- Transfer to nearest hospital.

Clearing the airway from nose or from mouth to lung is necessary for artificial respiration. When head and neck are extended, the tongue does not fall back and a clear air passage is produced (Fig. 19.1).

By pulling jaw the airway can be enlarged.

Mouth-to-Mouth Respiration

See the pictorial representations given in Figure 19.2.

Steps

While giving mouth-to-mouth respiration, the following steps should be followed:
- With one hand, hold the jaw forward with the mouth open. The thumb should not be placed inside the mouth (it may be bitten at recovery).
- Thumb and forefinger of other hand are used to keep the nostril closed, while the wrist steadies the extended head.

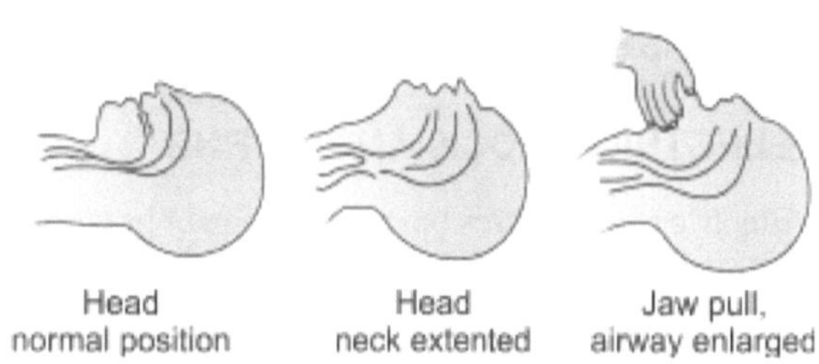

Fig. 19.1: Clearing the airway

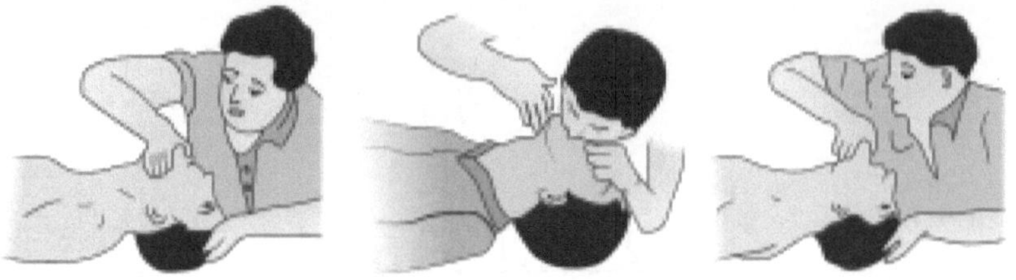

Fig. 19.2: Mouth-to-mouth respiration

- A fairly deep breath is taken
- Open mouth is placed round that of drowned and steadily blowed into his mouth. If air enters, the chest rises
- Mouth is removed and a further breath is taken When air comes out, chest is seen falling back.
- The action is repeated till natural breathing is restored.

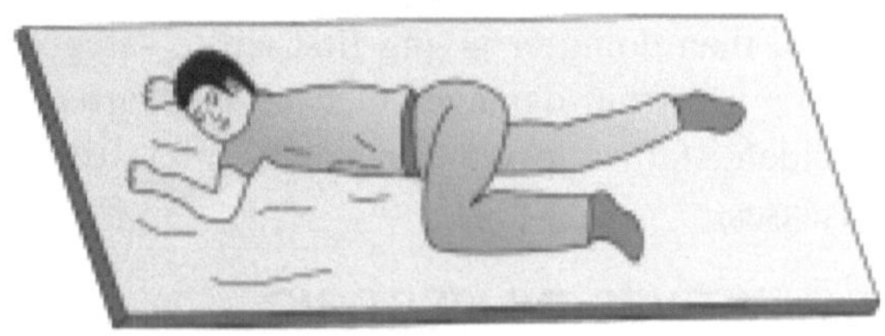

Fig. 19.3: Position to be maintained after recovery

Recovery Position

When normal breathing starts, he is turned into recovery position (Fig. 19.3).

Manual Resuscitation

Steps

While giving the manual resuscitation, the following steps should be observed (Fig. 19.4):

- The patient is placed on his back
- Cushion or mound of sand is kept between shoulder-blade
- Sitting behind head, forearms are grasped
- Draw arms upwards, outwards and backwards
- Sweep back arms to ribs and squeeze chest
- Repeated till breathing recovers
- Put to recovery position.

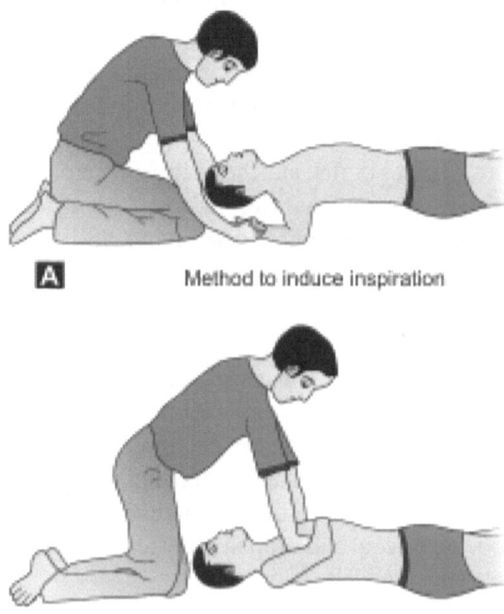

Figs 19.4A and B: Sylvester-Brosche's method of manual resuscitation

ELECTRIC SHOCK AND BURNS

Electric shock causes burns, stoppage of breathing, stoppage of heartbeat.

Signs

The signs of electric shock will be:

- Patient is unconscious
- Patient is in contact with a source of electricity.

First Aid

- Shut off the current
- Free the person from source of electricity by using a piece of wood, paper, rubber to push or to pull him away
- Mouth-to-mouth respiration is given till the pulse returns

  After recovery, the skin is examined for burns.

Community Education

Educate the community on how to avoid electric shock by taking the following points:

- Ensure safe electric points
- Ensure no live wires are exposed
- Prevent children playing with sockets and switches
- Prevent children from climbing up electric poles.

HEATSTROKE

This results from exposure to excessive heat and sun and may occur during the hot summer months. It is more likely to occur in those who have been drinking alcohol and those who are weak.

Signs and Symptoms

The early signs and symptoms of heatstroke are:

- High body temperature (up to 42°C)
- Headache
- Dizziness
- Nausea and vomiting
- Cramps in the limbs
- Dry flushed hot skin.

  The patient may become unconscious later on.

When this happens, he usually dies.

First Aid

- Put him in the shade in the coolest and most airy place
- Undress him
- Pour cold water over him or apply cold clothes
- If conscious, give cold drinks.

Community Education

Educate the community on how to avoid heatstroke by adopting the following steps:

- Avoid exposure to direct sunlight
- Drink plenty of cold water with lime juice and salt if possible, during the hot season
- Cover head and back of neck with turban or towel when exposed to the sun for long periods
- Avoid drinking alcohol.

ANIMAL BITES

Snake bite

Snake bite produces punctured wound caused by fangs of a snake. Wound seems small. But most of the snakes are poisonous. Hence, unless you see the snake and know that it is not poisonous, you should always treat the snake bite as poisonous.

Signs and Symptoms

- The person may tell you that he has seen the snake that has bitten him
- The two wounds produced by the snake's fangs are visible
- The person may show bleeding as a sign of poisoning
- The person may show paralysis as a sign of poisoning
- There may be signs of shock.

First Aid

- Tie a piece of cloth tightly above the bite to prevent the blood from returning to the heart

- With clean razor blade, make 4 to 6 cuts 1 cm deep over the bite area
- Squeeze the part hard so that blood flows out of the cuts
- Apply potassium permanganate crystals in the cuts
- Apply a piece of clean gauze or cloth on the cuts
- Rush him to hospital for getting antivenom.

The piece of cloth tied above the bite should be removed for a few minutes every half an hour. The requirements of cloth tying do not occur after 3 hours of bite.

Except for simple drug like APC for pain, no other drug or injection is allowed in first aid.

Scorpion Bite

The person stung by a scorpion, usually a child, complains of severe pain at the site of the sting and shows signs of shock (Table 19.1). A scorpion sting is poisonous and if the child is small and weak, it may produce serious results.

Insect Bite

Honeybee, wasp and hornet stings occur in rural areas, especially if the nests of insects are disturbed (Table 19.2).

Dog Bite

In India, dog bite causing hydrophobia or rabies alarms the concern for any dog bite. It should be considered seriously.

Table 19.1: Signs and symptoms and first aid for scorpion bite

Signs and symptoms	*First aid*
• Patient will tell that he is stung by a scorpion • The wound is red; there may be bleeding • Signs of shock are present particularly in children	• Cold compress to the site of sting • Treat shock • Give APC tablet • Refer to hospital at the earliest

Table 19.2: Signs and symptoms and first aid for insect bite

Signs and symptoms	*First aid*
• History of attack and stung by insect • Site of sting is red, swollen and painful	• Cold compress to the site of sting • APC tablet • Refer to hospital or PHC for advice

Dog bite will be invariably infected because dirt and germs are introduced into the wound from the teeth of the dog (Table 19.3).

ACCIDENTS

Accident is an event, which happens unexpectedly. The extent of injury depends on various factors. The injuries caused by accident are:

- Wound
- Sprain
- Dislocation
- Fracture
- Burns and
- Scalds.

Sometimes, there may be history of injury by accident but there may not be any visible injury. However, in these conditions, the patient may be unconscious, may show signs of shock or may complain of pain. In these circumstances, after

Table 19.3: Signs and symptoms and first aid for dog bite

Signs and symptoms	*First aid*
• History of dog bite • There may be one or more irregular wounds	• Clean the wound with soap and water • Swab the wound with antiseptic lotion • Apply mercurochrome to the wound • Refer to health centre or hospital for advice and ARV treatment

attending to first aid, at the earliest the case must be shifted to a hospital for required emergency treatment.

Primary Duty at First Aid

The primary duty at first aid will be:
- To provide medical aid as quickly as possible
- To prevent danger of death
- To prevent progress of seriousness.

Rules

Following are rules to be followed at every time of dealing with an accident:
- Stop any bleeding
- Give artificial respiration, if required
- Tight clothing around neck, chest, waist and foot must be undone
- Handle the patient as gently as possible
- Place the patient in a comfortable position
- Guard against shock
- Do not remove clothing unnecessarily
- Reassure the patient
- Relieve the pain
- Reassure the crowd
- Arrange for the required:
  - Positioning
  - Splints
  - Bandaging
  - Tourniquet

TRANSPORT OF THE INJURED

There are two methods that are used to carry the injured. This constitutes vital area of first aid. They are as follows:
1. Manual transport:
   - By one person:
     - The cradle carry
     - The human crutch
     - The pick-a-back
     - Dragging
     - The drag-carry
     - Fireman's lift and carry.
   - By more than one person:
     - The two-hand seat
     - The human stretcher
     - The three-hand seat
     - The four-hand seat.
2. Stretcher transport:

   This includes stretcher bearing and an ambulance, found very useful for shock, haemorrhage and fractures.

Rules

General rules to be followed in transport while at first aid:
- Safety
- Steadiness
- Speed
- Continuous observation

Manual Transport

Cradle Carry

The first aider stoops by the side of patient, places one arm under his knees and the other well round his back, rises and carries the patient. This is very useful for children and lightweight patients (Fig. 19.5).

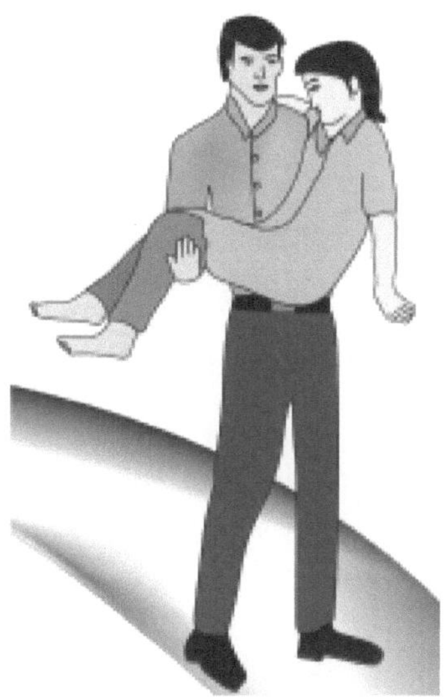

Fig. 19.5: Child carrying (Cradle carry)

Human Crutch

This is useful for adults who have slight injury. The patient must be able to help by placing lightweight on the injured foot and supporting himself against the first aider's body (Fig. 19.6).

Pick-a-Back

This is useful to carry a conscious adult patient. Here the patient is able to support himself on the first aider's back (Fig. 19.7).

Fireman's Lift and Carry

This is a useful method of carrying an adult patient where first aider will have one free hand (Fig. 19.8).

The first aider lifts the patient into upright position and grasps the patient's right wrist with his left hand; then, bending down with his head under the patient's extended right arm, places his right arm around or between the patient's legs. Taking the body weight to right shoulder, he rises to erect position, pulls the patient across both shoulders, transfers patient's right wrist to his right hand, which will allow his left hand free.

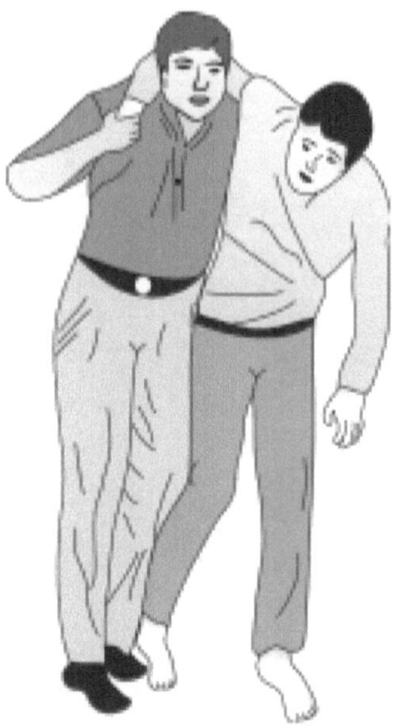

Fig. 19.6: Adult carrying (human crutch)

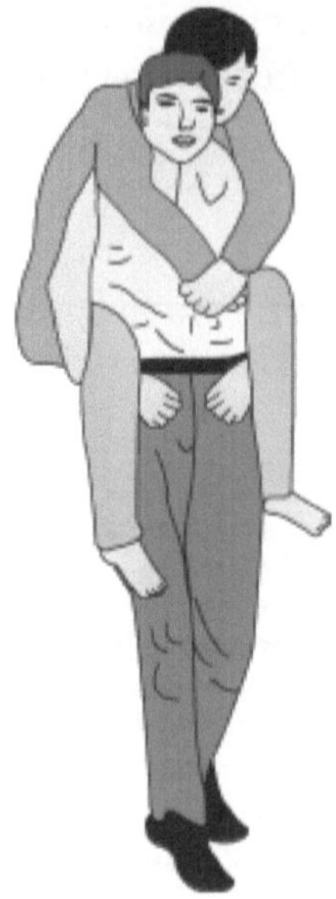

Fig. 19.7: Adult carrying (pick-a-back)

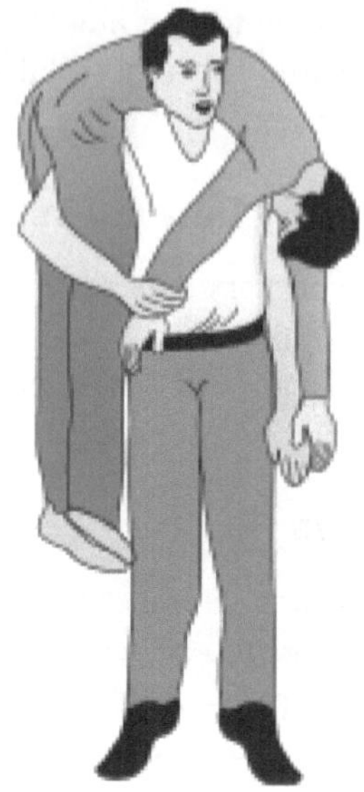

Fig. 19.8: Fireman's lift

The 2-Hand and 4-Hand Seats

Figures 19.9 and 19.10 show how to make a hook grip by 2 hands and a fix grip by four hands.

These are useful when the patient is conscious.

Stretcher Transport

St. John Ambulance Association has formulated many types of stretchers among which the following are widely used:

- Ordinary
- Telescopic
- Metal
- Mark-2 (army).

They are called Furley stretchers named after the late Sir John Furley (Fig. 19.11).

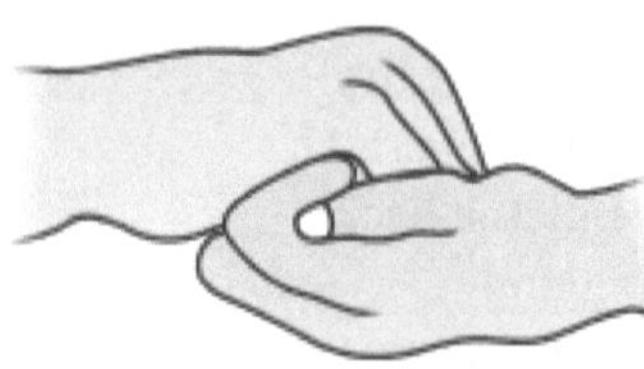

Fig. 19.9: Hook grip to carry sick patient (2 hands)

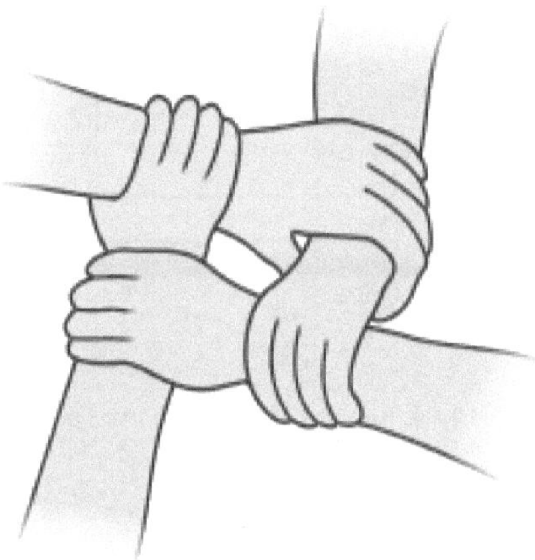

Fig. 19.10: Fix grip with 4 hands

Preparation

Preparation of a stretcher includes:

1. Opening of a stretcher
2. Testing the stretcher
3. Blanketing of stretcher.

Loading

Loading the stretcher needs 4 bearers who work as a team (Fig. 19.12). They are numbered 1, 2, 3, and 4 and shown for learning or practice purpose. No. 2 and 4 should be stronger who carry the patient. Loading includes:

- Lifting
- Lowering

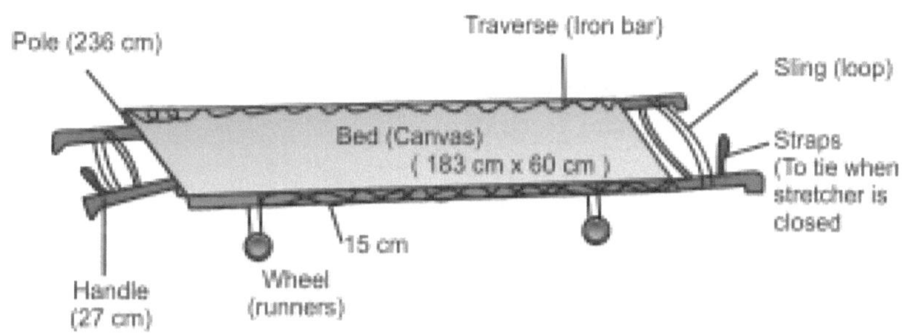

Fig. 19.11: Structure of a stretcher

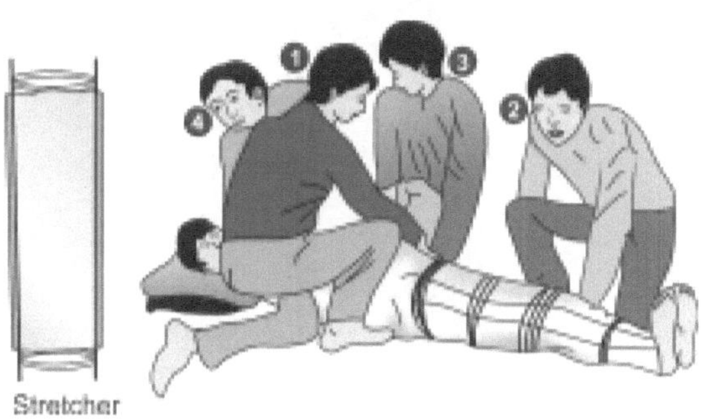

Fig. 19.12: Lifting patient to stretcher positions of stretcher bearers

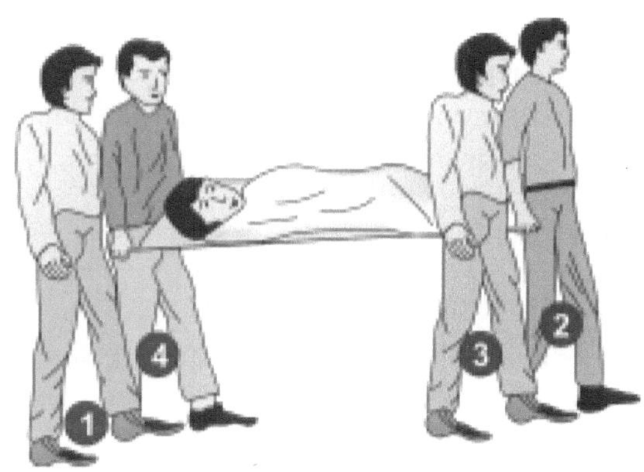

Fig. 19.13: Advancing (bearers carrying 2 and 4, 1 and 3 walking on right)

- Wrapping
- Patient arrangement.

Advancing

Advancing stage includes (Fig. 19.13):
- Lifting
- Adjustment
- Carrying
- Observing throughout
- Shoulder carry.

BANDAGING

It is a part of first aid. Art of bandaging hallmarks the aid giving at accidents and emergencies.

Triangular Bandage

Very commonly used is a special kind of bandage called triangular bandage which is normally prepared by cutting diagonally a square piece of calico cloth (Fig. 19.14).

Parts

Parts of triangular bandage and its use are depicted in Figure 19.15.

Advantages

Advantages of triangular bandage are:
- Can prepare broad and narrow bandages
- Can fit any part of body without any discomfort
- It is an emergency tool.

Uses

Uses of triangular bandages are:
- Help to secure dressings
- Slings can be prepared
- Help in fixing splints
- Help to secure pads
- Can be used as a roller bandage (Fig. 19.16).

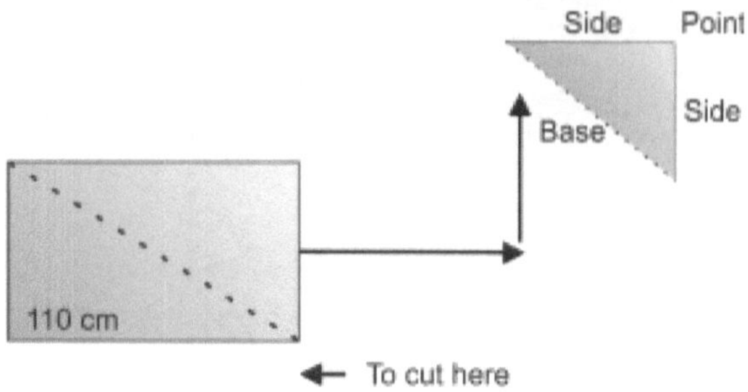

Fig. 19.14: Triangular bandage from calico cloth

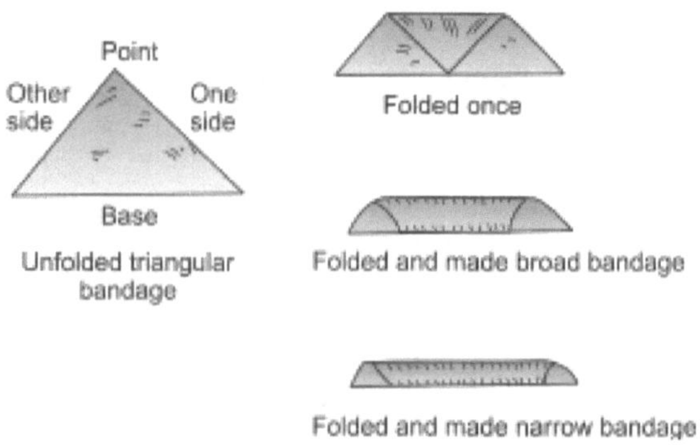

Fig. 19.15: Use of triangular bandage

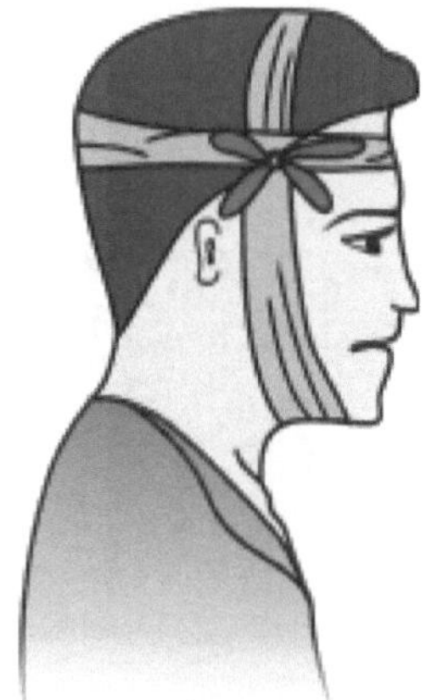

Fig. 19.16: Support of lower jaw by narrow bandage

Wrist Bandage

It is used to retain a dressing on the palm of the hand. It is also useful for sprains of the wrist (Fig. 19.17).

Ankle Bandage

It is helpful in ankle sprain. It can be made wet after application to make it tighter (Fig. 19.18).

For chest, place the point of the bandage over the shoulder of the affected side of the chest, allowing the remainder of the bandage to hand downwards (Fig. 19.19). For back, place the point of the bandage over the shoulder of the affected side of the back so that it touches the collar bone, and allow the remainder of the bandage to hand downwards across the back (Fig. 19.20).

Spiral Bandage

It is a pattern of bandaging. It is useful for a limb, for a finger where there is little increase in thickness (Fig. 19.21).

Fracture

Triangular Sling to Support

Collar bone fracture: Direct violence; fall on the hand causes fracture of collar bone which needs

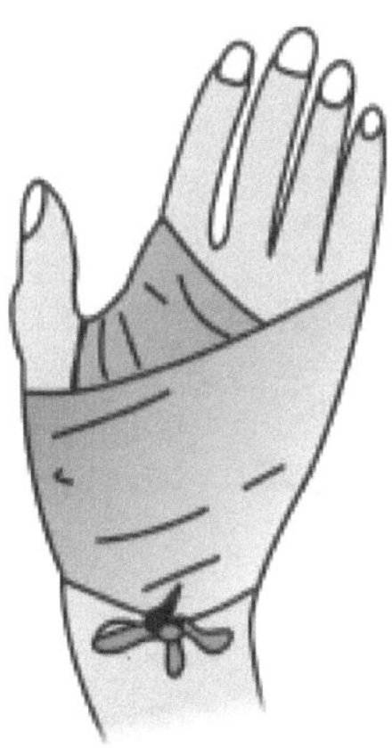

Fig. 19.17: Bandage for wrist

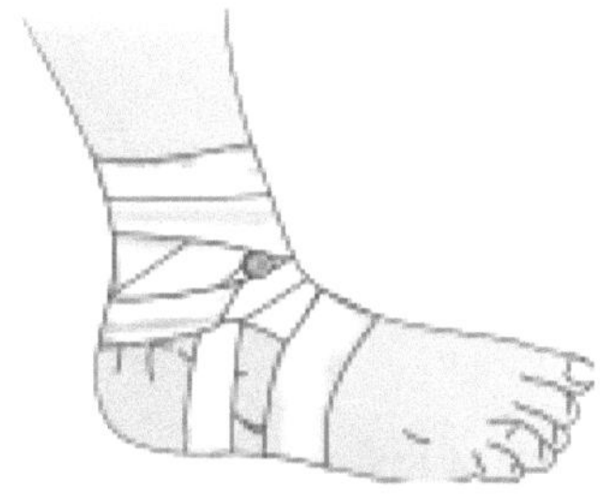

Fig. 19.18: Ankle bandage

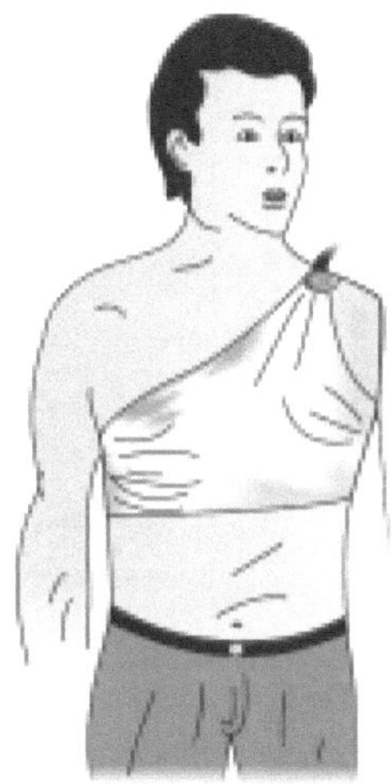

Fig. 19.19: Bandage for chest

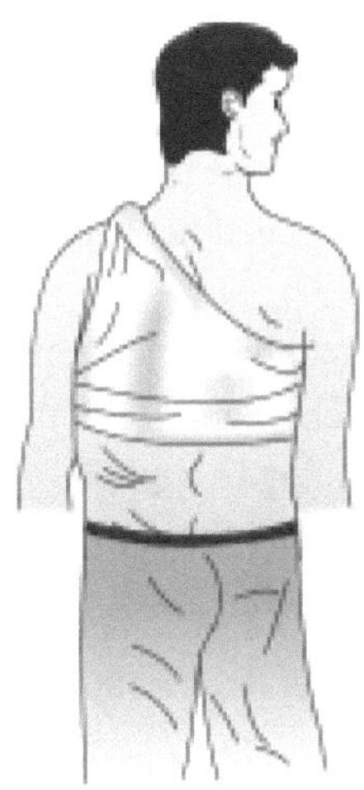

Fig. 19.20: Bandage for back

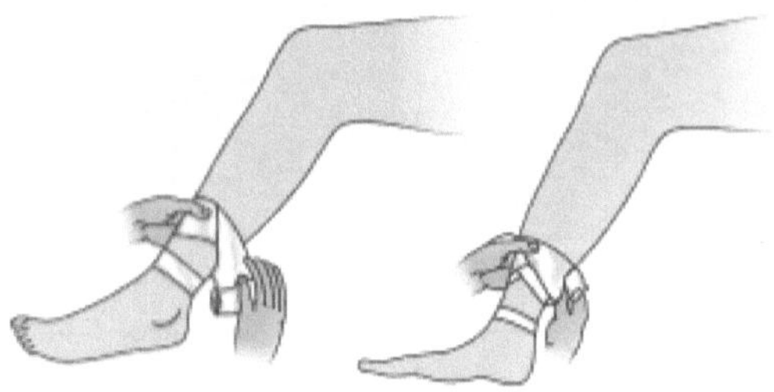

Fig. 19.21: Method of putting the spiral bandage

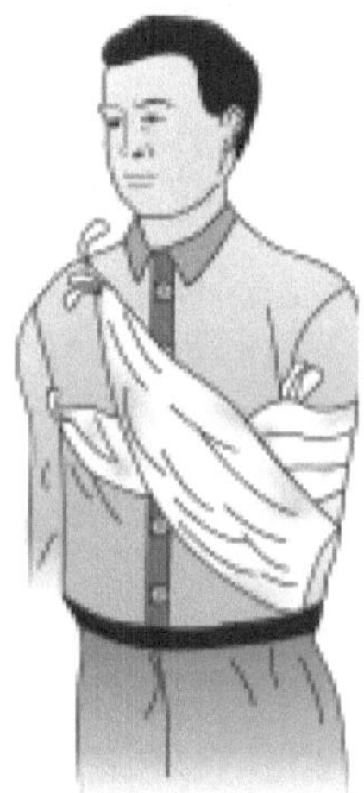

Fig. 19.22: Triangular sling to support fractured collar bone

immediate immobilization by sling method (Fig. 19.22).

The procedure involves:

- Immediate support to arm on the injured side
- Padding is applied between upper arm and the chest
- Using a broad bandage secures the arm to the side of the chest and leave the forearm free
- Triangular sling is applied
- Pulse is checked for active circulation.

Small Arm Sling

It is intended to supply support to wrist and hand, which leaves elbow free. It is made from a broad bandage and the knot is tied on the injured side (Fig. 19.23).

Collar- and-cuff Sling

When we want to restrict the movement of elbow joint, this type of sling is found very useful (Fig. 19.24).

This is made out of a roller bandage by forming a clove hitch (Fig. 19.25).

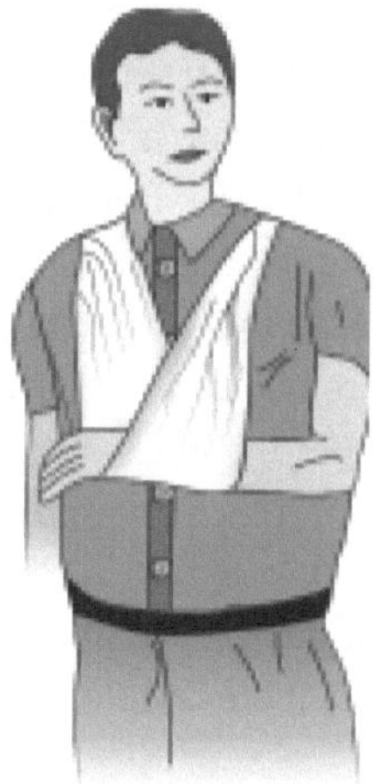

Fig. 19.23: Small arm sling for support to wrist and hand

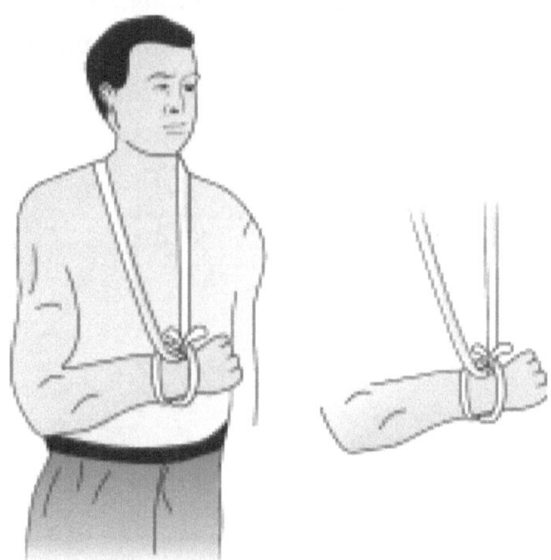

Fig. 19.24: Collar-and-cuff sling to restrict movement of elbow

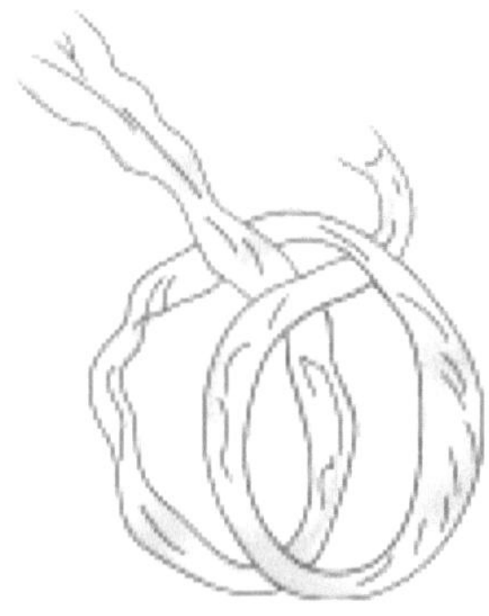

Fig. 19.25: Clove hitch from a roller bandage

Splint for Arm Bone Fracture

When shaft of arm bone is fractured, it requires splint for support. The affected arm should be put in a small arm sling. Guide one bandage through armpit and allow its upper end to hang over the shoulder. The second bandage is placed through the bend of the elbow. Three splints of suitable length are applied to the arm (front, outside and back). The bandages are collected round the arm and splints and tied (Fig. 19.26).

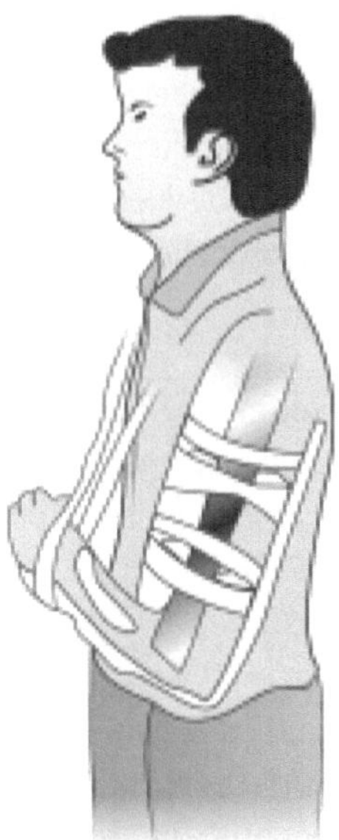

Fig. 19.26: Splint for arm bone fracture

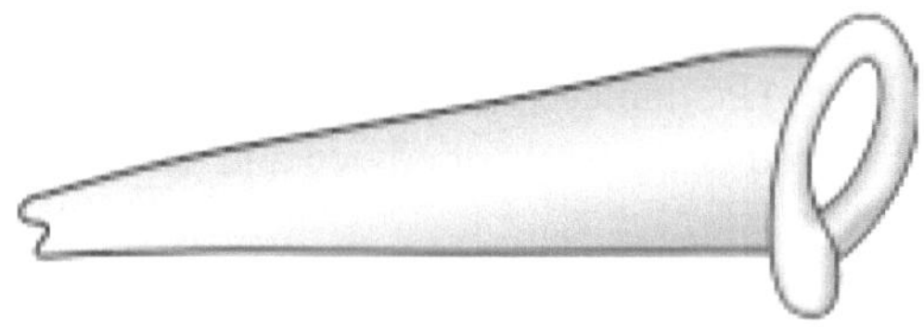

Fig. 19.27: Thomas splint for thigh bone

Thomas splint: It is a well-known splint for fracture of thigh bone (Fig. 19.27).

Thomas' splint is readily available. It can be applied without removing shoes. Since it fixes lower limb, fractured bone does not jolt during transport.

WOUNDS

Wound is a break or tear in the skin following an accident. The deeper the wound, the more likely it is to bleed and get infected, as it cannot be properly cleaned. First aid allows control of bleeding and infection.

Types of Wound

The types of wound are:

- Grazed
- Cut
- Torn
- Punctured.

First Aid

- The patient is allowed to sit or lie down
- Gentle handling is required
- Cleaned with water and soap. Cleaning must be always away from the wound
- Washed with antiseptic solution
- Dirt and foreign matter are removed
- Bleeding is controlled by pressure or by tourniquet
- Mercurochrome and sulphonamide powder are applied
- If gaping, adhesive plaster helps
- Needs dressing and bandage

- If necessary, shock is treated
- Given APC tablet
- Referred to hospital for advice and action

Sprains

This occurs when a muscle is twisted or contracted.

Dislocations

This occurs when a joint is twisted or by a sudden wrench (Table 19.4).

Fractures

Fracture is a broken bone. It may be a crack (hairline), broken to 2 pieces or splintered (Table 19.5).

Types of Fractures

Open: There is wound reaching from skin right down to the broken bone or the broken bone may protrude through the wound.

Closed: There is no wound leading down to the bone and there is no bone protruding through the skin.

Table 19.4: Signs and symptoms and first aid for sprains and dislocations

Signs and symptoms	*First aid*
	Sprain
• Severe pain	• Rest
• Swelling	• Support
• Bruising around	• Cold compress
• Reduced movement	• Bandage (elastic)
• Deformity in dislocation	• Referred to health centre or hospital
• Signs of shock may be present	
	Dislocation
	• Rest
	• Support
	• Keep in comfortable position
	• Treat shock if present
	• Shift to health centre or hospital

Table 19.5: Signs and symptoms and first aid for fractures

Signs and symptoms	*First aid*
• History of fall or accident	• Make comfortable and give support
• Pain at the site	• Do not remove clothing
• Tenderness present	• Immobilise by splint or bandage
• Inability to move the part	• Treat shock if present
• Deformity may be present	• Stop bleeding if present
• Swelling at the site	• Arrange transport
• Fracture may be felt	• Referral at the earliest
• Movement at a place where there should be no movement	
• Broken end of bone may be seen protruded	

Specific First Aid

All fractures need the following specific first aid:

- Immobilise
- Arrange transport
- Give first aid
- Shift to hospital or health centre.

Burns and Scalds

Burns are caused by dry heat (fire, explosive, petrol burn, hot metal or electricity).

Scalds are caused by wet heat (boiling water, steam, hot oil, hot ghee, heated tar) (Table 19.6).

Shock

Severe injury, bleeding, pain, emotional upset can cause shock. It can occur immediately after injury. If it occurs after a few hours, it could be due to bleeding (Table 19.7).

BLEEDING

Wound, fracture and damage to organs by accident cause bleeding. If there is oozing, it can be controlled by direct pressure. If severe, it may need tourniquet.

Table 19.6: Signs and symptoms and first aid for burns and scalds

Signs and symptoms	*First aid*
Skin intact or partly destroyed – Red skin, blisters, severe pain	Apply sulphonamide ointment Dressing done Plenty of fluid given
Skin completely destroyed – Raw look – Severe shock – Severe pain	Covered with autoclaved gauze or clean cloth Allow fluids to drink Rush to hospital or centre

Table 19.7: Signs and symptoms and first aid for shock

Signs and symptoms	*First aid*
• Pallor face, lips	• Allow to lay down
• Beads of sweat on forehead	• Raise foot to about 22 cm off the ground
• Sticky moist skin	• Cover with blanket, keep warm
• Cold hand, feet	• Avoid unnecessary handling
• Shallow breathing	• Stop bleeding if any
• Rapid feeble pulse	• Allow hot tea and sugar if conscious
• Vomiting	• Splint fractures
• Restlessness	• Cover wounds
• Vacant expression	• Transfer to hospital or centre at the earliest
• Unconsciousness	

Materials

The materials available on the spot like:

- Narrow triangular bandage
- Handkerchief
- Necktie
- Broad belt
- Piece of cloth, etc. can be used.

Methods of Tourniquet Application

- Fold the triangular bandage to a width of 5 cm
- Apply it on clothing at the level of the middle of the limb (upper or lower)
- Tie the free ends of the bandage in a half knot on the outer side of the limb
- Place a pencil or wood piece on the half knot
- Complete the knot to hold the pencil or wood in position
- Twist the pencil or wood gradually so as to tighten the bandage until the bleeding stops
- Use a second bandage to tie around the limb to keep the pencil or wood in the tightened up position
- Leave the tourniquet but loosen it gently every fifteen minutes
- If bleeding has stopped, leave the tourniquet in place, but do not tighten it up again
- If bleeding starts, again tighten the tourniquet
- Move with patient, helping stop bleeding up to hospital or centre
- Attach label or a piece of paper to the patient's shirt showing the time when the tourniquet was applied.

Special note: A tourniquet is a very useful appliance for use in the presence of open fractures of a limb.

Bleeding from the Nose

Small vessels in the walls of nostrils cause bleeding when rupture. This is called epistaxis. Other causes are injury, growth, high BP, high altitude and foreign body.

First Aid

- Reassurance is given
- Slightly forward position of the head is maintained
- Tight clothing around neck, chest and waist are loosened
- Allowed mouth breathing
- Instructed not to blow his nose
- Kept at comfortably warm
- The bleeding can often be controlled by firmly compressing the nostrils with the thumb and forefinger against septum of the nose
- Early medical assistance is sought.

20

Public Health Administration

SUPERVISORY DUTIES

Health Inspectors are Health Supervisors and Health Assistants and hence they are expected to know their day-to-day supervisory duties at Primary Health Centre, at Primary Health Unit, at Corporation, at Railway Hospital, or any other hospital, which depends on their place of postings.

Supervisory Activities

While working with the community and the health team, the Health Inspector has to carryout the following supervisory activities by checking the health activities carried out by Multipurpose Workers (Health workers Male and Female) in their areas.

The supervisory activities are grouped as under for easy comprehension:

- Village survey for the village records
- Household survey for family records
- Use of record for health education purpose
- Use of records for service programme
- Preparation of map of the area on:
  - Communities
  - Resources
  - Wells
  - Latrines
  - Other facilities
- Activity charts for subcentre:
  - FP acceptors
  - Child immunisation
  - Vitamin A administration
  - ANC registration
  - Deliveries conducted
  - *Dais* trained
  - TB cases detected and treated
  - Leprosy cases detected and treated
  - Blood smear taken for MP smear
  - Blood smear positive
  - Village leaders identification
- Group meetings, OTC camps
- Approaches used to health education:
  - Individual approaches
  - Group approaches
  - Mass approaches
- Staff meetings
- Coordination in team work
- Guidance to subordinates
- Camps and campaigns:
  - Health check-up
  - Cancer detection
  - Family planning

EVOLUTION OF HEALTH SERVICES WITH PARTICULAR REFERENCE TO INDIA

Brief History

Health services in India are known since the period of *Vedas*. In the Indian history, Harappa-Mahenjodaro discovery has showed the practices of health and sanitation.

During the period of Buddhism, hospital system was started for the man and also for animals. This got expanded in the era of king Ashoka.

During the Mughal Empire, the Unani system was developed.

Before Independence

Following milestones were observed up to the Independence of India:

- The Quarantine Act 1825
- Sanitary Commission appointed 1864
- The Birth and Death Registration Act 1873
- The Vaccination Act 1880
- The Indian Factory Act 1881
- The Epidemic Disease Act
- ICMR started in old name 1911
- The Madras Public Health Act was passed 1939
- The Drug Act 1940
- The Bhore Committee appointed 1943
- The Bhore Committee Report 1946

After Independence

Following milestones are observed after the Independence of the country:

- India became WHO Member 1948
- India became Republic 1950
- Five Year Plan started 1951
- Primary Health Centre with many National Health Programmes was set up 1952
- School Health Committee 1960
- MTP Act 1972
- Smallpox Eradication Declared 1977
- National Health Policy amended 1982
- Pulse Polio Immunisation (now IPPI) started 1996
- RCH started 1997
- Present **five year plan** ongoing 2007 to 2012.

Current Status of India (Table 20.1)

Table 20.1: Current status of India

Population	1112 million
Rural population	72.18 per cent
Literacy rate	65.38 per cent
IMR	58
MMR	3.01
Birth rate	23.8
Death rate	7.6
Growth rate	1.62 per cent
Family size	3.0

CENTRAL, STATE AND LOCAL ORGANISATIONS IN INDIA

India is a vast country with 17 major States, 12 smaller States and 6 Union Territories. Health organisation network is through 3910 community Health Centres, 22669 primary health centres and 144988 subcentres.

Central Health Organisation (Fig. 20.1)

Functions

Central Health Organisation looks after the following functions:

- Health administration
- Drug standard
- Coordination with States
- Power of legislation on the control of diseases, drug, food.

State Health Organisation

In State Health Organisation, regional directors help administration (Fig. 20.2). In the field of RCH, FP, Nutrition, Tuberculosis, Leprosy and Health Education, Concerned functional directors will coordinate. Public Health Engineering also joins in public health administration and activities.

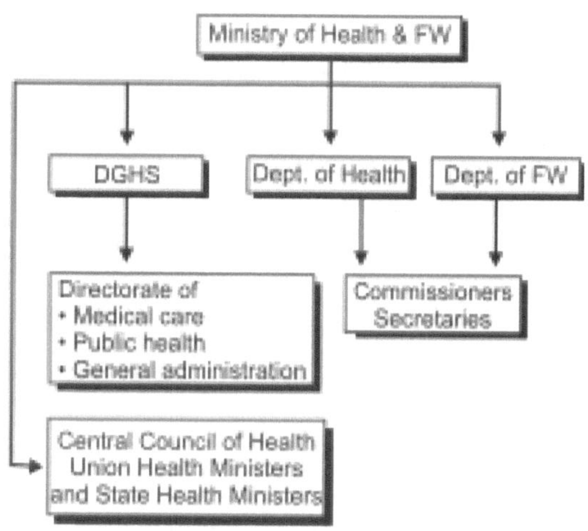

Fig. 20.1: Health organisation at centre

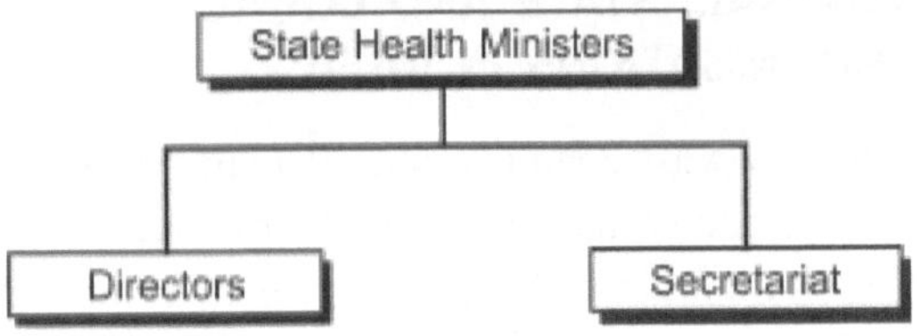

Fig. 20.2: Health organisation at state

District Health Administration

In India, District is the unit for all Health and Family Welfare activities (Table 20.2). There are about 590 districts in India.

DH and FWO at district level heads district Organisation, by Taluka level MOH at Taluka level and PHC MOH at PHC level. PHC team will help to carry out all Health and FW services and National Health Programmes.

The district administration is helped and coordinated by Zilla Parishad, Mandal Panchayat and Village Panchayat, which are **Rural Self-government Organisations.**

District Health Organisation is also called Local Health Organisation because the District is considered as a unit of Health and FW activities in the country.

Table 20.2: District health administration

District	Dist. Health and FW Officer and District Surgeon
Taluka	Taluka Level Medical Officer
Block	Block Development for the Community (CBD)
PHC	PHC Medical Officer and PHC Staff, Local GPs
Subcentre	Multipurpose Worker — Male and Female, Local GPs

RELATION WITH OTHER DEPARTMENTS

Development of a country implies progressive improvements in the living conditions and quality of life enjoyed by society and shared by its members. It is a continuing process that takes place in all societies; few would claim that their development is complete.

Health department alone cannot get involved in socio-economic development in isolation. Activities of one department impinge on the goals of another; hence there is need for constant consultation between major social and economic sectors to ensure development and to promote health as part of it. Primary health care too requires the support of other sectors; these sectors can also serve as entry points for the development and implementation of primary health care.

Following sectors or departments need interdepartmental or inter-sectoral coordination for an effective implementation of administration and to reach the goal of achieving health for all:

- Agriculture sector
- Water
- Housing, public works and communications
- Educational sector
- Mass media
- Industries

Education Sector

It has an important part to play in the development and operation of Primary Health Care. Community education helps people to understand their health problems, possible solutions to them and the cost of different alternatives. Instructive literature can be developed and distributed through the educational system. Associations of parents and teachers can assume certain responsibilities for primary health care activities within schools and the community, such as sanitation programmes, food for health campaigns or course on nutrition and first aid.

Education is an important factor responsible for an individual or family health. In India, mothers take full responsibilities in bringing up children. In this process of child upbringing if mother is literate or if she is educated, she can determine health status of growing children.

Thus, education and health are linked components. For healthy population, the following are found requisites:

- Proper nutrition
- Safe water for drinking
- Newborn care
- Immunisation

For creating conditions for equity and efficiencies, both health and education are germinated from the same root of:

- Accessibility
- Availability
- Affordability
- Accountability
- Acceptability

In Kerala, high literacy and education among female is one single factor, which has significant relation with socio-economic improvement.

Education gives knowledge for decision making towards conditions of health promotion. It also determines political awareness to say a right to health

Thus, education and health are interlinked with each other. Sometimes education creates demand for the health. At times, health promotion can create demand for education in the society.

Health and Agriculture

The agriculture sector is very important in most countries. It can ensure that production of food for family consumption becomes an integral part of agricultural polity and that food actually reaches those who produce it, which in some countries may require changes in the pattern of land tenure. Also, nutritional status can be improved through programmes in agriculture and home economics geared to meeting priority family and community needs. Women enjoy the benefits of agricultural development equal to men. In most developing countries the majority of women in rural areas are engaged simultaneously in agriculture, household management and the care of infants and children. They need appropriate technology to lighten their workload and increase their work productivity. They also require knowledge about nutrition that they can apply with the resources available, in particular, concerning the proper feeding of children and their own nutrition during pregnancy and lactation.

Agricultural development of a country helps in poverty alleviation. Poverty is the root cause of hunger and malnutrition. Increase in agricultural produce can make family enjoy high income, good assets, high education, good housing and good sanitation, whereby none succumb to infection.

India is aware of the link between agriculture and health. Nearly about 78 per cent of the rural community are depending on agriculture. Major improvements in well-being are within our grasp through high agricultural produce.

Agricultural development leads to better nutrition of the community and helps in socio-economic development.

The fact remains that famine and malnutrition are not acceptable in the world. Hence, all countries that are members of the UN adopt strategies to promote food and agriculture development on a sustainable basis with economic and social equity to ensure positive health of individual in the society.

Ministry of Health and FW has understood that primary health care; RCH and family welfare are greatly associated with food production and food grain storage in the country.

Ministry of agriculture in close cooperation with Health and FW Ministry has been pursuing the following schemes to bring greater link between agriculture and health:

- *Krishi Vigyan Kendra*: To train farmers for agricultural technology and increase food production.

- *National Rural Employment Programme*: To improve nutrition status of rural poor by providing part of wage in the form of food grains.
- *Rural Landless Employment Guarantee Programme*: To provide 100 days of labour by agricultural ways for unskilled workers.
- *Integrated Rural Development Programme*: To achieve high income by agriculture including animal husbandry, fishery and horticulture.
- *Training of Rural Youth for Self-employment*: To encourage youth to engage in agriculture produce.

The relation of health and agriculture is seen by the following aims of the Food and Agriculture Organisation.

- Help raising living standard
- To improve nutrition
- To increase efficiency of farming, forestry and fisheries
- To increase food production
- To keep pace with population

Thus, ensuring that food is consumed by people is of good quality and quantity, can maintain a better health status.

Communication and Health

Aspects of communications are of strategic importance to primary health care, particularly for dispersed population.

Feeder roads not only connect the farmers to the market but also make it easier for people to reach villages, bringing new ideas together with the supplies needed for health and other sectors. Two-way radio communication, where this can be afforded, puts isolated areas in contact with more centrally located administrative levels, at the same time serving as a vehicle for learning. Low-cost pedal operated radio communication has been successfully used in primary health care in some of the developing countries.

Health is in full swing of progress by advanced communication system in the world. Roadways, Railways, Airways are known physical transport, which can make the health service accessible to the community or common man. Transport system is an accepted inbuilt structure for health care services. Doctors, paramedical workers like health inspectors, nurses, etc. can reach the community for active and passive surveillance, survey, screening and treatment for minor ailments. Emergency care, essential obstetric care and essential paediatric care depend on physical transport, and the department of transport can integrate and coordinate for a better community health.

Of late, communication does involve distant communication system like telephone, telegraphy and teleconference, which can work as intersectoral coordination body for providing better health of the community.

OTHER DEPARTMENTS

Water and Health

Water for household use is as important as water for cattle, irrigation, energy and industry. Plentiful supplies of clean water help to decrease mortality and morbidity, in particular among infants and children as well as making life easier for women. Countrywide plans are required to bring urban and rural water supplies within easy reach of the majority of people.

Housing

Housing is a physical and physiological need of man for positive health. Houses help in food storage, prevent insect bite, rodent bite, help in food sanitation.

Mass Media

This is very helpful in the development and operation of primary health care. Mass media helps to offer valid information on health and ways of attaining it and by depicting the benefits to be derived from improved health practices within primary health care.

Intersectoral coordination requires political will for good and sustained effort. Without duplication of actions, if all sectors work together, achieving health for all is not difficult.

INTERNATIONAL ORGANISATIONS AND THEIR COOPERATION IN THE FIELD OF HEALTH

To check disease spread and to isolate infected persons specific actions are required. Quarantine and isolation are two major such specific actions to maintain positive health of the people of a country. Efficient and fast travel through land, air and water has increased the mobility of population between countries and hence need inter regional cooperation to apply quarantine measure.

International organisations cooperation is required in the following health measures:

- Control of dreaded diseases like cholera, plague, SARS, anthrax
- Health notification
- Control of other communicable diseases
- For drug standardisation
- For training of health personnel
- For research activities

WHO (World Health Organisation)

This came into existence in 1948. The headquarters is in Geneva. Most of the countries are WHO members.

Functions

Following are the functions of WHO:

- Prevention and control of specific diseases
- Development of comprehensive health care
- Improvement of family health
- Promotion of environment health
- Provides health strategies
- Stimulates research
- Provides literature

For South-East Asia, the headquarter is New Delhi in India. This covers a wide range of health actions like malaria eradication, TB control, laboratory service set up, vaccine production, improving rural health services, encouraging RCH, helping health education and quality control of drugs.

WHO Day Themes of Recent Years

2000: Safe Blood starts with me—blood saves lives.
2001: Stop Exclusion—dare to care.
2002: Move for Health
2003: Shape the future of life—healthy environments for children.
2004: Road safety is no accident.
2005: Make every mother and child count
2006: Working together for health
2007: Invest in health, build a safer future
2008: Protecting health from climate change.

UNICEF (United Nation Children's Fund)

UNICEF collaborates with WHO, FAO, UNDP, UNESCO, and other international organisations. Its regional office is in New Delhi.

Functions

Chief functions are:

- Child health
- Child nutrition and family planning
- Health education

UNDP (United Nation Development Programme)

This organisation helps poor nations for the development of their own resources.

FAO (Food and Agriculture Organisation)

To improve nutrition of people of the world, FAO helps and coordinates various functions, through increasing efficiency of agricultural production.
ILO (International Labour Organisation)

This organisation helps in solving problems of industry and industry workers.

World Bank

It is an agency of United Nation. It helps fewer developing countries to raise their living standards.

VOLUNTARY AGENCIES IN HEALTH PROGRAMMES

They are key agencies in all public health activities. They collect the fund from private source and spend for public health activities.

Achievements

In the history of medicine, voluntary health agencies have shown the following achievements:

- Help government organisation
- Do new discovery
- Provide health education without expectations
- They demonstrate the useful items in public health
- Help to make legislation

VOLUNTARY HEALTH AGENCIES IN INDIA

In India, the following are noted Voluntary Health Agencies.

IMA (Indian Medical Association)

It conducts and sets up standard education, organises relief camps in earthquake, floods, and famine.

FPAI (Family Planning Association of India)

It propagates family planning in India.

TAI (Tuberculosis Association of India)

It organises TB control, TB campaigns, and training for better health services.

Indian Council for Child Welfare

It helps in the proper development of physical, mental, spiritual and social health of children.

Indian Red Cross

It is a greater, accessible and all-round voluntary health agency available at suffering of people anywhere in the country.

Functions: Following functions highlight its role in health care services:

- Relief work in natural disaster
- Relief work in war affected area
- Medicine supplies
- First aid training of men and women

RURAL DEVELOPMENT

Concept

It is an active process where conditions are created for an economic and social progress of the rural population who are the mainstream of the society constituting 78 per cent of population of the country.

In recent days, rural development is called "community development". In community development, people are united with government agencies to improve their economic, social and cultural conditions to contribute to nation's progress.

Organisation

Under rural development, community development blocks (CDBs) are established for every 100 villages with a population of 1 lakh. Now, there are about 6000 CDBs in the country.

This is headed by BDO (Block Development Officer). Community development blocks are permanent units of rural planning and development.

Under rural development, the following National Programmes are carried out:

- Improvement of agriculture
- Improvement of communication
- Improvement of education
- Improvement of health
- Improvement of sanitation
- Improvement of housing

Under rural development, IRDP (Integrated Rural Development Programme is an another innovation. For bank loans, assistance is provided to:

- Agricultural labourers
- Small cultivators
- Handicrafts men

The Government of India through following network takes up rural developments:

- TRYSEM (Training of Rural Youth for Self-employment)
- SITRA (Supply of Improved Toolkits to Rural Artisans)
- DWACRA (Development of Women and Children in Rural Areas)
- GKY (Ganga Kalyan Yojana).

Under rural development, Gram Sevaks are appointed who help and take care of rural socio-economic development. Every 10 villages with 6000 populations is covered by a Gram Sevak.

Panchayat Raj

It is a rural local self-government structure with 3 tiers, linking the following:

- Village (Panchayat)
- Block (Panchayat Samiti)
- District (Zilla Parishat).

Panchayat Raj system is a democratic accepted institution in India for the public welfare.

In Panchayat Raj, the following points are to be noted:

- Better public cooperation
- Effective cooperative movement
- It is self-government
- Ensure effective public participation
- All development activities are channelled through ZP, Panchayat Samiti, and Panchayat of village.

HEALTH CENTRE

Concept

By the recommendation of the Bhore Committee, a basic health unit is provided in rural areas to provide integrated health care (integration of curative and preventive health care).

PHC is a proper health infrastructure, which can provide basic health services to rural India.

Definition

It is a basic peripheral health unit for curative and preventive health care services to rural India. It is reorganised on the basis of one PHC for 30,000 rural population; one PHC for 20,000 tribal/hilly/backward areas. By definition, PHC gives Primary Health Care to the population of covering areas.

Organisation

PHC has the following staff:

- MO – One
- Pharmacist – One
- Nurse Midwife – One
- Health Worker (F)/ANM – One
- BEE – One
- Health Assistant (M) – One
- Health Assistant (F)/LHV – One
- UDC – One
- LDC – One
- Lab Technician – One
- Driver – One
- Class IV – Four

Every PHC will have 4 to 6 subcentres as outposts for health care delivery.

Staff at Subcentre

- HW (F)/ANM/MPW (F) – One
- HW (M)/MPW (M) – One
- Voluntary worker/VHG – One

Functions

Following functions of PHC will cover all Primary Health Care essentials. They are:

- Medical care
- MCH and FP
- Safe water supply and basic sanitation
- Prevention and control of local endemic diseases
- Collection and reporting of vital statistics
- Health education
- National health programme
- Referral of cases to CHC or District Hospitals
- Training of VHG, TBA and other health workers
- Basic laboratory services

ROLE OF HEALTH CENTRE IN HEALTH PROGRAMME

NMEP (National Malaria Eradication Programme)

- Case diagnosis and case treatment
- Health education of the community
- Active surveillance
- Passive surveillance
- MP smear, PT and RT
- OTC camps
- Mosquito control measures

NFCP (National Filaria Control Programme)

- Case diagnosis and case treatment
- Health education of the community
- Mosquito control measures
- DEC mass therapy, DEC selective therapy

NLEP (National Leprosy Eradication Programme)

- Early case detection
- Confirmation of diagnosis
- MDT
- Health education in the area
- Social support by rehabilitation

NTCP (National TB Control Programme)

- Case finding by sputum examination
- MMR (X-ray)
- Tuberculin test
- DOTS under RNTCP (Directly Observed Treatment Schedule under Revised National TB Control Programme)
- BCG vaccination
- Rehabilitation

World TB Day Themes since 2000 AD

2000: Forging new partnerships to stop TB
2001: DOTS: TB cure for all
2002: Stop TB, flight poverty
2003: DOTs cured me—it will cure you too
2004: Every breath counts—stop TB now
2005: Frontline TB care providers: heroes in the fight against TB
2006: Action for life—towards a world free of TB
2007: TB anywhere is TB everywhere
2008: I am stopping TB

NDDCP (National Diarrhoeal Disease Control Programme)

- Case management
- Health education
- ORS guidelines
- Better RCH
- Sanitation

ROLE OF HEALTH INSPECTOR IN A PHC

The Health Inspector is expected to cover 1 PHC with 6 Subcentres (total 30,000 population). He plays the following role:

- Supervises the activities of MPW (M)
- Guides the MPW (M)
- Coordinates PHC functions
- Attends staff meetings
- Takes care of indent and supplies of PHC
- Maintains PHC records
- MP smear, PT and RT
- Action in epidemic

- Helps in the construction of soakage pit, kitchen garden, manure pit, compost pit, RCA latrine and smokeless *chulhas*
- UIP work
- Motivation of eligible couple
- Treatment advice on malnutrition
- Registration of births and deaths
- Health education of the community.

Legal Consideration

Details of Public Health Acts and Rules are detailed in Chapter 23. The health Inspector has the power of designation to act on the following situations:
- Selective isolation of cases
- Action and measures on epidemic
- Use of Municipal Act
- Prevention of food adulteration
- ESI Act
- Public health analysis of water, milk, and drug.

IMPACT OF SICKNESS ON INDIVIDUAL, THE FAMILY AND COMMUNITY

Sickness influences production, socio-economic status, level of living, standard of living and quality of life at individual, family and community levels.

Individual

Individual is affected to become non-ambulatory, dependent, morbid and incapable of carrying out routine. When his earning comes down, he becomes impoverished, malnourished and condition deviates further. If early diagnosis and prompt treatment is not done, progress of illness may cause organ damage; sometimes, inevitable organ failure and even death.

Family

Family is affected by the sickness of a member. It is obvious if the sick is the sole earner. Per capita may become zero. Accessibility for health care for nutrition may become remote. Death due to sickness may bring about broken family, or even problem family.

Loss of income and loss of status of a member may cause family damage in terms of psychological damage and social damage.

Community

Community is affected by the sickness to produce lowered socio-economic development of the community. Death rates, IMR, MMR, Life expectancy — all are influenced by sickness, which determine the community health. Mortality (death) and morbidity (sickness) indicate the level of community diagnosis and hence are called the health indicators.

21

School Health

In India, raising children health is made possible by the powerful tool of group health through organised school health activities.

School age forms a high proportion of general population; and hence, the health care services by health authorities are relevant. Early socialisation in school child for a good habit, good personal hygiene, clean surrounding, good nutrition, relevant sports activities, relevant recreation will be long lasting and is responsible for future healthy citizen of the country.

School Health Committee Report by the Government of India helps departments like education and health to assess standard of health and level of nutrition among schoolchildren.

Majority of states in the country have adopted mid-day meal, which provides half of calorie and nutrient requirement of the school-going child. This is also helping in bringing out positive health among school children.

SCHOOL HEALTH : OBJECTIVES

- Help children to adopt health measures to be healthy
- To allow them to make best use of educational facilities
- To involve in SUPW at home and in society
- To develop concern for others

SCHOOL HEALTH : COMPONENTS

- Regular health check-up at schools
- Detection of chronic defects
- Prompt referral to further treatment
- Good immunisation coverage
- Teachers' training on school health
- Teacher-parent counselling
- Health education
- Population education
- Healthy environment with:
  a. Safe drinking water
  b. Good sanitation
  c. Accident prevention
  d. Food hygiene
- School mid-day meal

TEACHERS' TRAINING

Plan and arrange one-time teachers' training for all schools in your area. Training programmes should help teachers to identify the following:

- Teachers can differentiate normal and abnormal aspect of schoolchildren
- Teachers can detect and differentiate normal and abnormal aspect of schoolchildren
- They can detect chronic defects like poor vision, hard of hearing, physical disability, etc.
- Able to guide children for a clean personal habits
- Can convey message to children for healthful living and to their parents the need for small families
- Can ensure healthy environment by available measures
- Will be in a position to give first aid in case of emergencies

For teacher's training, help of MOH PHC, BEE and staff of DH and FWO are taken to make the effort fruitful.

CHECKLIST FOR OBSERVATIONS AT SCHOOL HEALTH CHECK-UP

Clean drinking water	Available/not available
Sanitary toilet	Present/absent
If present	Sufficient/not sufficient
If present	Maintained/not maintained
Hand wash facility	Available/not available
Refuse collection	Made/not made
Refuse disposal	Done/not done
Classroom	Ventilated/not ventilated
Classroom light	Sufficient light/insufficient light
Seating arrangements	Good/not good
Accident hazards (for example, pond, defective wiring, building cracked, fire hazard, etc.)	Present/absent
Bucket of sand (for first aid)	Present/not present
Bucket of water (for first aid)	Present/not present
First aid kit	Present/not present
Playground	Yes/No
Space for sitting and eating	Present/not present

Health inspector should discuss above items with Headmaster of the school for action. Later, he should intimate the same to MOH in his inspection report.

IMMUNISATION

Class-wise list of unprotected children is made. Arrangement of necessary immunisation to the unprotected is done. Parents' cooperation is very necessary in this venture.

Otherwise, school-age child has the following immunisation schedule, which is to be attended (Table 21.1).

Table 21.1: Immunisation schedule for school-age children

Age	*Vaccine*
5 to 6 years	DT (booster dose)
10 years	TT
16 years	TT
Nutrition	

Nutrition

Observe the following at midday meal feeding:

- Meal item provided
- Method of storage of food
- Method of handling of food
- Method of preparations of food
- Method of cleaning utensil
- Method of serving and distribution
- Personal hygiene of food handlers

Above items are discussed with Headmaster and later report is submitted to the MOH of PHC.

Since midday meal in a school has become part of Minimum Need Programme (MNP) in India, the Health Inspector is expected to know the model menu suggested by the School Health Committee (per day per child is given) (Table 21.2).

Above requirements are attended at least for 250 days in a year to bring out the good effect of mid-day meal school programme

HEALTH EDUCATION

Involvement of schoolchildren, teachers and parents is necessary for giving health education. Here learning by doing is allowed in creating awareness of the following:

Table 21.2: Model menu for mid-day meal

Cereal and millet	75 g
Pulses	30 g
Oil	8 g
Leafy vegetable	30 g
Other vegetable	30 g

- Personal hygiene
- Safe drinking water
- Clean surroundings
- Nutritious food
- Prevention of communicable disease
- Growing up
- Tomorrow citizen
- Accident prevention
- First aid

Arrangement of the following by the Health Inspector will help in appropriate health education:

- Cleanliness campaign
- Health parade
- Competitions among children
- Exhibition
- Film show

POPULATION EDUCATION

It is an educational programme (health education on benefits of small family norm). This provides an idea about current situation of society, community and nation with regard to socio-economic, productive and progress of the country.

Population education inculcates a rational, positive and responsible attitude towards population control. This also tells them the effect of population explosion in the country. Population education during health education involves the following major topics that interests students, teachers and parents:

- Economics
- Sociology
- Statistics
- Health

The topic coverage during population education can be:

- Demography of district, state and the country
- Information on census
- Benefits of small family
- Effects of overpopulation
- Burden of nation on population explosion

School health check-up involves the following areas:

1. Medical examination of schoolchildren should be annual after initial health check-up at admission. Every child should have a cumulative health record maintained by the school. This Cumulative Health Record contains the following sections:
   - History on health and disease (family history)
   - Immunisation record till date
   - Findings of medical examination carried out

It is preferred that parents are requested at each health check-up of their ward. This builds up rapport. Simultaneously, all teachers are involved for assistance, history taking and writing, recording height, weight and vision, etc.

2. Examination of each child should contain the following:
   - General condition — Good/fair/sick
   - Physical growth — Good/not good
   - Height — ....cm
   - Weight — ....kg
   - Vision — Normal/short sight/long sight/others
   - *Eyes*:
     - Squint — No/Yes
     - Vitamin deficiency — No/Yes
     - Eye infection (Redness) — No/Yes
     - Pallor — No/Yes
   - *Teeth*:
     - Caries — Present/absent
     - Gums — Normal/bleeding/pus
   - *Throat*:
     - Tonsils — Normal/enlarged
   - *Ear*:
     - Hearing — good/impaired
     - Discharge — present/absent

- *Chest*: Chest examination is done by MOH
- *Abdomen*:
  - Liver examination
  - Spleen examination
  - Lump
  - Testes (any undescended)
- *Limbs, spine*:
  - Any residual paralysis (lameness)
  - Defects (bent, clubfoot, etc.)
  - Rickets
- *Skin*:
  - Normal/any patch/any infection
- *Hair*:
  - Normal/colour change/head louse

SUMMARY REPORT BY HEALTH INSPECTOR

- Health Inspector is expected to do simple diagnosis of minor ailments and give treatment for minor ailments.
- For major ailments, the child is referred to MOH of PHC.
- The report should mention:
  - Number of children examined
  - Number of minor ailments diagnosed and treated
  - Number of children referred.

COMMON HEALTH PROBLEMS OF SCHOOLCHILDREN

- Malnutrition
- Infections like common cold, measles, chickenpox, ARI, diarrhoea, skin infection
- Injuries by fall, accident and sports
- Intestinal infections like amoebiasis, roundworm, hookworm, threadworm
- Eye infections with redness, watering
- Ear infections with pain and discharge
- Tooth ache by caries

During every health check-up, the following items should be checked:

- Swelling in the face
- Colour change in the face
- Skin rashes on the body
- Running in the nose
- Cough
- Fever
- Headache
- Depression
- Loose motion
- Scabies
- Not playing with children

SCHOOL ENVIRONMENT

For the development of mental, social and emotional health, a healthful school environment should be created in every school. During inspection by the Health Inspector under his jurisdiction, he has to inspect the following:

- Location – Place of school
- Land – Good or any dampness
- Building – Single-storeyed/multi-storeyed
- Classroom – Sufficient/not sufficient (40 students per class)
- Seat and desk (Figs 21.1 and 21.2)
- Water supply – Yes/No

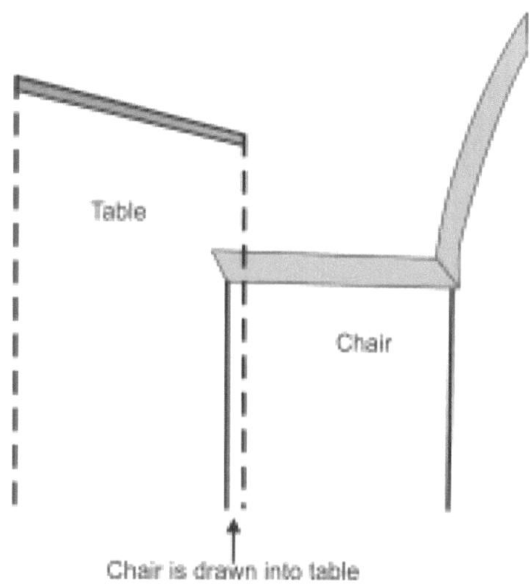

Fig. 21.1: Minus (negative) desk

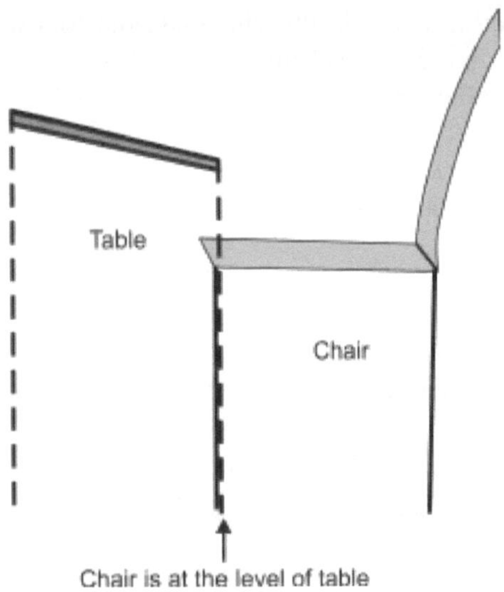

Fig. 21.2: Zero desk

- Toilet – Yes/No
- Eating place – Yes/No
- Lavatory – Yes/No
- Cross-ventilation – Yes/No

Following first aid facilities are made available at school and teachers are trained in first aid:

- Injury by fall
- Injury by accident
- Bleeding by cut or injury
- Severe loose motion
- Fits (convulsion or epilepsy)
- Fainting
- Drowning
- Artificial respiration.

22

Essential Drugs and Treatment of Minor Ailments

ESSENTIAL DRUGS

Essential drugs are those drugs that satisfy the health care needs of the entire population of a country. They should be available in adequate amount, in appropriate dosage and at all times.

The choice of essential drugs depends on prevalence of diseases, treatment facilities, training and experience of health workers and budget. Now the term "health care needs of the majority" is specified for the term essential drug.

Other requirements are:
- Safety
- Efficiency
- Storage
- Price
- Availability
- Single compound

Drugs for Primary Health Care

It is determined at national level. If the health worker is well-trained, he can use a wide range of drugs appropriate to his skill and acceptable safety. In India, the drug use for primary health care depends on:
- Indian systems of medicine
- Available trained health workers
- Training facilities of health workers
- Supplies
- Pattern of local diseases

Examples of essential drugs:
- APC
- Paracetemol
- Codeine
- CPM
- Phenobarbitone
- Piperazine
- Chloroquine
- Ampicillin
- Metronidazole
- Cotrimoxazole
- Dapsone
- INH
- Aluminium hydroxide
- Benzyl benzoate
- Antiseptic lotion
- Whitefield ointment

GUIDE TO HEALTH INSPECTORS FOR THE USE AND ADMINISTRATION OF DRUGS

Internal Use

- *APC tablet* for common cold, sore throat, fever, headache, backache, joint pain, toothache, and earache
  - *Infants*: One-fourth tablet dissolved in honey or water, given after feed, 3 times a day
  - 1 *to* 4 *years*: Half tablet dissolved in honey or water 3 times a day

- *5 to 9 years*: One tablet 3 times a day
- *10 to 14 years:* One and half tablet 3 times a day
- *15 years and above*: Two tablets 3 times a day.

Caution: Tablets should not be taken on an empty stomach.

- *Chloroquine tablet* for malaria presumptive treatment
  - Infants: Half tablet with honey
  - *1 to 4 years*: One tablet with honey
  - 5 *to 9 years*: Two tablets
  - 10 *to* 14 *years*: Three tablets
  - 15 *years and above*: Four tablets

Caution: Tablets should be given single dose after taking thick and thin blood films. Tablets should not be taken on an empty stomach.

- *Cough mixture (supplied from PHC)* for cough and sore throat
  - Infants: Half teaspoon 3 times a day
  - 1 to 4 years: One teaspoon 3 times a day
  - 5 to 9 years: Two spoon 3 times a day
  - 10 to 14 years: Two spoon 3 times a day
  - 15 years and above: Three to 4 spoon 3 times a day
- *Kaolin powder (from PHC taken)* for diarrhoea
  Powder is mixed with water and given to drink.
  - Half spoon to infant
  - One spoon to 1 to 4 year and 5 to 9 years
  - Two spoon to 10 years and above
  - All 3 to 4 times a day
- *ORS (from PHC)* for dehydration
  Dissolve in 1 litre of water; give small quantity at each item, after every bout of diarrhoea. Child is given 1 spoon every 10 minutes for hydration.
- *Magnesium hydroxide* for burning sensation in stomach.
  Advised to chew the tablet slowly.
- *To follow guidelines given at PHC for*
  - ARI
  - Tuberculosis
  - Leprosy
  - Worm infection.

External Use

- *Antiseptic lotion for:* Wound clean and ulcer clean.
  - Half spoon in ***boiled and cooled*** water. With cotton swab, swab the wound or ulcer from within outwards.
- *Benzyl benzoate for* Scabies or lice
  Follow PHC instructions
- *Menthol and eucalyptus oil for:* Cold and cough
  Apply over nostrils; rub ointment on throat, chest, back. Cover with warm cloth.
- *Mercurochrome 2% for*: Cuts, scratches and dog bite.
  Wash wound with clean water and with antiseptic lotion. Mercurochrome is applied by a cotton swab. Then clean dressing is applied.
- *Methyl salicylate ointment for:* Headache, backache, joint pain and sprain
  Rub gently on painful area as and when needed.
- *Spirit for:* Wound clean, before smear taking or before immunisation.
  For MP smear taking—take spirit swab. Press left ring finger of fever case so that blood collects at the tip, swab the tip of finger and prick the clean finger with Hagedorn's needle.
  Caution: Always keep Hagedorn's needle used for pricking finger in a bottle containing spirit.
- *Potassium permanganate for*:
  - Snake bite — incise site of bite, suck or squeeze the site, apply crystals to the wound
  - Sore throat — solution prepared is used as mouthwash or gargle.
- *Sulphacetamide eye drops for:*
  - Sore eye — after cleaning affected eye, instil 2 drops to space of lower lid, 4 times a day for 2 days.
  - Ear discharge — after cleaning affected ear, instil 2 drops 3 times a day for 2 days.
- *Sulphanilamide ointment for:* Infected wound, burn and scalds
  Clean, apply ointment, put clean dressing.

- *Sulphanilamide dusting powder for:* Wound and ulcer
  Clean with antiseptic lotion, dry with cotton swab, dust the powder, cover with dressing.
- *Whitefield ointment for:* Ringworm
  Advice bath with soap and water. Dry the skin well. Apply ointment on affected area, 4 times a day for one week.

TREATMENT OF MINOR AILMENTS

Since you are available as first contact, the care given by you is called ***first contact care***. You are living in PHC area and people will come to you for the treatment. Hence, it is important that the Health Inspector shall know the treatment of minor ailments.

One should take care to refer cases in time according to the instructions. In spite of your first line of treatment, instruct them to visit subcentre or PHC where service of MOH is available.

Common Ailments

Following are common ailments that need immediate treatment and advice.

Fever

Fever can occur with many diseases and is important to look for other signs and symptoms. In a child fever can produce convulsions (fits) and hence need immediate treatment.

Elicit history and follow the steps as under:

- Enquire how fever started and how it progressed?
- Ask about other accompanying signs and symptoms such as headache, nausea, vomiting, diarrhoea, cough or running nose
- Look for skin rashes
- Enquire any shivering
- Ask any pain in specific part of the body
- In children, note for rapid and difficult breathing
- Take body temperature by clinical thermometer.

If fever is with rigors and sweating or without any accompanying symptoms, always presume it as malaria, take thick and thin blood smear and give presumptive treatment (PT) with chloroquine.

In addition to the above:

- Ask the patient to remain in bed
- Give APC or paracetemol
- Tell him to drink plenty of water
- Advice cold sponge to forehead
- Visit next day for follow-up

Refer the case, if:

- The fever has not come down.
- Other signs or symptoms developed.
- Stiff neck, vomiting, convulsion or unconsciousness are seen.

Headache

Since many causes are there for headache, it is better to look for other signs.

- Ask for sore throat, earache, toothache, dizziness
- Look for fever, rash, stiff neck, ear discharge, running nose, sore eyes or vomiting

Treat with:

- Give APC tablet
- Rub forehead with methyl salicylate ointment, apply tight band around forehead
- Sore eye, earache, toothache, cough, cold are treated

Always refer, if:

Stiff neck, dizziness, vomiting, swelling of feet, if patient is pregnant woman

Backache and Joint Pain

They are caused by sprain, strain or injury. Some diseases also cause backache and joint pain.

- Ask how long the pain has been present
- Ask whether the patient has any injury
- Any symptoms like fever and joint pain
- See for deformity of spine

Treat by:
- Rest the joint as much as possible
- APC tablets are given
- Rub the back or joint with methyl salicylate ointment

Refer the case: If deformity is present, pain is lasting for 3 days, or if it is getting worse.

Joint pain is due to injury, infection, and ageing. An enquiry for duration of pain is made. The person is examined for red, hot, swollen, or tender joint and for fever.

Treat by:
- APC tablet
- Local methyl salicylate ointment application
- Giving hot fomentation

A child with fever and joint pain should be referred to PHC for advice.

Cough, Cold

It is a common condition which is associated with diseases of throat and lung.
- Ask the duration of cough
- Dry? With sputum? Whooping cough?
- Check history of fever, sore throat, chest pain, difficulty in breathing, vomiting or blood-stained sputum
- Any history of weight loss

Treat with:
- APC
- Cough mixture
- Mouth gargling for sore throat by potassium permanganate in water or salt in water
- External application of menthol and eucalyptus oil to throat, chest and back, cover with warm clothes.
- If whooping cough allows rest, keep away from other children, give frequent liquid feed, and refer.

Always refer, if:
- Chronic cough of 15 days
- Blood-stained sputum
- Loss of weight
- Chest pain
- Difficulty in breathing
- Vomiting

Common cold occurs in the rainy season and winter months. This is common in weak and ill-nourished. Symptoms are:
- Running nose
- Blocked nose
- Watering eyes
- Headache
- Body ache
- Fever.

The patient may also have sore throat and ear discharge.

Treatment:
- APC tablets
- Steam inhalation with menthol and eucalyptus oil
- External application of menthol and eucalyptus oil on chest and back
- Plenty of fluids allowed
- Nourishment is continued
- Rest is advised till the patient is free from symptoms.

Referral is done, if:
- Severe headache
- Severe ear infection
- High fever and rigors
- Child patient refuse to eat
- Child patient has difficulty in breathing

Diarrhoea

It is frequent loose stool. This is caused by contaminated water, food and by poor personal hygiene.
- Ask the duration, frequency, consistency of stool

- Ask any associated fever, vomiting, pain abdomen
- Ask whether passed any worms
- Look for sunken eyes, dry mouth, wrinkled skin

Treat the case with:

- Bismuth kaolin mixture in water
- Plenty of oral fluids
- Give soft diet like banana, buttermilk, arrowroot juice, and rice gruel.
- Give ORS
- If there is no ORS packet, then prepare home-made ORS as follows.

Add a pinch of salt and a handful of sugar to little over 1 litre clean potable water. Boil the mixture for 10 minutes. If available, add the juice of half a sour lime to the solution and mix. Keep the container covered and cool the mixture until it can be given without the risk of burning lips or mouth. Give this mixture at frequent intervals.

Refer if:

- There is sign of dehydration.
- If the stool is rice watery.
- If stool contains blood, mucus.
- If worms are passed.
- If fever and vomiting are present.
- If there is no improvement within 24 hours.

Vomiting

Eating infected food, overeating and excessive drinking can cause vomiting. In children, fatty food, spicy food, uncooked food, and improper feeding techniques can cause vomiting.

- Ask frequency of vomiting, nature of vomit (blood, bile, undigested food, watery)
- Ask any abdominal pain, constipation, fever, history of amenorrhoea in women
- Look for skin rash, yellow skin, yellow eyes, signs of dehydration, signs of malnutrition

Treat with:

- Antacid (magnesium hydroxide)
- Oral rehydration fluid

Always refer, if:

- Vomit contains blood
- Severe dehydration
- Unable to retain taken food
- Stool is rice watery
- No improvement within 24 hours

Pain Abdomen

Disease and discomfort of stomach, intestine, liver, spleen, kidney, bladder, uterus (women) can cause abdominal pain. Location of pain refers to organ involved in the patient (Table 22.1).

- Ask the duration of pain
- Ask the place of pain felt over abdomen
- Pain is continuous or not continuous
- Is it related to taking food, passing urine, menstruation (women)
- Any injury or blow on the abdomen
- Check associated fever, nausea, vomiting, diarrhoea, and constipation
- Check skin and eyes for yellow colour
- Check urine colour or blood stained
- Any worm in stool or vomit

Constipation

When the patient has not passed motion for the past 3 days, has discomfort, has staining while passing stool we use the term constipation. In rural areas, irregular bowel habit will be due to absence of privacy or absence of latrine. This is checked through history.

If vomiting and acute pain are present, the case is referred to PHC and no treatment is advisable at visit.

In case of mild symptoms treatment include:

- Magnesium hydroxide tablet
- Plenty of water
- Fresh fruits, leafy vegetables
- Follow-up on next day

Table 22.1: Pain abdomen and treatment

Pain abdomen	*Treatment*
• When no other symptoms	– Milk, soft diet advised – Avoid spices – Avoid raw vegetables – Give APC tablets – Can give ginger juice – Can give garlic juice
• When diarrhoea is associated	– ORS – Plenty of oral fluids – Referral
• When constipation is associated	– Liquid paraffin 1 teaspoon at bed – Time (if PHC supplied) – Referral
• When nausea, vomiting is associated	– Refer
• Passing worms	– Refer the case
• Fever and vomiting are associated	– Refer at the earliest to PHC
• Pregnant women	– Take help of TBA – Refer
• Vaginal bleeding associated	– Give APC tablet – Refer at the earliest to – PHC
• Signs of shock are associated	– Give first aid to see respiration and heart rate is OK – Refer at the earliest to PHC

Toothache

It is common when oral hygiene is poor. History of fever, duration of pain, presence of tooth decay, redness of gums are observed.

Treatment include:
- APC tablet
- Mouthwash with salt water or potassium permanganate water
- Clove is boiled and the oil is applied to affected tooth
- Referred to PHC

Earache

Both ear infection and throat infection cause pain in the ear. Presence of earwax, foreign body in the ear also cause earache.
- Duration of pain is elicited
- Foreign body, insect, a solid object are checked in the ear
- Checked for ear discharge
- Checked for sore throat
- Ask for dizziness or hearing disturbances
- Check for fever

Treatment: Ear discharge is cleaned with sterile swab before putting eardrops. Sulphacetamide eardrops added to the affected ear. APC tablet is given.

Referral: In case of foreign body, high fever, dizziness, hearing disturbances, refer the case.

Sore Eyes

Infections of eye cause soreness of eye. Dust and chemical irritation or injury to eye can lead to sore eyes. Measles in children is looked for. Redness, watering and burning sensation are manifestation of sore eyes. If many people are affected, we should suspect epidemic conjunctivitis.

A check on duration of sore eye, injury, foreign body, fever, skin rash is done.

Treatment:
- Clean outer eye with sterile swab
- Apply sulphacetamide eye drops
- Sunlight, bright light avoided
- APC tablet given

Referral is done: if injury is present and if foreign body is present.

Boil, Abscess

Skin infection leading to red painful swelling of the skin is called boil. The neglected boil develops to an abscess. Abscess contains pus, which is opened-up. This is common in children who are malnourished and who has poor personal hygiene.

Treatment: Boil is given hot fomentation (cloth wrung out of hot water in which neem leaves have been boiled) part is given rest. APC given.

Abscess is dusted with boric powder dressed and referred.

Ulcers

Skin sore due to injury, infection, malnutrition, leprosy, and STD are considered. It shows a broken skin, raw, red, discharge may be watery or pus, painful, may be associated with fever and headache.

Steps taken are:
- Ask how long patient has ulcer
- Any signs of malnutrition
- Any other symptoms like fever, headache and skin rash, getting tired easily.

Treatment:
- Ulcer is cleaned with swab dipped in antiseptic lotion. Cleaning is done away from the ulcer.
- Mercurochrome is applied
- Sulphanilamide powder dusted
- Clean dressing done

Referral is a must when:
- Fever
- Chronic ulcer
- On genitalia
- No improvement

Scabies

This infection is caused by itch mite producing cracks in finger webs, front of the wrist, elbow, armpit, waistline, thigh and external genitalia. Itching is severe especially at night.

No personal hygiene, no daily bath, influence scabies spread. It is common to find all the members of the family are affected.

Steps of treatment:
- Bath with soap and water using brush to open all cracks
- While the skin is slightly wet, apply benzyl benzoate emulsion over the whole body except head and neck
- Allow the body to partly dry
- Apply second layer of benzyl benzoate on the whole body again
- Leave the emulsion on the body for 24 hours
- Next day bath thoroughly with soap and water
- Put on clean washed cloths
- The treatment is repeated for 3 days

Caution: Clothing and bedding are washed well after immersing in boiling water.

Referral: It is done when no improvement is seen.

Ringworm

It is flat, ring-shaped skin infection caused by fungus. They show red border and a lightly coloured scaly centre. It can occur anywhere on the body including scalp. It is accompanied by itching.

Treatment include:

- Bath with soap and water
- Break the scaly centre with a brush
- Apply Whitfield ointment
- Wear clean washed cloth

Referral: It is done when there is no improvement.

RECORD MAINTENANCE BY HEALTH INSPECTOR

Health inspector should maintain a register called "Medical Care Register" which should give the following information.

- Date of visit
- Name of the patient
- Age of the patient
- House number, street, area and village
- Symptoms recorded
- Signs observed
- Treatment given (drug, dose and duration)
- Advice given
- Referral done to whom, to which place.

Medical care register will help the Health Inspector in the following way:

- Reporting to PHC Medical Officer
- Follow-up of case
- To take instructions and to discharge such instructions
- Surveillance of diseases in the service area.

23

Basic Legal Medicine

For the past one century, we know the area of health law, which combines health staff and legal profession. It is concerned with application of knowledge of health and law for the benefit of society.

DEFINITIONS

1. 1942 — *Alan R Moritz* (Harvard University) "The application of medical knowledge to the needs of justice, although by definition this would appear to be a broad and scientifically heterogeneous field, the practice of legal medicine is concerned chiefly with what might be most adequately described as Forensic Pathology".
2. 1975 — *William J Curran* (Boston University) "Area of medicine concerned with relation to Law".

TERMS IN BASIC LEGAL MEDICINE

Affidavit

A written declaration under oath, made without notice to the adverse party.

Allegation

The assertion or statement of a party to an action, made in a pleading, setting out what he expects to prove.

Appeal

The complaint to a superior court of an injustice done by inferior court.

Argument

An effort to establish belief by a course of reasoning, by speeches in the court.

Attachment

A proceeding to take a defendant's property into legal custody.

Case

Generally, it refers to a suit in the court. Case at Bar is the particular case which is before the court.

Common Law

It is a body of law, which is originated, developed and formulated and is administered in a country.

Complaint

It is the first pleading on the part of the plaintiff in a civil action.

Compromise

It is an arrangement for settling a dispute.

Contempt

It is the disobedience of the court's orders.

Court

It is the judicial department that applies the laws to controversies brought before it.

Deposition

It is the testimony of a witness taken in writing under oath.

Evidence

They are witness, record, and document, concrete objects for inducing beliefs in the minds of Jury. They may be (i) direct evidence or (ii) circumstantial evidence.

Execution

It is a judicial writ issued from the court where a judgement is rendered.

Ex parte

Proceedings by and for one party without notice to opposition.

Indemnity

It is a collateral contract when a person engages to secure another person.

Injunction

It is a prohibitive writ issued by the court.

Judgement

Decision given by a court.

Jury

Persons selected to enquire matters of fact to declare truth.

Justice

When a person is disposed to render him his due.

Liability

A state of oblige in law.

Negligence

It is the omission to do something, which a reasonable man does.

Summon

It is notification to inform that a person is required to appear before court.

Surety

When a person binds himself for the payment of a sum of money for another person.

Testimony

Evidence given by witness under oath.

Verdict

A definite answer by Jury to the court.

Will

A written instrument, executed with the formalities of law, whereby a person makes disposition of his property to take effect after his death.

HEALTH INSPECTOR AND PATIENT INTERACTIONS

Very commonly there are two areas, which a Health Inspector comes across. They are:
- Damages
- Dying declaration

Damages

When a person suffers detriment to his person, property or rights from the unlawful act or omission of another; can recover from the person in fault a compensation in money is called *damages*.

Dying Declaration

They are statements made by a person who is at the point of death and who is conscious of his approaching dissolution in reference to the manner in which he received the injuries of which he is dying and in reference to the person who inflicted the injuries.

They are admissible in evidence in a trial.

Area of Legal Medicine

Here, principles of medicine are applied for law. The Health Inspector during the course of his professional duties, comes across certain situations like:

- Examination of case for age
- Examination of injury on human body
- Help MOH in medical examination of sexual offences
- Help MOH in medical examination of poisoning
- In the examination of a case regarding mentally healthy (sane or insanity)
- Help MOH in MLC/autopsies
- Birth registration
- Birth certificate
- Death registration
- Death certificate
- Medico-legal issues
- Community health care as paramedical
  - Check of commercial advertisement
  - Compulsory vaccinations
  - Notification of diseases
  - Isolation of infectious cases
- MTP and related issues
- Use of medicinal drugs
- Major Public Health Acts implementation.

Types of Law

There are three types of law in the country, which are used in Legal medicine. They are:

- *Criminal law*: They are statutes enacted to maintain order in the society.
- *Civil law*: It pertains to compensating individuals who have been injured physically or economically.
- *Administrative law*: This refers to promulgation and enforcement of regulations by Administrative Agencies.

General Public Health Laws

The legal authorities to protect the health and safety of the community define public health. When a condition encounters and threatens the health of the community, then the public health staff has to extend the use of authority to protect the health of the public.

These specify the area of epidemic and spread of acute infections. Reporting, quarantine, isolation, food sanitation, environmental health form main issues in the legal medicine.

Following public health laws are pertinent to note by the Health Inspector, in his day-to-day duties. They go hand in hand as Legal Medicine.

- The Quarantine Act (1825)
- The Birth and Death Registration Act (1973)
- The Vaccination Act (1880)
- The Indian Factory Act (1948)
- The Epidemic Disease Act (1897)
- The Municipal Act (1964)
- The Drug Act (1940)
- The Prevention of Food Adulteration Act (1954)
- The Suppression of Immoral Traffic Act (1956)
- The Population Law (1974)
- The Medical Termination of Pregnancy Act (1971)
- The Karnataka State Nursing Home Act (1976)
- The Employee State Insurance Act (1948)
- The Environment Protection Act (1986)
- The Panchayat Raj Act (1994)
- The Organ Donation Act (1995)
- The Prenatal Diagnostic Technique Act (1996)

Courts of Law (Table 23.1)

- Criminal Court
  - Supreme Court

- High court
- Courts of Session
- Magistrate court
  - Judicial Magistrate's court
  - Additional District Magistrate's court

HEALTH INSPECTOR IN PRIMARY HEALTH CARE

Basic Medico-legal Issues

Health care worker like Health Inspector and his relationship with patient arises from State Statutes and Common Law Rules. By his training and power of designation, the Health Inspector commands status in implementing health care under jurisdiction of basic medico-legal issues.

The courts have reviewed the constitutionality of laws that protect public health and safety. They have developed standards for defining an acceptable exercise of Public Health Authority.

Through District Magistrate, the Health Inspector has the power of designation through DH and FWO or the City Health Officer of the Corporation to exercise power in the interest of public. Particular reference is made on the specific functions as given here:

- Epidemic disease control
- Prevention of food adulteration

Table 23.1: Punishment power and jurisdiction

Punishment power jurisdiction	*Judge/Magistrate*
Death	Judge of Supreme Court
Transportation	Judge of high court
Solitary confinement	Sessions Judge
Fine	Asstt. Sessions Judge
Whipping	Magistrate
All offence	Session courts
2-year imprisonment and solitary confinement with or without fine	I class Magistrate
6-month imprisonment and fine	II class Magistrate
1-month imprisonment and fine	III class Magistrate

Table 23.2: Three-tier system in India

Professional cadre	*Doctors*
Middle level cadre	Health Inspector
Peripheral cadre	Village Health guide and community leaders

- Control of spread of diseases
- Birth and death registration
- Birth and death certification
- Notification of diseases

Today we have the technology and it does not require a high degree of technology to bring appropriate medical care to majority of population that can improve the health status of the family, community and society.

Reorientation of existing concepts of job responsibilities in health system has given us the legislation that defines the health rights of the community, the ongoing National Health Programmes in tackling national health problems.

The Health Inspector stands as Middle Level Cadre in *Three-Tier system (delivery system)* in India.

Legal medicine has provided the following job responsibilities to the Health Inspector in community health care by Primary Health Care:

- Simple diagnosis and simple treatment under doctor's supervision.
- Selection, training and authorisation to do the job are given to Paramedicals under present circumstances.
- Adequate legal recognition and authorisation are given through the Public Health Law and District Magistrate.

CONCLUSION

A number of laws, rules and regulations specifically concerning health professionals also affected the roles of Health Inspector, nurse, pharmacist, physiotherapist and ANM. The rationale for these laws are two-fold:

- One—to ensure that people received safe care

- Two—provision of health care professionals with professional safeguards

The law governing the use of medicinal drugs affects the role of Paramedicals like the Health Inspectors in their duties and responsibilities as health care workers.

No legal medicine is complete without a discussion of:

- Indian Food and Civil Supplies
- The Drug Administration
- Regulation of Food and Drug Products.

Public Health Laboratories and District PH Labs are jointly figuring out the issues and the following assistance are provided in the Public Health Legal Medicine:

- Water analysis
- Milk analysis
- Drug analysis
- Bacteriological analysis.

The public health issues are assisted by:

- Medical Jurisprudence
- Forensic Medicine
- Toxicology.

Appendices

I. Recommended Teaching Hours
II. Scheme of Examination for Health Inspector's Course
III. Paramedical Board Ordinance
IV. Health Inspector's Course
V. Syllabus for the First Year of Certificate Course in Paramedical Subjects for SSLC Passed Candidates (Condensed Course of I and II PUC)
VI. Inspection and Preparation of Fair and Festival
VII. Inspection of Factory
VIII. PFA Act
IX. Proforma for the Food Catering Establishment
X. Malaria Smear Staining
XI. Method of Giving Injection
XII. Camp Organisation (OTC Camp)
XIII. Minimum Information of a Village Record
XIV. Drug List with Health Inspector for Minor Illness Treatment
XV. Job Responsibilities of Health Assistant (Male)
XVI. Sanitary Survey of Village/Town
XVII. The Municipality Act 1964 (Specific Sections Relevant to Health Inspectors)
XVIII. Drugs to be known by Health Inspector in his Daily Routines from Other Systems of Medicine
XIX. Universal Precaution against HIV/AIDS
XX. Hospital Waste Management
XXI. Health Care Establishments Covered under Biomedical Waste (BMW) Rules 1998
XXII. Procedure of Killing the Stray Dogs
XXIII. Emergency Measures in Public Health
XXIV. Time Table for First Year HIT Course
XXV. Theory Coverage for First Year HIT Course
XXVI. Practical Coverage for First Year HIT Course
XXVII. Time Table for Second Year HIT Course
XXVIII. Theory Coverage for Second Year HIT Course
XXIX. Practical Coverage for Second Year HIT Course

Appendix I
Recommended Teaching Hours

Recommended teaching hours for Health Inspector Diploma 2 years' course

	Theory	*Practical/Field Visitors*	*Total*
First year	175 hrs	125 hrs	300 hrs
Second year	45 hrs	255 hrs	300 hrs
Total	220 hrs	380 hrs	600 hrs

Appendix II
Scheme of Examination for Health Inspector's Course

There shall be two examinations—one at the end of the first year called as the Preliminary Examination and the other at the end of the second year called the Final Examination to be conducted by the Paramedical Board.

No student shall be allowed to take up the Preliminary Examination if he has not put in 75% of attendance both in Theory and Practical during the First Year.

No student shall be allowed to take up Final Examination who has not put in 75% of attendance both in Theory and Practical during the II year of the course and also who has not completed successfully all the papers of the I year. However, a student can be permitted to the II year if the attendance is satisfactory during the I year though he has completed all the subjects of the I year.

Qualified Examiners for the Preliminary and Final Examinations will be appointed by the Paramedical Board.

A Certificate will be issued to the successful candidates after the final examination by the Paramedical Board.

Scheme of Examination for Diploma in Health Inspector's Course Preliminary Examination (Part I) at the End of First Year

Grand Total	—	**450 marks**
Theory	—	300
Practical	—	100
Viva Voce	—	50

Theory (Total Marks 300)

Papers	*Subjects*	*Internal assessment*	*Board examination*	*Total*
I.	a. Concepts in community health, sociological concepts of health and diseases b. Behavioural science and its importance in health	10 marks	90 marks	100 marks
II.	a. Nutritional and health b. Elementary microbiology and paracytology with particular emphasis on public health aspects c. Rate of environment in health and disease	10 marks	90 marks	100 marks
III.	a. Basic epidemiology dynamics of disease transmission, concepts of disease prevention and control b. Medical entomology c. Elementary statistics and its role in health sciences	10 marks	90 marks	100 marks

Practical (Total Marks 100)

Board of Examination (3 hr)	*Internal assessment*	*Practical record*	*Total*
80 marks	*10 marks*	*10 marks*	*100 marks*

a. Spotters. 10 slides—20 marks
b. Statistics calculation of vital rates and diagrammatic representation—25 marks
c. Stool examination—15 marks
d. Staining (Basic and special)—20 marks

Viva Voce Examination (Total Marks 50)

Diploma Health Inspector's Course
Final Examination (At the End of the Second Year)

Grand Total	—	**450 Marks**
Theory	—	300
Practical	—	100
Viva Voce	—	50

Theory (Total Marks 300)

Papers	*Subjects*	*Internal assessment*	*Board examination*	*Total*
I.	a. Epidemiology of important communicable and non-communicable disease (National Programme) b. Investigation of epidemics c. Concepts of primary health care	10 marks	90 marks	100 marks
II.	a. MCH and Family Planning b. Health Education and Communication c. Essential drugs and treatment of minor ailment	10 marks	90 marks	100 marks
III.	a. First aid b. Organization and delivery of health care services in India including principles of administration health legislation c. Basics of legal medicine	10 marks	90 marks	100 marks

Practical (Total Marks 100)

Board Examination (3 Hr)	*Internal assessment*	*Practical record*	*Total marks*
80 marks	*10 marks*	*10 marks*	*100*

a. Field inspection and report—40 marks
b. Practical exercise—40 marks
(Communicable disease, FP, PHA)

Viva Voce Examination (Total Marks 50)

Appendix III
Paramedical Board Ordinance

Health Inspector's Course

Name of the course: Diploma in Health Inspector's Course.

Eligibility for admission: A pass in PUC II or equivalent examination with a minimum of 40% marks in optional under Science faculty—such as PCB, PCMB, or CBZ. However, the minimum percentage or marks required can be relaxed to 35% in case of SC/ST students.

Age limit: The candidate should have attained a minimum age of 17 years as on 31st December of the year of admissions. Upper age limit is 40 years for in service candidates and candidates belonging to SC/ST groups. For others upper age limit is 35 years.

Duration of the course: Two year from the commencement of the term.

Infrastructure and Facilities:

a. This course must be run in the Department of P and SM of the Medical College only.
b. A library collecting adequate number of textbooks and reference books or latest edition pertaining to the concerned subjects.

Teaching Personnel

1. A qualified Principal with MBBS degree and PG Qualification in P and SM and having 5 years of teaching experience.
2. One Assistant Professor with MBBS and PG qualification having 3 years of teaching experience.
3. Two qualified Health workers qualified in HEALTH INSPECTOR'S COURSE.
4. The faculty members of attached Medical College or teaching Hospitals on part time basis can teach all the medical subjects.

Appendix IV
Health Inspector's Course

Following is the proposed syllabus for 2 years course for Health Inspector—after 10 + 2:

TOPICS TO BE COVERED DURING PHASE-I, FIRST YEAR

- Elementary concepts of applied anatomy and physiology.
- Sociological concepts of health and disease.
- Behavioural science and its importance in health, disease, administration and management.
- Concepts in community health.
- Elementary statistics and its role in health sciences.
- Elementary microbiology and parasitology with particular emphasis on public health aspects.
- Nutrition and health.
- Role of environment in health and disease.
- Concepts of health and diseases.
- Basic epidemiology.
- Basics of legal medicine.
- Dynamics of disease transmission.
- Concepts of disease prevention and control.
- Medical entomology.
- Concepts of Primary Health Care.

TOPICS TO BE COVERED DURING PHASE-II, SECOND YEAR

- Epidemiology of important communicable and noncommunicable disease (National Programme).
- Investigation of epidemics.
- MCH and Family Planning.
- Health education and communication.
- First aid.
- Organization and delivery of health care services in India including principles of administration, health legislations.
- Essential drugs and treatment for minor ailments.
- Basics of legal medicine.

ELEMENTS OF APPLIED ANATOMY AND PHYSIOLOGY

Understanding of the structure and functions of human body as a foundation to the principles underlying nutrition and disease process.

Practical

- Models, charts and slides related to structure and functions of the human body.
- How to take the blood pressure, pulse rate, respiration rate.
- Films showing the formation of human body.

ELEMENTS OF ENTOMOLOGY

Objectives

To identify the insects of public health importance and its control.

Contents

a. *Morphology:* Life history, bionomics, public health importance and control of the following vectors;
   - Housefly
   - Louse
   - Ticks/Mites
   - Sandfly
   - Rat flea
   - Mosquitoes
   - Cyclops.

b. *Practical:*
   - Demonstration of different stages in life history of above-mentioned vectors.
   - Demonstration of breeding places of the above-mentioned vectors.
   - Demonstration of control measures for the different stages of the above-mentioned vectors.
   - Collection of larva and adult mosquito.

Methods

Lectures, group discussions, films.

ELEMENTS OF MEDICAL MICROBIOLOGY AND PARASITOLOGY

Objectives

To be able to understand by acquiring sufficient knowledge regarding microbiological aspects of infectious disease, Lab and field methods of its diagnosis and principle of control of these infectious agents with particular reference to Public Health Microbiology and Parasitology.

Contents

Introduction to Microbiology: Characterisation including classification, morphology, staining/cultural characteristics, viability, virulence, pathogenicity, sensitivity, resistance, Lab-methods of diagnosis, field investigations.

Immunity
- Concepts
- Classification
- Importance
- Immunizing agents
- Adverse reaction

Disinfection
- Concepts/terminologies
- Principles
- Procedures

Parasitology
- Parasites of public health importance (Locally relevant)
- Including life history, lab diagnosis, field investigations and control measures.

Practical

- Use of microscope
- Demonstration of infectious agents and parasites as relevant locally.

- Methods of field investigations:
  - Specimen collection: Stool, urine, blood, sputum, etc.
- Stool examination: for ova/cysts, hanging drop.
- Blood smear collection, staining and examination.
- Sputum collection, staining and examination.
- Split skin smears collection, staining examination.
- Staining methods: Gram's, Albert's, ZN, JSB and Leishman's.

ENVIRONMENTAL SANITATION

Objectives

To acquire sufficient knowledge to understand the:
- Impact of environment on health.
- Impact of sanitation on health and to take preventive/promotive measures.

Contents

Water supply
- Source: Physical and Chemical
- Quality: Bacteriological indicators
- Conservation of sources, collection, storage and distribution.

With respect to:
Urban areas
- Steps in purification of water, storage, filtration, chlorination
- Purification of water on large scale with particular reference to rapid sand filter.

Rural areas
- Sanitary well: Concept, principles
- Purification of water in small scale: Bore well.

Practical

- Demonstration of purification of water on small scale.
- Visit to water treatment plant and a brief report.
- Collection of water samples.
- Demonstration of physical, chemical, bacterial quality of water.
- Estimating chlorine demand, steps in disinfection, estimating residual chlorine.
- Interpreting a water analysis.

WASTE DISPOSAL

Characterisation

- Solid/Liquid
- General—household/special circumstance including aspects of managements with emphasis on: Points of generation, storage. Collection, transportation and different options available for management (in terms of reducing, recycling, composting, landfill, soakage pit, sanitary latrine, septic tank, biogassification).
- Hazards due to improper/inappropriate management.
- Protective devices/universal precautions.
- Sewage treatment methods.

Practical

- Undertake waste survey in market area, hotel, health care settings (preferably a 30 bed institution).
- Demonstration of composting, incineration, sanitary landfill.
- Demonstration of Trench latrine, Sanitary latrine (including its maintenance). Septic tank, Biogas plant.
- Visit to a sewage treatment plant.

RESIDENTIAL ENVIRONMENT

General principles of healthy housing in terms of:

- Site, foundation, material and constructions.
- Walls, roof, floor, rooms, ventilators, lighting.
- Facilities/methods for waste disposal both solid/liquid.
- Codes/Regulations and legislations pertaining to scrutiny of buildings.

Practical

- Visit/observe at least 4 residences (2 urban and 2 rural); report and suggest practical, solution.
- Interact with Municipal authorities regarding legislative provisions.

AIR AND VENTILATION

- Concepts, importance of adequate ventilation.
- Ill effects of inadequate ventilation.
- Type of ventilation.
- Indicators of air pollution.
- Measures to reduce air pollution.

INDUSTRIES AND TRADE

- Location, ventilation, water supply, sanitation, lighting.
- Control of dust and other hazards substances.
- Occupational risk factor and safety measures.
- Legislative provisions.

Practical

- Visit to an industry and report.

PUBLIC GATHERINGS

- Selection of place
- Provision of:
  - — Safe water supply
  - — Sanitary disposal of waste — Solid / Liquid
  - — Construction of trench latrine
- Provision for emergency medical help
- Disaster planning

Practical

Visit/observe a weakly fair report with practical suggestions.

SCHOOL ENVIRONMENT

Standards of space, walls, roofs, floor, furniture, lighting, ventilation, water supply, playground, latrine.

Practical

- Disinfection of wells, testing for residual
- Water sampling
- Construction of latrine plates and pans
- Building of superstructure
- Construction of simple septic tanks
- Construction of bathing facilities, cattle drinking troughs and laundering platforms.
- Construction of smokeless chulhas
- Residual spraying
- Preparation of chemical solution for spraying and larvicides.
- Construction of compost pits and soakage pits.

NUTRITION

Objectives

To acquire sufficient knowledge regarding:
- Nutritional requirement of the body in maintenance of health including those for special groups like infants, pregnant and lactating women.
- Preventing nutritional deficiencies
- Promoting adequate nutrition.

Contents

- Concepts in nutrition like:
  - Classification of food
  - Nutrients—carbohydrates, proteins, fats, vitamins minerals—their daily requirement
  - Nutritive values of common food articles.
  - Balanced diet
  - Nutritional requirement for special group infants, weaning, pregnancy, lactation, pre-school, school going.
  - Assessment of nutritional status for family/individual.
  - Cultural factors/nutrition.
  - Nutrition education.
  - Malnutrition concepts:
    - Characterisation
    - Home management
    - Follow-up, therapeutic diet.

Practical

- Demonstration of food articles and their nutritive values.
- Planning a balanced diet
- Demonstration of kitchen garden for mother in community.
- Diet survey—3 families with nutrition education.

FOOD SANITATION

Objectives

- To acquire knowledge regarding the importance of maintenance and promotion of food sanitation.
- To acquire practical skills in detecting adulteration of food articles.
- To be conversant with legislative provisions.

Contents

- Disease transmitted through food including milk.
- Food poisoning, food adulterants, food toxins, food additives, food fortification, food safety.
- Concepts of food preservation—storage/transportation
- Mass catering—concepts, hazards, preventive measures.
- Legislations regarding promoting food sanitation with particular reference to FPA Act and Local bodies statutory requirements.
- Food processing centres including slaughterhouses, cottage industries in food (e.g. pickles, potato chips, etc.), public hazards, health importance, preventive measures.
- Food vending centres including markets, supermarkets, wholesales/Retail outlets.

Practical

- Visits and observation.
- Daily, marketplace, hotel, supermarket, wholesalers, retailers, slaughterhouse, food-processing factory.
- Common tests to detect food adulteration.
- Procedure for food sampling, dispatching and interpretation of results.
- Inspect and report on food establishment, marketplace and slaughterhouse.
- Interaction with a food analyst, visit to a Public Health Institute.

GENERAL EPIDEMIOLOGY

General Concepts of Control

- Selected definitions (e.g. Endemicity, Epidemic, Epizootic, Incubation period, etc.).
- *Concepts in disease:*
  - Causation, levels of prevention, modes of intervention, spectrum of illness, epidemiological triad, web of causation.
- Dynamics of disease transmission, including modes of transmission.
- Identification of the week link in chain of disease transmission.
- Different control measures—(e.g. protection of susceptible, immunisation, chemoprophylaxis, prompt treatment).
- Investigation of an outbreak.

Study of Communicable Disease

- *Airborne/Droplet infections*: Chickenpox, measles, diphtheria, mumps, measles, whooping cough, influenza, meningitis, TB, ARI
- *Water/food-borne infections*: Diarrhoeal diseases, polio, HAB, Guinea worm.
- *Zoonotic*: Rabies, anthrax
- *Contact*: Scabies, pediculosis.
- Tetanus; leprosy, arthropod-borne diseases.

Practical

- Outbreak investigation/reporting/practical suggestions.
- Visit to isolation hospital
- Demonstration of disinfection procedures for body fluids/discharges of persons suffering from the communicable diseases.
- Involve in planning, conducting an immunization session. Comment on the cold chain. Report and recommended practical solutions.

NONCOMMUNICABLE DISEASES

- Definitions/terminologies
- Public health importance of DM, HT, blindness, cancer, CHD.
- Health education.

ELEMENTS OF SOCIAL SCIENCE, RURAL COMMUNITY AND CHARACTERISTICS

Contents

- Family structures, relationships and responsibilities of individual.
- Community structure. Functioning of the community, its privileges and responsibilities, maintenance of law and order. Collection and expenditure of revenues. Services provided.
- Types of social institutions, religion, state, family marriage, inheritance of property, social rites on marriages and deaths, etc. regulated human behaviour in the society, difference and similarly in the institutions of primitive and advanced societies.
- Duties and responsibilities, citizenship, development of desirable social attitudes, ideals and abilities, Community organization for self-help, cooperative society.
- Comparative idea of the Indian and rural society, characteristics of the people and habitats, urban society in India; economic, educational and social difference between urban and rural society, caste, religion and nationality.
- Improvements in the standards of health and life expectancy; social customs and forms; resistance to adoption of new practices and things. Problem social order; economic aspects of family life; income and budget.
- Rural community and characteristics.

PERSONAL HYGIENE

Contents

- Habits and customs affecting personal hygiene.
- Cleanliness of body, habits, diet, clothing, exercise, and sleep, public baths, care of special senses.

CLIMATOLOGY

- General effects of climate on health
- Prevention of effects of cold climate
- Prevention of effects of hot climate
- Demonstrations 4 hours
- Visit to meteorological department 3 hours.

VITAL STATISTICS

Contents

- Definition, value and objectives.
- Population census, estimate of population.

- Rates—birth rate, death rate, infant mortality rate, stillbirth rate, neonatal rate; maternal mortality and morbidity rates—significance.
- Importance and use of vital statistics—informants, collections, compilation and presentation.
- Registration—rural, urban objects, machinery, checking.
- Notification records, use of:
  - Record keeping and reporting, definitions, purpose, application, classification, service, records, sanitation, village health record—sanitary survey, form spot maps.

Practical

- Calculation of rates
- Presentation of vital statistics.

PUBLIC HEALTH ADMINISTRATION

Contents

- Evaluation of health services with particular reference to India.
- Central, state and local organizations.
- Relationships with other departments. Education, agriculture, communications.
- International organisations and their co-operation in the field of health.
- Voluntary agencies in health programme.
- Rural development, concept, organisation, local self-government, Panchayat, Co-operatives.
- Health Centre: Concept, definition, organisation, functions.
- Role of Health Centre in health programme.
- Role of Health Inspector in a PHC.
- Legal consideration: Public health acts, rules.
- Impact of sickness on the individual, the family and the community.

HEALTH EDUCATION

Contents

- Introduction of health education, definitions, philosophy, scope.
- Education in relation to environmental sanitation programme
- Sanitary inspectors approach to village health problems for organising educational programme.
- Sanitary inspectors approach to village health problems for organising educational programme.
- Principles underlying use of visual aids.
- Place of visual aids in education programme; importance of using visual aids.
- Tools and techniques in health education.
- Utilising community resources for educational programme.
- Education through Primary Health Centre.

Practical

- Demonstration of audio-visual aids; posters, flip-charts, flannel graphs, *khaddar* graphs, film strips, films, puppet shows, etc.
- Preparing: Bulletin/Boards, charts, flannel graph.
- Evaluation of teaching aids, organising meetings.
- Collecting information about resources available in the region.

MATERNAL AND CHILD HEALTH AND FAMILY PLANNING

Contents

- History of MCH movement; present organisation, other agencies
- Pre-natal services, maternity hospitals and pre-natal clinics, MCH centre, clinics, private clinics, etc.
- Diet supplements
- Home visiting
- Delivery services, maternity hospitals and homes
- Domiciliary midwifery, salaried midwifery service, private midwife practice
- Infant and pre-school services
- Family welfare
- Role of Health Inspectors in MCH Programme.

DRUGS

- Source of drug, western, Ayurvedic, Unani and others
- Mode of action
- Hazards in prescribing drugs without expert medical advice
- Drugs commonly used by health inspectors
  - Anti-malarial and anti-filariasis, sulphones, drugs for dysentery and diarrhoea and deworming drugs.
- Treatment of minor ailments and injuries.

MANAGEMENT OF HEALTH CARE WASTE

1. Public health importance
2. Disease transmitted due to improper waste management
3. Definitions/classifications
4. *Concepts in waste management*:
   - Point of generation
   - Segregation
   - Sanitary landfill
   - Incineration.

   } Periodic Medical Examination
5. Universal precautions to prevent HBV/HIV infection
6. M*ethods of waste management*:
   a. Different types of waste and their recommended methods of management
   b. Three hierarchies
      - Reduction and recycling
      - Final disposal including deep burial
      - Sanitary landfill, Incineration
7. Occupational hazards of waste handlers
8. Importance of monitoring/recording.

Practical

- *Educating Session*: Pourakarmikas/Labourers regarding
  - Universal precautions
  - Use of protective devices
  - Hazards of improper waste managements.

Appendix V
Syllabus for the First Year of Certificate Course in Paramedical Subjects for SSLC Passed Candidates (Condensed Course of I and II PUC)

Paper	*Subjects*	*Teaching (Hr)*		*Examination (Marks)*		
		Theory	*Practical*	*Int. Ass.*	*Board Exam*	*Total*
I.	English	60	–	10	90	100
II.	Physics	60	10	10	90	100
III.	Chemistry	50	10	10	90	100
IV.	Biology	50	10	10	90	100
						400

ENGLISH

Articles

There are two types of articles. They are:

1. **Indefinite articles** are 'a' and 'an'. They are used to denote the singularity of an object. A is used before a consonant and 'An' is used before a vowel. Vowel sounds are a, e, i, o, and u.

   Examples

   a. Indefinite article 'A'—A ball, a village, a school, a cat, a dog, a yatch, a woman, a man, etc. (Consonants are Ka, Cha, ta, tha, Pa)

   b. 'An'—used before vowel sounds.
      i. An aunt
      ii. An apple
      iii. An European
      iv. An egg
      v. An inkbottle
      vi. An ox
      vii. An umbrella.

2. **Definite article**—The

   It is not used before proper nouns. But it is used before famous rivers, mountains and epics.

   Examples

   a. Rivers—the Ganges, the Amazon
   b. Mountains—the Himalayas, the Vindya, the Alps.
   c. Epics—the Ramayana, the Mahabharata, the Allied, the Odyssey, the Quran.

Tense

1. *Present Tense*

   i. Simple present or present indefinite:

      Examples

      I teach He teaches They teach

      I swim He swims They swim

   ii. Present continuous:

      He is teaching
      She is teaching
      They are teaching

   iii. Present perfect:

      He is taught
      She is taught
      They are taught

   iv. Present perfect continuous:

      He has been teaching
      She has been teaching
      They have been teaching

2. *Past tense*

   i. Simple past:

      He taught

She taught
They taught

ii. Past continuous:
He was teaching
She teaching
They were teaching

iii. Past perfect:
He had taught
She had taught
They had taught

iv. Past perfect continuous:
He had been teaching
She had been teaching
They had been teaching

3. *Future tense*
   i. Simple future:
   He will teach
   She will teach
   They will teach

   ii. Future continuous:
   He will be teaching
   She will be teaching
   They will be teaching

   iii. Future perfect:
   He will have taught
   She will have taught
   They will have taught

   iv. Future perfect continuous:
   He will have been teaching
   She will have been teaching
   They will have been teaching

4. *Active voice and passive voice*
   No details
   Simple sentences to transform from active to passive

5. *Direct and indirect speeches*
   a. Direct: The teacher said to the students "I am not well"
   Indirect: The teacher told the students that he was not well.

   Note:
   - In reported speech verb 'say' of direct speech becomes 'tell' in indirect speech.
   - 'I' becomes 'he'
   - Tense is changed to its corresponding past.

   b. The teacher said to the student, "Are you not keeping well?"
   ID: The teacher enquired the student if he was keeping well.

   c. The teacher said to the student, "Get out of the class".
   Indirect Speech: The teacher ordered the student to get out of the class.

   d. Indirect Speech: Mary said to John "Please lend me your books"
   Direct Speech: "Mary requested John to lend her his book".

   e. Mary said, "What a surprise!"
   Mary exclaimed that it was a surprise.

f. Direct speech: The Police asked the stranger, "Where are you going? "
Indirect speech: The police enquired the stranger as to where he was going.
Direct speech: The police said to the thief, " Where did you steal the scooter?"
Indirect speech: The police interrogated the thief as to where he stole the scooter?

Linkers

- In addition to
- Besides
- Moreover
- However
- Because
- Either, or, Neither, nor.

Examples:

1. Rama is very obedient
   Rama is a loving husband
   Rama, in addition to being obedient, is a loving husband also.
2. John is good in studies
   John is good in sports
   John besides being good in studies is good in sports as well.
3. James is a successful businessman.
   James is hardworking.
   James is a successful businessman. Moreover, he is hardworking.
4. Mary did not study well.
   Mary passed the exam.
   Mary did not study well. However, she passed the exam.
5. Suresh is honest.
   Suresh is respected.
   Because Suresh is honest, he is respected.
6. You study.
   You go to sleep
   Either you study or go to sleep.
7. The doctor was not present in the hospital
   The nurse was not present in the hospital
   Neither the doctor nor the nurse was present in the hospital.

Example of using Linkers in Paragraph

Taking photographs of birds is more difficult than wild animals. Because, the wild animals pose at least for a few minutes. But birds camera shy, and do not stay in one place for long. Moreover, any slight noise or movement is enough to distract the birds. Hence, a great deal of patience is required for a wild life photograph.

This passage also can be used as an example for paragraph writing.

Paragraph writing

A. A paragraph can be begun with a topic.
   Sentence: e.g. elephant is a useful animal.
   After this topic sentence, show how an elephant is useful to man.

OR

B. Write uses of an elephant and finally end, with the topic sentence that ' Elephant is a useful animal'.

Letter writing

Formal letter or official letter (Format)

Bangalore–41
03.02.2004

From address
TK Suresh
176, 36 'A' Cross,
18th Main Road
4–T Block, Jayanagar,
BANGALORE – 560041

To
The Principal
The National College
Basavangudi
BANGALORE – 560004
Sub: Request for TC [Transfer Certificate]

Sir,

I am a student of your college, studying in II BSc II (computers). I have passed I BSc with Reg. No..... due to unexpected circumstances, I am going to continue my studies in Karnataka Science College, Dharwar. Therefore, I request you send my TC to the Principal, Karnataka Science College, Dharwar.

Thanking you,
Yours faithfully,
TK SURESH

Letter of application (Format)

Bangalore
03.02.2004

From Address

Gopinath C
127, Shirur Park Road
Sheshadripuram
BANGALORE – 560009

To
The Headmaster
Gandhinagar High school
Gandhinagar
BANGALORE – 560009

Dear Sir,

Yours advertisement in Deccan Herald 15.10.99.

In response to the reference cited above, I am submitting my application for the post of a typist in your school. I have passed the senior typewriting exams both Kannada and in English after PUC. I have worked for a private finance company as a typist. I am enclosing the required documents.

Kindly consider my application favourably.

With regards,
Yours faithfully,
Signature.

Report Writing

Students must be told to pay attention to factual details. Passive sentences to be used while reporting (If it is a medical report – appropriate method should be followed).

Telegrams

- Learners must be instructed to write the address of the person in detail. Message must be brief.
  Sender's name should be brief, and short if it is going to be charged.

- Sender's address must be given at the bottom of the application.

- E-mail.

PHYSICS

Theory: 60 hours **Practical: 10 hours**

For I year paramedical course for students who have passed their X Standard (SSLC) examination.

UNIT-1: UNITS AND DIMENSIONS

1.1 Definition of Unit CGS and SI units. Definition of dimension. Dimensions of certain physical quantities (10 examples) Mention of uses of dimensions.

UNIT-2: DYNAMICS

2.1 Motion of a particle, definitions of speed, uniform speed and variable speed, velocity, uniform and variable velocity, acceleration, uniform and variable equations of motion for a uniformly accelerated particle (no derivation). Acceleration due to gravity corresponding equations. Newton's law of gravitation. Artificial satellite, orbital and escape velocity, expressions (no derivation) 3 hours

Problems (direct substitution problems) 1 hour

2.2 Newton's laws of motion. Mention of F = ma. Law of conservation of momentum (Statement and explanation) 1 hour

Problems 1 hour

2.3 Work, power and energy—definition. Units, expressions for potential and kinetic energies (no derivation). Law of conservation of energy statement. Explanation with respect to a freely falling body (qualitative) SHM definition examples. 3 hours

Problems 1 hour

UNIT-3: STATICS

3.1 *Scalars and vectors*. Concurrent co-planar forces. Resultant law of parallelogram of forces. Expression for resultant (no derivation) special cases, law of triangle of forces Lami's theorem. Components of a force. Resolution—rectangular components. 3 hours

Problems 1 hour

UNIT-4

4.1 Surface tension, phenomenon, definition, unit viscosity—definition and unit 1 hour

UNIT-5: HEAT

5.1 Heat and temperature units—mention of different types of thermometers 1 hour

5.2 Expansion of solids, liquids and gases. Gas laws—Boyle's and Charles's. law Statement—explanation. Mention perfect gas equation and problems. 2 hours

5.3 Thermal radiation—properties and uses 1 hour

UNIT-6: GEOMETRICAL OPTICS

6.1 Introduction to light. Optical medium. Rectilinear propagation of light—illustration 1 hour

6.2 Laws of reflection. Plane mirror. Image formation. Spherical mirrors. Definitions of pole, centre of curvature, focal length—aperture, radius of curvature. Mention of mirror formula, magnification and formula for magnification (no derivation) 2 hours

Simple problems 1 hour

6.3 Refraction—laws, refractive index (relative and absolute). Critical angle and total internal reflection. 1 hour

6.4 Refraction through a lens. Image formation in a lens. Mention of lens formula. Magnification and formula for magnification 2 hours

Problems 1 hour

6.5 Dispersion—definition, refraction through a prism—spectrum—pure and impure spectrum. 1 hour

6.6 Simple microscope, compound microscope, telescope (Astronomical and Galilean). Description without ray diagram. Formula for magnifying power (no derivation). Spectrometer. Description (without diagram). Simple problems. 5 hours

UNIT-7: WAVES AND SOUND

7.1 Wave, wave motion, longitudinal and transverse waves, characteristics of wave motion. Mention of $V = F\lambda$. Propagation of waves from one medium to another medium.

Problems

7.2 Sound-introduction—properties. Newton-Laplace equation (no derivation), variation of velocity of sound with respect to pressure, temperature and humidity (quantitative).

Problems

7.3 Ultrasonic, infrasonic and audible frequency, ultrasonic properties and uses.

UNIT-8: ELECTRONICS

8.1 Friction, charges types of charges. Electroscope and electrometer (derivation description). Coulomb's law (statement and equation). Electric field, electric intensity and potential units and expressions. Important applications of static electricity. 2 hours

Simple problems 1 hour

8.2 Capacitance, definition, unit, capacitor. Mention of different types of capacitors, uses. 1 hour

UNIT-9: CURRENT ELECTRICITY

9.1 Introduction, definition of current unit, potential difference, Ohm's law, statement, explanation, resistance, conductance units—limitations of Ohm's law. Variation of resistance with respect to dimensions and temperature. Specific resistance (resistivity) and temperature co-efficient of resistance. Combination of resistances in series and in parallel. Effective resistance in series and in parallel—expressions (without derivation), branch currents in parallel circuit (expressions only).

Emf of a cell, internal resistance, terminal PD (expressions to be mentioned). 4 hours

Ohm's law applied to a circuit.

Problems 1 hour

9.2 Brief description of ammeter and voltmeter and mode of connection in an electrical circuit. 1 hour

9.3 Electromagnetic induction—phenomenon laws—statement and mention of applications. 1 hour

9.4 DC and AC—generation of AC (principle only), peak value rms value of current and voltage and expression. Definition of impedance. Brief description of transformer. 2 hours

UNIT-10: MODERN PHYSICS

10.1 Introduction—Cathode rays properties, uses photoelectric effect and its application and uses. X-rays—production and uses 3 hours

10.2 Radioactivity—properties of nuclear radiations. Radioisotopes and their uses. Nuclear fission, nuclear fusion. Nuclear reactor and its uses. 3 hours

10.3 Semiconductors, p-type, n-type, p-n junction diode. Transistor and its uses.

Note: Only SI units should be given for all physical quantities.

PRACTICAL WORK [DIMENSION] **10 hours**

- Measurements with slide callipers and screw Gauge.
- Focal length of a concave mirror.
- Focal length and refractive index of the material of a convex lens.
- Refractive index of the material of the prism using a spectrometer.
- Resonance column experiment—to find $V_{\_}$ and V_0
- Verification of Ohm's law and calculation of resistance.
- Verification of law of resistance in series and parallel.
- Determination of specific resistance of the material of a wire using Wheatstone's bridge or Metre–bridge.

Note:

1. Use of logarithm should be explained in calculation.
2. Elements of trigonometry should be taught. 10 hours
   10 marks from internal examinations.

PATTERN OF THE QUESTION PAPER FOR FINAL EXAMINATION

Time: 3 hours Max. Marks 90

Part A: 18 questions of 1 mark each to be given
16 questions to be answered (16)

Part B: 10 questions of 2 marks each to be given
8 questions to be answered (16)

Part C: 8 questions of 4 marks each to be given
7 questions to be answered (28)

Part D: 6 Problems of 5 mark each to be given
4 questions to be answered (20)

Part E: a. (Practical experiments) 2 questions of 6 marks each to be given 1 question to be answered (6)
b. 1 question—two or three experimental readings to be given from which the required quantity can be calculated—4 marks.

Total Marks 90

CHEMISTRY

Theory: 50 hours | Practical: 10 hours

I. Hydrogen peroxide—preparation, properties and uses — 1 hour

II. Sulphuric acid—manufacture by contact process—properties and uses. — 2 hours

III. Nitric acid—manufacture by Oswald's process—properties and uses — 2 hours

IV. *Halogens*:
- Fluorine—preparation, properties and uses
- Chlorine—preparation, properties and uses
- Bromine—preparation, properties and uses
- Iodine—preparation, properties and uses — 3 hours

V. Structure of an atom, atomic weight, molecular weight. Equivalent weight of an element—definition, methods of determination—to determine the equivalent weight of magnesium by hydrogen displacement method—to determine the equivalent weight of copper by oxide—method.
To determine the equivalent weight of lead by chloride method—problems — 3 hours

VI. Acids, bases and salts, indicators. Equivalent weight of an acid, base, oxidizing and reducing agent. Normality, molarity, molality, volumetric analysis—problems — 3 hours

VI. Hydrocarbons—saturated and unsaturated
Alkanes—methane, ethane—preparation, properties and uses.
Alkenes—ethylene—preparation, properties and uses.
Alkynes—acetylene—preparation, properties and uses. — 3 hours

VIII. Colloids—difference between colloids and crystalloids—classification of colloids—methods of preparation of sols—dialysis—applications of colloids in medicine, food, Cottrell's electrical precipitator.

IX. *Electrochemistry*:
- Arhenius theory of electrolytic dissociation—merits and demerits.
- Acids and bases—Lowry and Brousted concept hydrogen ion concentration—pH, pOH of a solution.
- pH values of biological fluids.
- Buffer solutions—definition—different types of buffer solutions.
- To determine the pH of a solution using buffer solutions.
- To determine the pH of a solution using buffer solution (Indicator method).
- Henderson's equation
- Importance of buffer solutions in medicine — 6 hours

X. Radioactivity—natural radioactivity—properties of alpha, beta and gamma particles—Half-life period—Isotopes—applications of CO^{60}, P^{32}, I^{131}, Na^{24}. — 3 hours

XI. Sodium hydroxide—method of manufacture (Nelson cell)—properties and uses.
Sodium carbonate—method of manufacture—properties and uses. — 3 hours

XII. a. Ethyl alcohol—manufacture from molasses—properties and uses.
Benzyl alcohol—preparation—properties and uses.
b. Phenol—manufacture from coal tar—properties and uses.
c. Aldehydes—formaldehyde, acetaldehyde, benzaldehyde—preparation properties and uses.
d. Ketones—acetones—preparation, properties and uses.
e. Acids—formic, acetic, benzoic and salicylic acids.
f. Esters—ethyl acetate—preparation, properties and uses.
g. Diethyl ether—preparation, properties and uses. Amines classification. — 10 hours

XIII. *Carbohydrates*:
- Classification, open and ring structures of glucose, fructose.
- Ring structure of maltose, sucrose and lactose.
- Partial representation of structure of cellulose, starch, glycogen.
- Carbohydrates as a source of energy. 3 hours

XIV. Proteins—amino acids—formulae of amino acids such as glycine, alanine, serine, cystiene, aspartic acid, lysine, tyrosine.
Peptide linkage—functional properties of proteins such as enzymes, antibodies, transport agents, biochemical messengers—hormones (insulin, oxytocin) 3 hours

XV. Nucleic acids—DNA and RNA—purine and pyrimidine bases—biological importance of nucleic acids. 2 hours

PRACTICAL **10 hours**

Titrations

- Estimation of sodium carbohydrate using standard hydrochloric acid.
- Estimation of sodium hydroxide using standard hydrochloric acid.
- Estimation of oxalic acid using standard potassium permanganate.
- Estimation of iodine using standard sodium through sulphate.
- Tests for carbohydrates and proteins.

BIOLOGY

Theory: 50 hours Practical: 10 hours

I. A. Study of cell—Ultra structure of cell membranes, cell organelles, endoplasmic reticulum, mitochondria, Golgi bodies, ribosome, lysosomes and nucleus.
Cell division—mitosis and meiosis 2 hours

B. Ultra structure of a typical chromosome. Branches of biology—cell biology, physiology, anatomy, histology and biochemistry—fundamentals.

II. A. Viruses—general structure of a virus. Diseases caused by viruses—encephalitis, polio, mumps, measles, smallpox, AIDS. 1½ hours

B. Bacteria—general structure of bacteria, types of bacteria—based on shape. Bacterial disease—diphtheria, cholera, gonorrhoea, syphilis, plague, pneumonia, tetanus, typhoid and tuberculosis. 1½ hours

III. A. Enzymes—nature classification and mechanism of its action.
B. Nucleic acids—occurrences, structures, functions of DNA and RNA. 1½ hours

IV. *Genetics:*
- Sex determination in man
- Human blood groups and Rh factors, genetic engineering 1½ hours

V. *Biotechnology:*
- Basics of gene—cloning 3 hours
- Basics of genetic finger printing
- Biological molecules—carbohydrates, proteins, lipids.

VI. Human histology—structure and functions of basic tissue.
- Epithelium 1½ hours
- Connective tissues—areolar tissue, adipose, cartilage, bone 2 hours
- Muscular 1 hour
- Blood and lymph 1 hour

• Nervous tissue.	1 hour
• TS of small intestine, liver and pancreas	2 hours
VII. *Human anatomy and physiology:*	
• Digestive system—digestion of proteins, lipids and carbohydrates.	3 hours
• Circulatory system—structure of heart, artery and vein.	
Mechanism of working of heart, blood pressure	1 hour
• Respiratory system + Mechanism of breathing.	1½ hours
Brief account of cellular respiration glycolysis and Kreb's cycle	1½ hours
• a. Excretory system + Ultrastructure of nephron.	1½ hours
b. Urine formation.	
c. Important nitrogenous wastes—urea, uric acid, NHB, creatine and creatinine	1 hour
• *Nervous system*: Main divisions	
a. Central nervous system.	
b. Peripheral nervous system.	
c. Autonomic nervous system	1½ hours
Main parts of the brain and their functions.	1½ hours
VIII. *Reproductive system and embryology:*	
• Male and female reproductive system	1 hour
• Structures of sperm and graafian follicle	1 hour
• Brief account of fertilisation	1 hour
• Cleavage and early development up to blastocyst stage	1 hour
• Germ layers and their derivative	1 hour
• Implantation	1 hour
• Placenta—structure and function	1 hour

IX. Endocrinology—Hormones of the following endocrine glands and their functions. Effects of their hypo- and hypersecretion.

- Pituitary
- Thyroid
- Adrenal
- Ovary
- Testes

X. *Cancer biology:*

Cancer characteristics and causes, listing of types of cancer and preventive measures.

PRACTICAL	**10 hours**
I. Microscopic study of typical cell, virus bacterium.	1 hour
II. Study of basic tissues.	4 hours
III. TS of liver and pancreas	1 hour
IV. Study of sperm and graafian follicle	1 hour
V. Physiology	3 hours

- Tests for protein—Biuret's test
- Test for carbohydrate—iodine test
- Test for fats—acroteic test
- Test for urine sugar—Benedict's test.

Appendix VI
Inspection and Preparation of Fair and Festival

Checklist to Health Inspector

1. Planning the arrangement—levelling, road poster, advertisements.
2. Accommodation—residence block with sanitary convenience.
3. In charge for 1 block for medical and sanitary arrangement.
4. Filtered water supply.
5. Conservancy—road sweeping, urinal cleaning, latrine cleaning.
   1 Sweepers per 2000 pilgrims
   2 Seats (Latrine) per 1000 people for 1 day fair
   1 Seat (Latrine) per 100 for 1 week fair.
6. Supervision on open food sale.
7. Cholera inoculation, if DH and FWO has notified
8. Inspection post to check sick person entry.
9. Handling prostitute problem.

Appendix VII
Inspection of Factory

Checklist to Health Inspector

Name of Factory ________ Production item ______ Number of marks ______________

Working hours ___________ Plant cleanliness

Water supply ______________ Food sanitation at canteen______________

Sanitary conveniences __________ Sufficient working place______________

Lighting ________ Cross-ventilation ______________

Medical treatment facility ______________

First aid training of workers ______________

Crèches/day nurses ______________

Maternity benefit to women workers ______________

Frequency of health check-up of workers ______________

Does the factory come under offensive trade?

Welfare activities existing in the factory

____

____

____

____

Remarks:

____

____

____

Signature of Inspector

Appendix VIII
PFA Act

PFA (Prevention of Food Adulteration Act) was enacted in 1954.
Later, it was amended twice in 1976 and the other 1986.
Present Act is called PFA (Amendment) Act 1986. ________

Published in Gazette of India Part II section I on 26.12.1986. ________

i. Adulterant—any material that could be employed for purpose of adulteration.
ii. Adulterated—an article is not of the nature, substance or quality demanded by the purchaser.
    - An article affect injuriously the quality thereof.
    - Cheaper substance has been substituted wholly or in part.
    - Wholly or in part abstracted so as to affect injuriously the quality thereof.
    - Prepared, packed, under insanitary condition.
    - Article is putrid
    - Content injurious to health obtained from diseased animal
    - Contain poisonous ingredient.
    - Colour not within the prescribed limit.
    - Contain prohibited preservative.
    - Quality falls below the prescribed standard.

Food—means any article used as food or drink for human consumption other than drugs and water.

Misbranded—when imitated, falsely stated, sold in others' name, made to appear better, false claim on label, not conspicuously stated.

General Provisions as a Food

- Prohibition of import of certain article of food
- Application of law relating to sea customs and powers of customs officers.
- Prohibition of manufacture, sale, etc. of certain article of food.

Analysis of Food

- Public analysist—government (Centre or State) by notification appoints persons with prescribed qualifications.
- Food inspectors
  - The Central or State Government, by notification appoints person with prescribed qualification who do not have any financial interest in manufacture, import or sale of article of foods.
  - Every food inspector shall be deemed to be public servant within the meaning of section 21 of IPC 1860 (45 of 1860)
- Powers of food inspectors:
  - To take samples of any article of food at selling or at course of conveying and after selling.
  - To send such sample for analysis to the public analyst for the local area within which sample has been taken.
  - Prohibit sale of article of food with the previous approval of Local Health Authorities.
  - Inspect and collect suspected sample of article of food.
  - Can seize, carry away and keep in safe custody of the vendor
  - Has power to break open package or break open door of any premises

- But follow provisions of code of criminal procedure 1973 (2 of 1974)
- Can seize documents
- Can ascertain true name and residence of person (sec 57 of CCP 1973) (2 of 1974).

Procedure to be followed by Food Inspectors (Sec 11)

- Give notice in writing to person before collection.
- Divide to 3 parts, mark and seal
- Send 1 part to Public Analyst
- Send 2 parts to Local Health Authority.

Sec 15—Notification of food poisoning

Sec 16—penalties

Sec 22—protection of action taken in good faith—no suit, prosecution or other legal proceedings shall lie against any person for anything which is in good faith done or intended to be done under this Act.

Appendix IX
Proforma for the Food Catering Establishment

I. *General information*
  1. Authority to inspect:
  2. Date of inspection:
  3. Name and Address of Catering Establishment:
  4. Name of the owner:
  5. License No. and is it renewed for Current year.
  6. Boundaries
     On east:
     On west:
     On south:
     On north:
  7. Location:
  8. Any housefly breeding: Present/Absent
     Place
  9. Water supply source:
  10. Fuel used for cooking:
  11. Accidents and its prevention measures:
      i. Fire extinguisher: Present/Absent
      ii. First aid kit: Present/Absent.

II. *Description of food catering establishment*: Kitchen Eating-place
  1. Floor
      i. Space
      ii. Pervious
          Impervious
  2. Walls: Pervious
            Impervious
  3. Lighting
  4. Ventilation
  5. Furniture
     Tables at eating-place
     covered with non-absorbent
     materials: Yes/No
  6. Water supply:
      i. Storage
      ii. Usage
  7. Houseflies: Present/Absent

III. 1. Storage of cooked food
  a. Glass cupboard: Present/Absent
  b. Fly proof: Present/Absent
2. Storage of raw food:
  a. Common for perishable and non-perishable foods: Yes/No
  b. Cold storage : Present/Absent
  c. Rodents : Present/Absent
  d. Fly proof : Present/Absent

IV. Sanitary Measures:
1. Washing utensils
2. Disposal of Refuse:
  a. Collection
  b. Disposal
3. No. of Toilets/Washbasins

V. Food Handlers
  a. No. of workers
  b. How many children below 14 years are working?
  c. Any Register maintained? Yes/No.
  d. Examination of food handlers:

Sl. No.	*Name*	*Age*	*Sex*	*Personal hygiene*	*Diseases if any*	*Type of work*	*KAP about food handling*
1.							
2.							
3.							
4.							
5.							
6.							
7.							
8.							
9.							
10.							

VI. Layout of the catering establishment:
VII. Remarks
VIII. Recommendations

Requirement for Food Catering Establishment as per column 343 of Municipal Act

1. Floor must be stone and washable.
2. Except coffee tea, rest are to be properly cooked in a separate kitchen
3. Wall and roof should be white-washed or distempered periodically
4. Safe and protected water should be supplied.
5. Food should be protected from flies by glass cage.
6. Tabletop must be covered with waterproof material
7. Food should be stored in a vessel, which has cover.
8. Vessels are washed in a separate wash room and hot water must be checked.

9. Glass vessels and used vessels should be thoroughly cleaned.
10. Copper and brass vessels should be alloy plated once in 2 months.
11. Workers should be free from infectious diseases.
12. Known infections persons should not be allowed to kitchen and dining hall.
13. Workers are supplied with neat clean wears.
14. Workers should have medical fitness certificate.
15. Any sudden close should be intimated to corporation.
16. License from corporation given should not be transferred to second person.
17. Dustbin with lid should be available for work refuse and garbage.
18. Workers should have minimum space of 25 sq ft floor space per person and 250 cu ft per person for residing or sleeping as accommodation.
19. Visitors and workers should have toilet, latrine, bathing facilities and workspace.
20. Hotel owner should allow inspection from city health officers at any point of time.
21. Premises given under license should not be changed.
22. Workers' name, address register must be maintained.

Appendix X
Malaria Smear Staining

MP SMEAR MAKING

A. For Thick Smear:

Step 1: Four drops of blood taken on slide (Fig. X1)

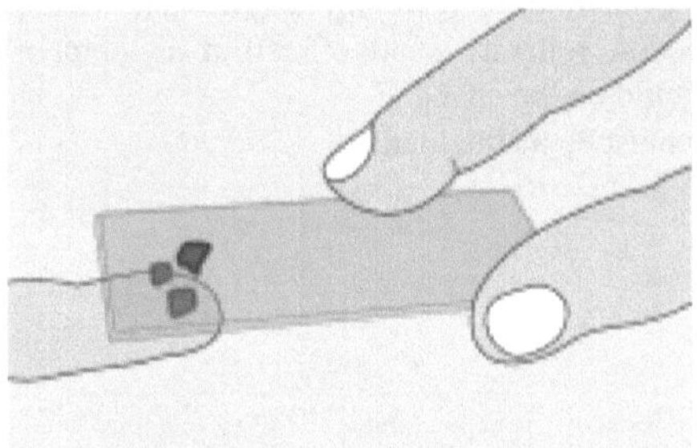

Fig. X1: Blood on slide

Step 2: By slide method with another slide, a smear is made which will be a thick smear (Fig. X2)

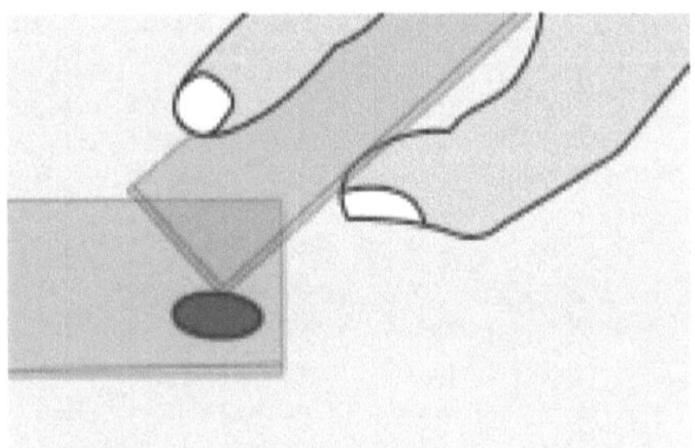

Fig. X2: Preparation of thick smear

B. For Thin Smear

Step 1: One drop of blood is taken on a slide (Fig. X3)

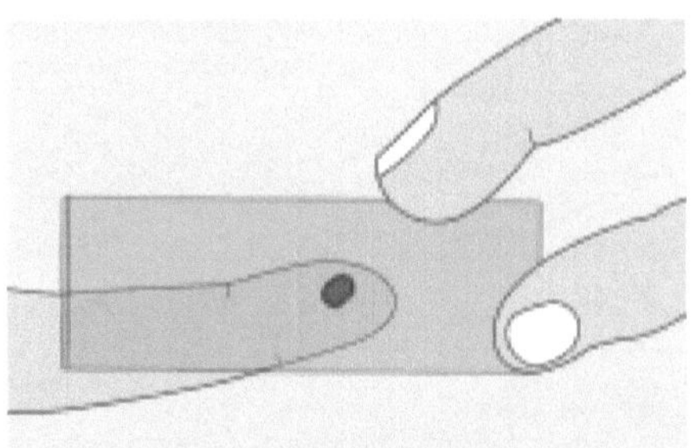

Fig. X3: Preparation of thin smear

Step 2: Spread by another slide (Fig. X4)

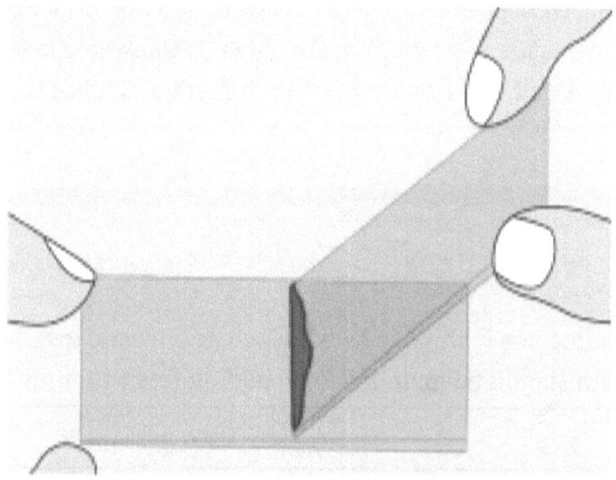

Fig. X4: Preparation of thin smear on another slide

C. For Both Thick and Thin Smear

Step 1: One small drop and one big drop of blood are taken on a slide (Fig. X5).

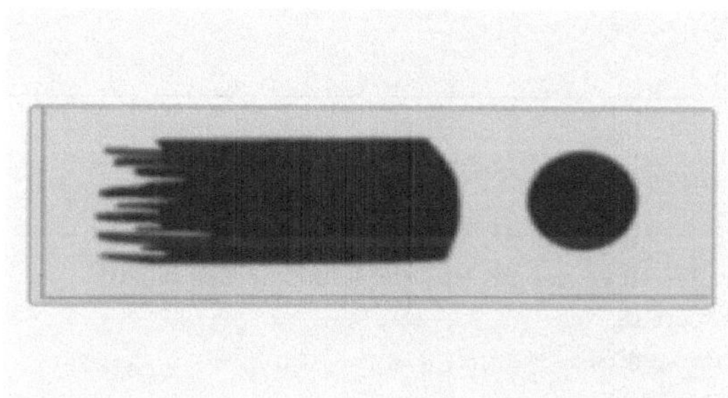

Fig. X5: Two drops on slide (one small and one big)

Step 2: With the help of another slide, the drop is spread to make thick and thin smears (Fig. X6)

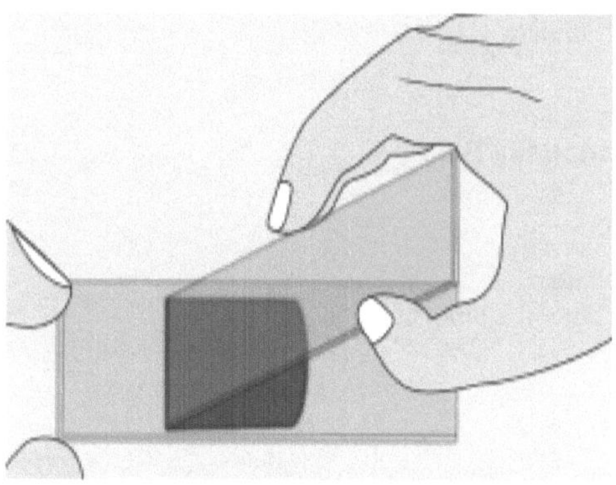

Fig. X6: Preparation of thick and thin smears

Procedure of MP Smear Making

Finger tip is cleaned with spirit swab. Skin is allowed to dry. Then by a blood Lancet, a firm quick stab is made. First drop which comes out is wiped off. A clean slide is taken to make either a) thick smear, b) thin smear or c) both.

The smear prepared is dried in air and fixed by immersing in methyl alcohol for 3 minutes (if ethyl alcohol, then for 15 min).

MP SMEAR STAINING

By Field Stain

Field stains A and B are kept in separate jars with wide neck, which permits the insertion of slide. The depth of field a stain should be 3 inches. The level of stain should be maintained by adding fresh solution periodically.

Field stain A	*Field stain B*
Methylene blue 0.8 g Azure I (Azure B) 0.5 g Disodium hydrogen phosphate (anhydrous) Potassium dihydrogen phosphate (anhydrous) 6.25 g Distilled water 500 ml	Eosin (yellow and water soluble) 1.0 g Disodium hydrogen phosphate (anhydrous) 5 g Potassium dihydrogen phosphate (anhydrous) 6.25 g Distilled water 500 ml

Steps

1. Smear is placed in field stain A—two seconds.
2. Removed, rinsed in clean water—few seconds (till glass slide is seen clean).
3. Placed in field stain B—one second.
4. Rinsed in clean water—three seconds.
5. Dried by holding in vertical position.

Leishmen Stain (Modified Romanousky Stain)

1. Undiluted Leishman stain is poured on blood smear—allowed 3 minutes.
2. Buffer solution added by pipette (equal quantity), Mixed by gentle blow—seven minutes
3. Washed in distilled water—half minute
4. Dried.

Giemsa Stain (Modified Romanousky Stain)

Quick Method by Giemsa Stain

1. Pour methyl alcohol—three minutes
2. Giemsa Stain (1: 2 dilution) is poured—three minutes
3. Wash with water—five minutes
4. Dried in air.

Slow Method by Giemsa Stain

1. Pour methyl alcohol—three minutes
2. Giemsa stain (1: 10 diluted) is taken in a dish
3. A glass rod is placed in the dish
4. Slide with smear is placed in the dish placing the film downwards, with support of rod left for 24 hours
5. Washed in water
6. Dried.

MP SMEAR EXAMINATION

Smear in the slide is examined under oil immersion and malaria parasite type is identified (Figs X7 to X10).

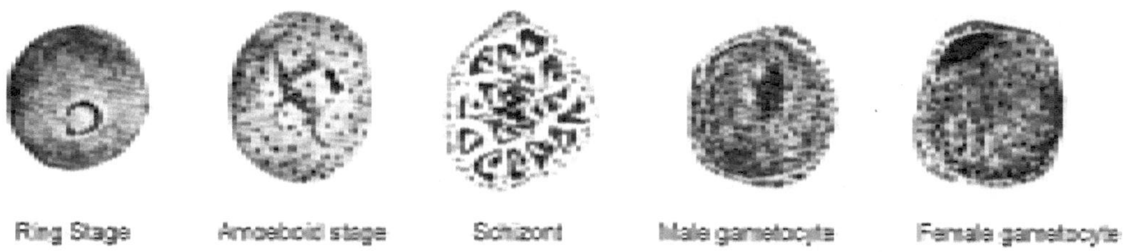

Fig. X7: *Pl. vivax* stage as seen under microscope

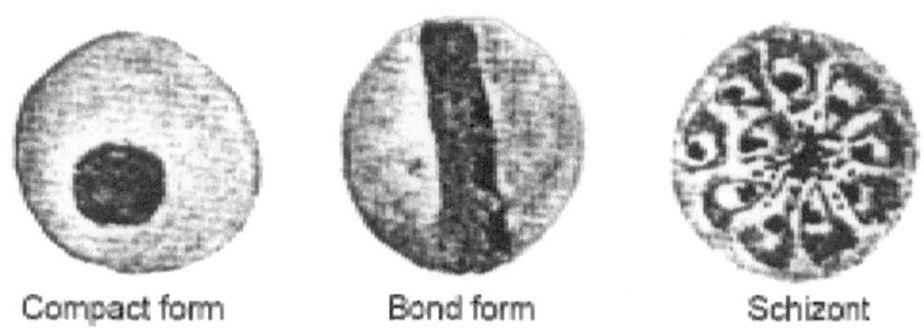

Fig. X8: *Pl. malariae* stage as seen under microscope

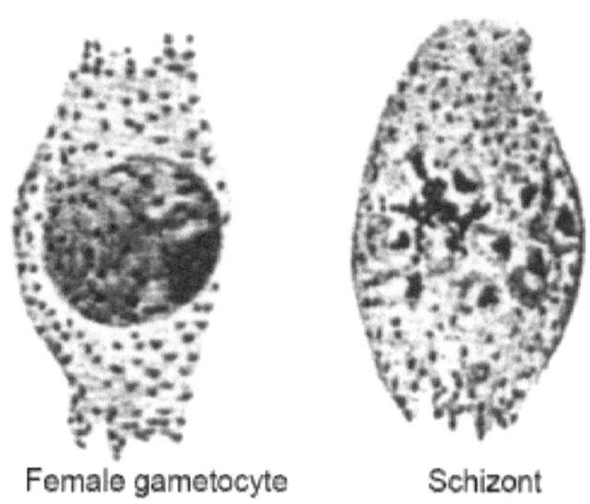

Fig. X9: *Pl. ovale* stage as seen under microscope

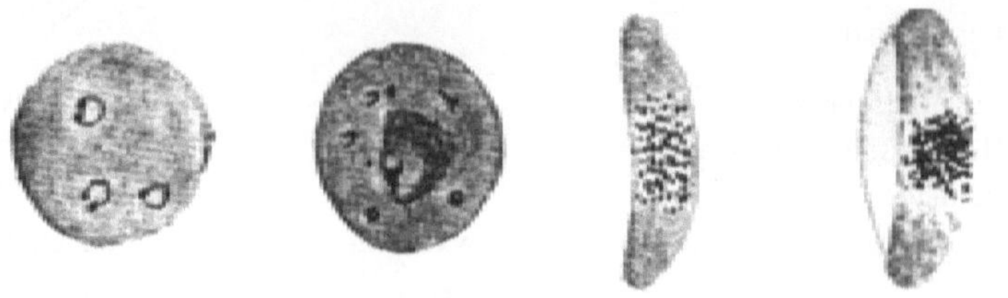

Fig. X10: *Pl. falciparum* stage as seen under microscope

Specific difference in Plasmodium Parasite Species

Pl. vivax	*Pl. malariae*	*Pl. ovale*	*Pl. falciparum*
Increase in size Schuffner's dots+ 30-40 merozoites	Not increase in size No Schuffner's dots Bond form + 15-20 merozoites	Oval or irregular Schuffner's dots+ 8-10 merozoites	Not increase in size No Schuffner's dots 8-10 merozoites Ring stage +

Appendix XI
Method of Giving Injection

The following figure illustrates the parts of a syringe viz, plunger, barrel and needle. Figure also gives the idea of how the syringe must be held at the time of giving injection (Fig. XI 1).

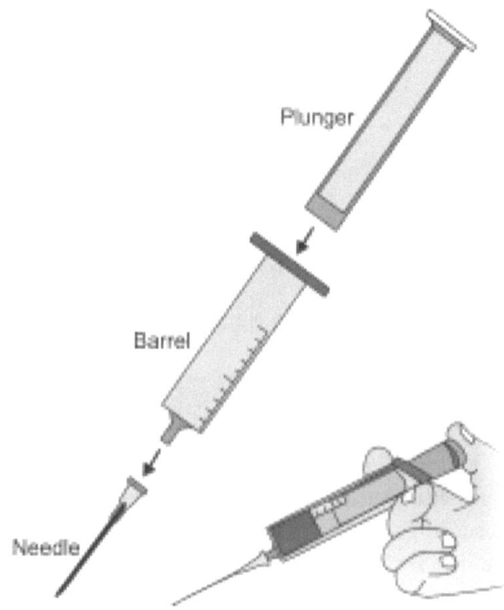

Fig. XI 1: Parts of a syringe

Size of syringe and needle:

For BCG	1 ml syringe	26-gauge needle
For other vaccine	2 ml syringe	23 gauges
For other drugs	5 ml or 10 ml	23 or 24 gauge

Injection Safety Checklist

- Wash hands to remove bacteria
- Use sterile forceps to pick up syringe and needle.
- Separate syringe for separate injection.
- Use forceps to remove band, plunger and needles from tray.

- Turn needles, fit it securely.
- Be careful that to break syringe.

Routes of Administration

- Intradermal
- Subcutaneous
- Intramuscular

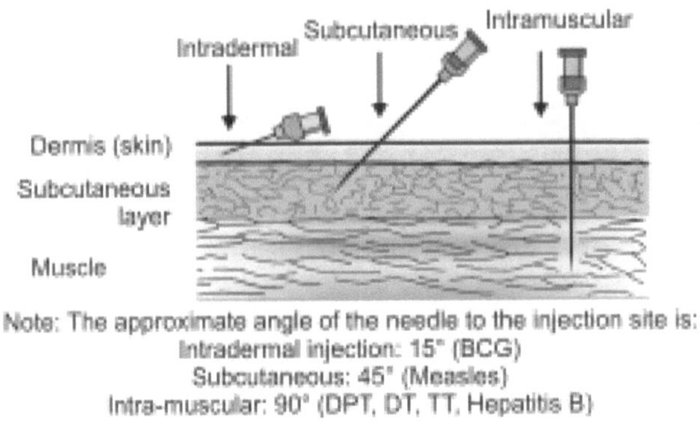

Fig. XI 2: Needle position in IM, SC and ID injections

PROCEDURE OF IM INJECTION

- Syringe, needle and forceps are sterilised as per specifications available in PHC manual.
- Hands are washed with water and soap.
- Lids of the vial are cleaned with spirited swab.

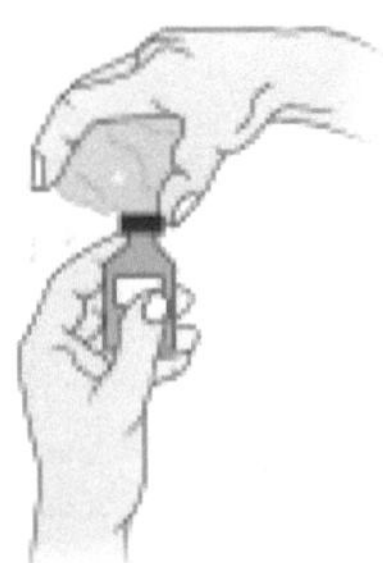

Fig. XI 3: Vial lid cleaning

Site of injection is marked, cleaned with spirited swab (Fig. XI 4).

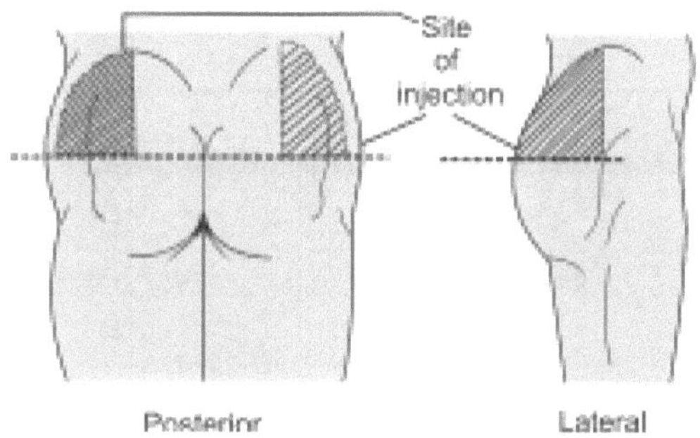

Fig. XI 4: Site of injection

Sterilised forceps is used to take barrel, to take plunger and to fix needles. Injectable liquid is collected to syringe as in Figure XI 5.

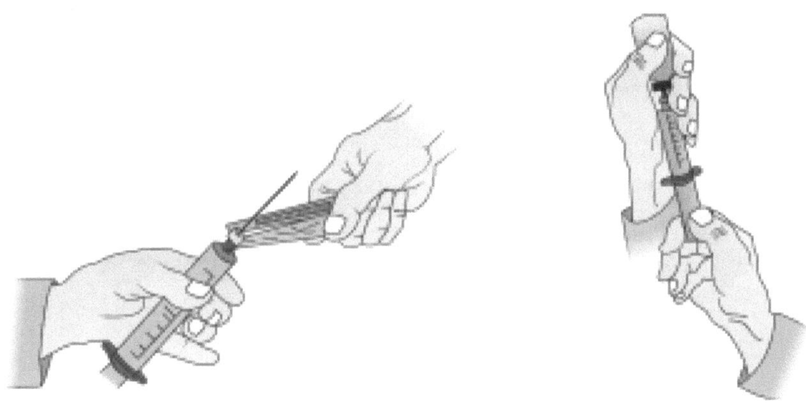

Fig. XI 5: Fixing needle and collecting injectable liquid

Syringe is held as shown in Figure XI 6. Injection is given. Needle is taken out.

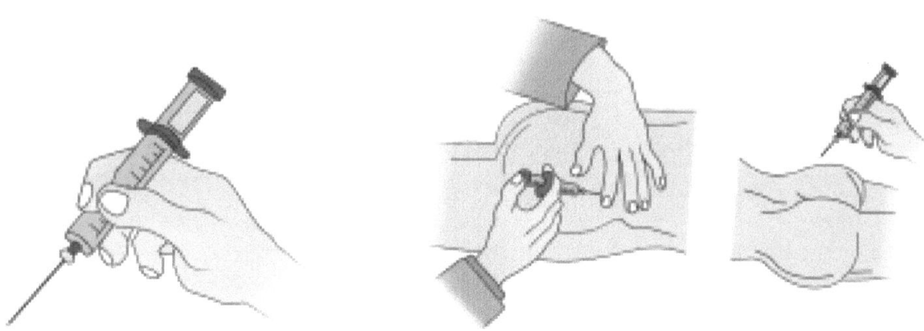

Fig. XI 6: Syringe holding, giving injection and taking out needle

METHOD OF GIVING SUBCUTANEOUS INJECTION

Common place for subcutaneous injection is shown in figure XI 7.

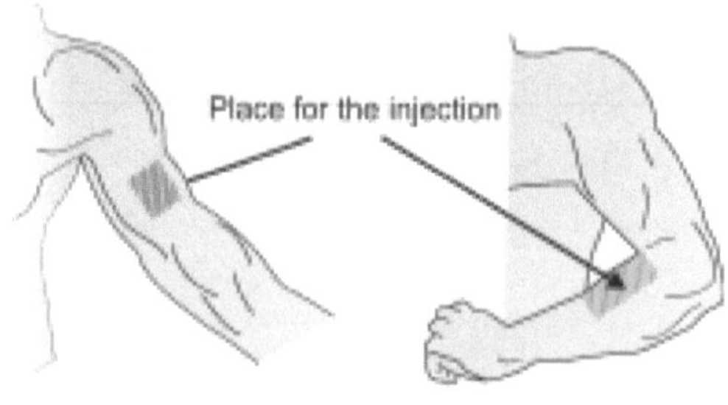

Fig. XI 7: Place for subcutaneous injection

Syringe is held as shown in Figure XI 8. Pick up the skin of the forearm or arm with the fingers of left hand. Push the needle into skin, which is pulled out, so that the needle goes in about 1 cm. Once the needle is under the skin, let go off the skin and press on the plunger of the syringe to make all liquid go in. Later, pull the needle out.

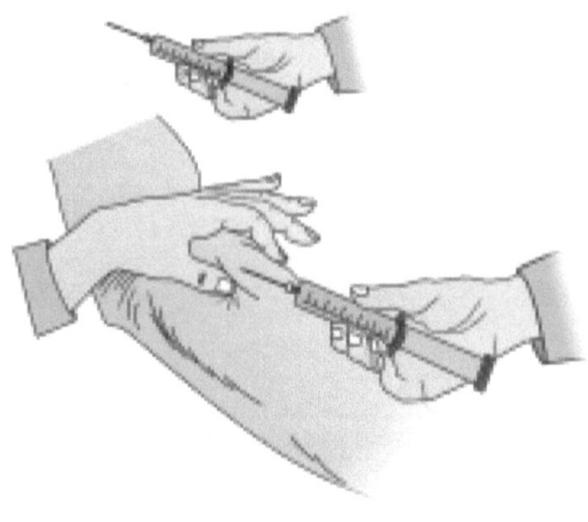

Fig. XI 8: Method of holding syringe and giving subcutaneous injection

Appendix XII
Camp Organisation (OTC Camp)

Village leaders or Community leaders have potential role in adopting health practices. Hence, OTC camps have great impact in H and FW activities. These camps help the people to achieve better health, clear their doubts and involve them in planning and in implementing programmes.

OTC are centres of support to the programme within community themselves.

OBJECTIVES OF OTC CAMPS

- It helps to enlist the active support of people.
- People appreciate the importance of health programme.
- People give priority.
- It clears doubts and misconceptions.
- Develop an action plan.

SELECTION OF PARTICIPANTS

For participation in 1 camp, 40 to 50 opinion leaders are invited. This includes formal and informal leaders. Formal leaders include:

- Mandal Pradhan
- Member of Village Panchayat
- Office bearers of cooperative societies
- Youth club
- Mahila Mandals
- CHV
- School teacher
- Postmen
- TBA
- Priest of village.

In a camp, it is better women leaders and minority group are included.

CAMP PLANNING

- Arrangement is made well in advance.
- Place can be PHC, Subcentre and BDO office.
- MOH, BDO and BEE should discuss early
- Rural development departments are involved like agriculture, animal husbandry, labour cooperative, cottage industry, education, social welfare, adult education, and voluntary organisations.
- Media and extension officers should supervise the camp.
- Suitable motivational materials are obtained in local language and distributed to participants.
- Sitting arrangements are properly made, usual expenditure is Rs. 5 per participants and should limit to 200 per camp.
- Participants are informed date, time and place of camp well in advance.

Content and schedule of OTC camp

Sessions	*Method*	*Duration*
Inauguration/ Introduction		30 minutes
Subject content of camp	Group discussion Q and A Lunch, Break	2 hours
Contd., discussion	Group discussion with Educational aids and participation	1 hour
Priority area of contact	Group discussion	30 minutes
Role of participation	Group discussion	30 minutes
Plan of action	Group discussion	1 hour
Conclusion		30 minutes

FOLLOW-UP OF OTC CAMP

- Contact with participants and follow-up are a must after OTC camp.
- Recording of follow-up helps in future plan of action or modification of activities in H and FW service.

Appendix XIII
Minimum Information of a Village Record

Name of village ______ Distance from PHC ______

Population ________

Births in one year ________

Birth (added) ________

Date of birth	*Name*	*Sex*	*Residence*	*Person assisted delivery*	*Alive/not*

Death in one year ________________

Deaths (added) ________________

Date of death	*Name*	*Sex*	*Age*	*Cause of death*	*Person reported death*

Number of cases:

Pregnant ___________ Lactating ___________ 0–6 child ___________

Eligible couple __________ Trained *dais* _____________

Tubectomy ___________ Leprosy _____________

Malaria treated _____________

Water supply system:

- Tank ______
- River ______
- Wells ______
- Piped ______

Waste disposal:

- Drainage ______________
- Solid waste ______________
- Number of sanitary latrine ______________
- Number of community latrine ______________
- Number of hotels ______ Number of entertainment place _____
- Fair and festival of village ______________
- *Village leaders:*
  - Number of formal leaders _____
  - Number of nonformal leaders _____
  - Number of religious leaders _____

Appendix XIV
Drug List with Health Inspector for Minor Illness Treatment

For Internal Use

1. Acetyl salicylic acid tablets
2. Belladonna and phenobarbitone tablets
3. Chloroquine phosphate tablets
4. Cough mixture
5. Dried aluminium hydroxide tablets
6. Ergometrine maleate tablets
7. Iron and folic acid tablets
8. Kaolin pectin suspension
9. Magnesium hydroxide tablets
10. Magnesium sulphate
11. Mepyramine (antihistamine) tablets
12. Mebendazole tablets (pantelmin)
13. Oral rehydration powder
14. Paracetamol tablets
15. Phthalyl sulphathiazole tablets
16. Piperazine citrate/Piperazine adipate tablets
17. Sulphadimidine tablets
18. Vitamin A solution

For External Use

19. Acriflavine ointment
20. Antiseptic lotion
21. Benzoic salicylic ointment
22. Benzyl benzoate emulsion
23. Chloromycetin eye ointment (Aplicaps)
24. Gentian violet 2%
25. Menthol and eucalyptus oil ointment
26. Mercurochrome 2%
27. Methyl salicylate liniment
28. Sulphacetamide eye and ear drops 10%
29. Tetracycline eye ointment
30. White Vaseline

Reagents

31. Chemistips (Miles India Ltd)
32. Litmus paper (blue and red)

MEDICINES TO BE KEPT AT SUBCENTRE

For External Use

1. Bephenium hydroxy naphthoate granules
2. Calcium gluconate
3. Liquid paraffin
4. Mist alkaline
5. Mist Carminative
6. Mist chloral hydrate
7. Mist sedative expectorant
8. Multivitamin tablet(A, B, C and D)
9. Prochlorperazine tab (Stemetil®)
10. Syrup ferric citrate
11. Vitamin C tab
12. Inj. methyl ergometrine maleate (Methargin®)
13. Boric acid powder
14. Calamine lotion
15. Methylated spirit
16. Tincture benzoin co.
17. Tincture iodine
18. Zinc boric dressing powder.

Appendix XV
Job Responsibilities of Health Assistant (Male)

Note: Under the Multipurpose Workers Scheme a Health Assistant (Male) is expected to cover a population of 20,000 in which there are four subcentres, each with one Health Worker (Male).

The Health Assistant (Male) will carry out the following functions:

SUPERVISION AND GUIDANCE

- Supervise and guide the Health Workers (Male) in delivery of health care services to the community.
- Strengthen the knowledge and skills of the Health Worker (Male).
- Help the Health Worker (Male) in improving his skills in working in the community.
- Help and guide Health Worker (Male) in planning and organising his programme of activities.
- Visit each Health Worker (Male) at least once a week on a fixed day to observe and guide him in his day-to-day activities.
- Assess periodically the progress of work of the Health Worker (Male) and submit an assessment report to the Medical Officer of the Primary Health Centre.
- Carry out supervisory home visits in the area of the Health Worker (Male).

TEAM WORK

- Help the Health Worker to work as part of the health team.
- Coordinate his activities with those of the Health Assistant (Female) and other health personnel.
- Coordinate the health activities in his area with the activities of workers of other departments and agencies and attend meetings at block level.
- Conduct regular staff meetings with the Health Workers in coordination with the Health Assistant (Female).
- Attend staff meetings at the primary Health Centre.
- Assist the Medical Officers of the Primary Health Centre in the organisation of the different health services in the area.
- Participate as a member of the health team in mass camps and campaigns in health programmes.

SUPPLIES AND EQUIPMENT

- In collaboration with the Health Assistant (Female), check at regular intervals the stores available at the subcentre and indent for and procure the supplies and equipment in good time.
- Check that the drugs at the subcentre are properly stored and that the equipment is well-maintained.
- Ensure that the Health Worker (Male) maintains his kit in the proper way.

RECORDS AND REPORTS

- Scrutinise the maintenance of records by the Health Worker (Male) and guide him in their proper maintenance.
- Maintain the prescribed records and prepare the necessary reports.
- Review reports received from the Health Workers (Male), consolidate them and submit periodical reports to the Medical Officer of the Primary Health Care.

MALARIA

- Give radical treatment to all cases when blood smears are positive for malaria.
- Supervise the spraying of insecticides during local spraying.

COMMUNICABLE DISEASES

- Be alert to the sudden outbreak of epidemics of diseases such as plague, diarrhoeal diseases or poliomyelitis and take all the necessary remedial measures.
- Take the necessary control measures when any notifiable disease is reported to him.
- In cases with continued fever, or prolonged cough, or spitting of blood, take sputum smears and send them for examination.
- In cases suspected of having leprosy, take skin smears and send them for examination.
- Carry out the destruction of stray dogs.

ENVIRONMENTAL SANITATION

- Help the community in the construction of:
  - Soakage pits;
  - Kitchen gardens;
  - Manure pits;
  - Compost pits;
  - Sanitary latrines;
  - Smokeless chulhas;

  And supervise their construction
- Supervise the chlorination of water sources including wells.

IMMUNISATION

- Conduct immunisation of all school-going children with the help of the Health Worker (Male)
- Supervise the immunisation of all children from one to five years.

FAMILY PLANNING

- Personally motivate resistant cases for family planning.
- Guide the Health Worker (Male) in establishing male depot holders for the distribution of conventional contraceptives and train the depot holders with the assistance of the Health Worker (Male).

NUTRITION

- Identify cases of malnutrition among infants and young children (zero to five years), give necessary treatment and advice and refer serious cases to the Primary Health Care.

VITAL EVENTS

- Report the birth and death occurring in his area to the HO of PHC

PRIMARY MEDICAL CARE

- Provide treatment for minor ailments, provide first aid for accidents and emergencies, and refer cases beyond his competence to the Primary Health Centre or nearest Hospital.
- Attend to cases referred by the Health Workers and refer cases beyond his competence to the Primary Health Centre or nearest Hospital.

HEALTH EDUCATION

- Carry out educational activities for control of communicable diseases, environmental sanitation, MCH, family planning, nutrition, immunisation and the need for registration of vital events.
- Arrange group meeting with leaders and involve them in spreading the message for various health programmes.
- Organise and conduct training of community leaders with the assistance of the Health Worker (Male).

Appendix XVI
Sanitary Survey of Village/Town

Name of Village/Town________________ Date of survey________

Population covered____________

Water Source: Well/pond/river/spring/pump/tap ____________

Chlorination frequency _____________

Sullage water disposal ______________

Soakage pits _____________ Kitchen garden __________ Drains_________

Solid waste disposal __________

Dustbin/land dumping/sanitary landfill/incineration/burning/burial/feeding to animal

Manure pit __________

Latrine: Sanitary __________ others __________

Community Latrine __________

Home sanitation ___________

Remarks on health hazards:

Unprotected electrical installations ____________

Breeding places __________

Polluted water ___________

Unhygienic eating place ___________

Dangerous occupation

Stable/cowshed/animal shed ___________

Name of Inspector

Appendix XVII
The Municipality Act 1964
(Specific Sections Relevant to Health Inspectors)

Section 222: Provision as to Dogs

Item 1: By public notice, shall be muzzled in such a way to allow dog free, while effectively preventing it from biting.
Item 2: Take possession of dog found wondering
Item 3: Licensed dog is not destroyed.
Item 4: Unclaimed dog be sold or destroyed after detaining for 3 clear days.
Item 5: All municipality expense of dog shall be borne by owner of the dog.
Item 6: No damage is payable to dog owner.

Section 223: Provision as to Keeping of Pigs

Item 1: Pigs cannot be kept without permission; if they cause nuisance or annoyance
Item 2: If kept without permission, owner is fined to the tune of Rs. 50.00.
Item 3: Pigs found straying may be forthwith destroyed and carcass be disposed off.

Section 243: Regulation of Markets, Sale of Goods, etc.

Item 1: License to market, sale of goods, etc.
Item 2: Use without license is punishable with fine of Rs. 25.00.
Item 3: Closure of market place forbidding sale and made punishable of deviant up to Rs. 5.00.

Section 244: Opening, Closing and Letting of Markets and Slaughterhouses

Item 1: Power to open or close
Item 2: Selling or exposing for sale without License is punishable up to Rs. 25.00
Item 3: Lease of place for 1 year.
Item 4: Vacating unauthorized occupation of stall.

Section 245: Power to Expel Lepers, Disturbers, etc. from Market

Section 246: Slaughterhouses, etc. beyond municipal limits (They are considered as if within limits).

Section 247: Unwholesome articles of food and drink

Item 1: Inspection of food, drink, animal food.
Item 2: Destroy and dispose of food, drink and animal food.
Item 3: Disposal of perishable items—power.
Item 4: This item takes care of poor hygiene of food.
Item 5: Seizing aforesaid food, drink and animal food.
Item 6: Concerned with food adulteration.

Item 7: Concerned with sale of butter, *ghee* and its adulteration.
Item 8: Punishment for adulteration of food.
Item 9: Summon for attendance of person accused.

PREVENTION OF DANGEROUS DISEASES

Section 248: Prevention of infections diseases
Item 1: Limitations, restrictions of conditions.
Item 2: Power on disease notification, punishment and prohibitions.
Item 3: Compensation of loss of property when destroyed for disease prevention.
Item 4: Punishment to disobey up to Rs. 200.00.

Section 249: Duties of Municipal Council on threatened or actual outbreak of infectious disease (it is dealt in investigation of epidemic chapter also).

Section 251: Duties of Municipal Council in respect of disease among horses, dogs, cattle, sheep or goats.

Section 252: Proceedings to abate the overcrowding of interiors of buildings.

Section 253: Special powers which may be conferred by Government in respect of overcrowded areas notified by Government.

Section 254: Prohibition of making vault or grave in place of worship.

Section 255: Closing places for disposal of the dead.

Appendix XVIII
Drugs to be known by Health Inspector in his Daily Routines from Other Systems of Medicine

AYURVEDA

It stresses diet, sleep, spiritual life, seasonal conduct and social conduct.

Illness	*Drug*
• Fever, cold, headache	Tribhuvana kirthi + Godanti 1 tablet 3 times daily
• Cough, sore throat	Sitopaladigudi 2 tablet 3 times daily
• Pain (any type)	Godanti pippali Mool 2 tablets 3 times daily
• Backache, urinary trouble	Chandraprabha vati 2 tablets 3 times daily
• Indigestion	Jatiphaladi 2 tablets 3 times daily
• Sprain	Panchaguna taila massage
• Scabies	Gandhakamalahara application

UNANI

Illness	*Drug*
• Fever	Qurs Mubarak
• Cold	Qurs nazla
• Cough	Qurs surfa
• Headache	Qurs shifa
• Backache	Qurs hudar
• Scabies	Marham kharish application
• Sprain	Roghan surkh application

SIDDA

It stresses diet, sleep, mental health, seasonal and social conduct.

Illness	*Drug*
• Fever	Sivanar Amirtham with honey
• Cough	Thalisathi vadakam for chewing
• Joint pain	Mayana thailam
• Headache	Neerkovai mathira with milk applied on forehead
• Sprain	Mayana thailam application
• Backache	Mayana thailam application
• Toothache	Chukku thailam in cotton plug to tooth.

HOMEOPATHY

Light food, rest, no other medicine, no coffee, no spices, no tobacco or no alcohol is advised.

Illness	*Drug*
• Fever	Aconite 6 X and combination I alternatively every one hour
• Headache	Mellilotus 30 and combination II alternatively every 2 hours
• Backache	Arnica 30 every 2 hours
• Joint pain	Bryonia 30 and combination III alternatively every 2 hours
• Cough	Arsemic albumb and Ipecac 30 alternatively every 2 hours
• Toothache	Staphysagria 200 and combination of No IX alternatively 2 hours
• Scabies	Calendula ointment apply

Appendix XIX
Universal Precaution against HIV/AIDS

This is impact to prevent skin and mucous membrane exposure when patient contact is expected.

- Gloves worn for touching blood and body fluids.
- Mask, eyewear worn during patient attending.
- Hands and skin-washed immediately after contact with contaminated blood.
- Care is taken to prevent injuries with needle, scalpel, sharp instruments at health work. Recapping of needle helps here.
- Minimise mouth-to-mouth respiration if he is known patient.
- If skin lesion is present better patient care is avoided.

Above statements are called *universal precaution* for blood and body fluids.

Appendix XX
Hospital Waste Management

Waste category	*Contents*	*Treatment and disposal options*	*Colour code*	*Type of container*
1. Human anatomical waste	Human tissues, organs, body parts	Incineration/deep burial	Yellow	Plastic bag
2. Animal waste	Animal tissues, organs, body parts, carcasses, bleeding parts, fluid, blood and experimental animals used in research. Waste generated by veterinary hospital colleges, discharge from hospitals, animal houses	Incineration/deep burial	Yellow	Plastic bag
3. Microbiology and biotechnology waste	Laboratory cultures, stocks, specimens of micro-organisms; live or attenuated vaccines, human and animal cell culture used in research and industrial laboratories, waste from production of biological, toxins, dishes and devices used for transfer of cultures	Local autoclaving/micro-waving/ incineration	Yellow/Red	Plastic bag/disinfected container
4. Waste sharps container/	Needles, syringes, scalpels, blades, glass, etc. that may cause puncture and cuts. This includes both used and unused sharps	Disinfections/chemical treatment /autoclaving/microwaving and mutilation/shredding	Blue/White translucent	Plastic bag puncture proof container
5. Discarded medicines and cytotoxic drugs	Waste comprising of outdated, contaminated and discarded medicines	Incineration/destruction and disposal in secured landfills	Black	Plastic bag
6. Soiled waste	Waste generated from disposable items other than the waste sharps such as tubing, catheters, intravenous sets, etc.	Incineration/autoclaving/microwaving	Yellow/Red	Disinfected container/ plastic bag
7. Solid waste	Waste generated from disposable items other than the waste sharps such as tubing, catheters, intravenous sets, etc.	Disinfections by chemical treatment/autoclaving/microwaving and mutilation/shredding	Red/Blue/ White translucent	Disinfected container/ plastic bag
8. Liquid waste	Waste generated from laboratory and washing, cleaning, housekeeping and disinfecting activities	Disinfections by chemical treatment and discharge into drains	Not applicable	Not applicable
9. Incineration ash	Ash from incineration of any biomedical waste	Disposal in municipal landfill	Black	Plastic bag
10. Chemical waste	Chemicals used in production of biologicals, chemicals used in disinfections, as insecticides, etc.	Chemical treatment and discharge into drains for liquids and secured landfill for solids	Black	Plastic bag

1. = There will be no chemical pre-treatment before incineration. Chlorinated plastics shall not be incinerated. 2. Deep burial shall be an option available only in towns with population less than 5 lakhs and in rural areas. 3. = Using at least 1% hypochlorite solution or any other equivalent chemical reagent. It must be ensured that chemical treatment ensures disinfection. 4. = Must be such so as to prevent unauthorised reuse. 5. = Liquid wastes do not require contains/bags. 6. = If disinfectioned locally need not be put into contains/bags.

Note: Colour coding of waste categories with multiple treatment options to depend on treatment option.

Appendix XXI
Health Care Establishments Covered under Biomedical Waste (BMW) Rules 1998

- Government hospitals
- Private hospitals
- Nursing homes
- Physician's office
- Dentist's office/clinics
- Dispensaries
- Primary health centres
- Medical research and training establishments
- Mortuaries
- Blood banks and collection centres
- Animal houses
- Slaughterhouses
- Laboratories
- Research organisation
- Vaccinating centres
- Biotechnology institutions/production units

Appendix XXII
Procedure of Killing the Stray Dogs

Pet dogs are manageable by vaccination. But in case of death of stray dogs caused by bite of infected stray dog, HI is expected to perform his duty, which is under Municipalities Act " Destruction of stray dogs".

Before the procedure, Health Inspector is expected to do the following:

a. Educate the person on rabies contact
b. Get cooperation of the person.

METHOD OF KILLING STRAY DOG

Strychnine a poison, which causes convulsion and death, is used to kill stray dogs.

Strychnine is supplied in bottle containing 25 gram of powder. There are two methods of preparing poison bait:

- 50 grams sugar is distributed in half litre milk
- 3 grams (one pinch) of strychnine pinch is taken and added to milk and mixed.
- This is sufficient for 6 dogs.
- A burfi is taken, upper position of burfi is cut. One pinch of strychnine powder is put in burfi. It is covered with cut portion of burfi.

PHC manual gives the method of feeding the bait, removal of dead dog and how to keep the record of killing stray dogs.

Monthly report includes the information about dog destruction in the area.

Appendix XXIII
Emergency Measures in Public Health

ANTHRAX EPIDEMIC

- Case reporting to DH and FWO is obligatory.
- Isolate case till skin lesion is cured
- Concurrent disinfection is done.
- Terminal disinfection is done.
- The body of animal died of anthrax should be buried deeply in a pit 6 feet (1.82 metres) in depth after plugging all the natural openings of the animal with a few of cotton saturated with disinfectants, surrounded by quicklime.
- No post-mortem exam is allowed of animal as the blood contains a large number of bacteria, which can get mixed-up with air.
- If fuel is available, burning the dead is preferred.
- Trade control in animal skin, hair, hides and bone meal are done.
- Health education of public.

SARS EPIDEMIC

- All suspected SARS cases are admitted and isolated. They are given N95 mask to wear.
- All visitors of case are given PPE (personal protective equipment)
- Notification done
- Health education is given to possible.
- Policy procedure (Local DC circulars) is enforced.
- Containment is selective isolation, home isolation, and segregation of suspected cases.
- All linen—detergent, bleaching done.
- All waste—hospital grade disinfectant 1:100 bleaching powder used.

POLIO EPIDEMIC

Emergency measures in polio epidemic are described under chapter Investigation of Epidemic (Chap 16)

GE EPIDEMIC

Emergency measures in GE epidemic is described under chapter Investigation of Epidemic (Chap 16)

NATURAL CALAMITIES

Common calamities are floods, earthquakes, fire, hurricane, cyclone, thunderstorm, tornados, snowstorm, volcano, landslide, famine and drought.

- Announce assurance through mike
- Assess requirement by quick emergency survey
- Shift people to shelter
- Monitor food supply
- Deal with disposal of dead bodies
- Arrange vaccination, sanitation and health education.

Appendix XXIV

Time Table for First Year HIT Course

	9-10 am	*10-11 am*	*11-12 noon*	*12-1 pm*	*9-1 pm*	*2-5 pm*
Mon	–	–	Theory	Tutorial	–	Field visit
Tue	Theory	Tutorial	–	–	–	–
Wed	Theory	Tutorial	–	–	–	–
Thurs	Theory	Tutorial	–	–	Practical	–
Fri	–	–	Theory	Tutorials	–	–
Sat	–	–	Theory	Tutorials	–	–

Note: Per week, theory 12 hours, practical 3 hours, field visit 6 hours

Appendix XXV
Theory Coverage for First Year HIT Course

Number of hours for theory and tutorial—subjectwise

	Theory (Hour)	*Tutorial (Hour)*
Topic		
Sociology	10	10
Behavioral science	10	10
Concept community medicine	10	5
Statistics	10	10
Microbe, parasite	5	5
Nutrition	10	5
Environment health	16	8
General epidemiology	16	8
Legal medicine	4	2
Entomology	10	5
Primary Health Care	4	2
Total	105	70

Grand Total 175 hours for Ist year course

Appendix XXVI
Practical Coverage for First Year HIT Course

Number of hours training practical, field visits—topicwise

Practical	*Hour*	*Field visit*	*Hour*
Anatomy museum	2	Water works	6
BP, Pulse, respiration		Sewage treatment	
Recording	2	Plant	6
Entomology 2 × 7	14	Milk diary	6
Microbiology lab	2	PHC 3 × 6	18
Slides on parasite	2	UHC 3 × 6	18
Slides on microbe	2	Epi OPD 3 × 6	18
Water Horrock's test	2	DTC	6
Water problem 2 × 2	4	ULC	6
Water spotters	2		
Statistics 2 × 5	10		
Total	42	Total	84

Grand total: 126 hours

Appendix XXVII
Time Table for Second Year HIT Course

	9-10 am	*10-11 am*	*11-12 noon*	*12-1 pm*	*9-1 pm*	*2-5 pm*
Mon	Theory	Tutorial	–	–	–	–
Tue	–	–	–	–	–	–
Wed	–	Theory	Tutorial	–	–	Field visit
Thurs	–	–	–	–	–	–
Fri	Theory	Tutorial	–	–	Practical	Practical
Sat	–	Theory	Tutorial	–	–	Field visit

Note: Per week, theory 8 hours, practical 6 hours, field visit 18 hour.

Appendix XXVIII
Theory Coverage for Second Year HIT Course

Number of hours for theory and tutorial—subjectwise

	Theory (Hour)	*Tutorial (Hour)*
Topic		
Communicable diseases	12	–
MCH and FP	10	4
Health education	4	4
First aid	2	1
Public health administration	6	–
Essential drug	1	–
Treatment of minor ailments	6	–
Total	37	10
Grand total	47 hours	

Appendix XXIX
Practical Coverage for Second Year HIT Course

Second Year HIT Course

Number of hours training practical, field visits—topicwise

Practical	*Hour*	*Field visit*	*Hour*
Epi OPD MP smear 3 × 4	12	Market survey	6
Epi OPD Imm. Clinic 384	12	Hotel inspection	6
Hosp. Incineration unit	6	Corporation 6 × 10	60
Epidemic investigation	8	Industry	6
Ward HE 2 × 10	20	Pilgrimage place	8
Pharmacy unit	6	School visit 2 × 6	12
AIDS cell study	6	UHC family visit 19 × 6	18
		PHC visit 10 × 6	60
		Sub centre visit	6
		FP Camp visit	8
Total	70		196
Grand total			266 hours

Index

J

L

M

U

V

W

Z